Quick Reference to Clinical Dietetics

Second Edition

Lucinda K. Lysen, RD, LD, RN, BSN

Registered Dietitian and
Registered Nurse Consultant
Chicago, Illinois

and

Medical Editor and Assistant Publisher
Southwest Messenger Press Newspapers
Midlothian, Illinois

JONES AND BARTLETT PUBLISHERS
Sudbury, Massachusetts
BOSTON   TORONTO   LONDON   SINGAPORE

World Headquarters
Jones and Bartlett Publishers
40 Tall Pine Drive
Sudbury, MA 01776
978-443-5000
info@jbpub.com
www.jbpub.com

Jones and Bartlett Publishers Canada
6339 Ormindale Way
Mississauga, Ontario L5V 1J2
CANADA

Jones and Bartlett Publishers International
Barb House, Barb Mews
London W6 7PA
UK

Jones and Bartlett's books and products are available through most bookstores and online booksellers. To contact Jones and Bartlett Publishers directly, call 800-832-0034, fax 978-443-8000, or visit our website, www.jbpub.com.

Substantial discounts on bulk quantities of Jones and Bartlett's publications are available to corporations, professional associations, and other qualified organizations. For details and specific discount information, contact the special sales department at Jones and Bartlett via the above contact information or send an email to specialsales@jbpub.com.

Library of Congress Cataloging-in-Publication Data
Quick reference to clinical dietetics / [edited by] Lucinda K. Lysen.
 —2nd ed.
  p. ; cm.
Includes bibliographical references and index.
ISBN 0-7637-3198-6 (pbk.)
1. Dietetics—Handbooks, manuals, etc.   2. Diet therapy—Handbooks, manuals, etc.   I. Lysen, Lucinda K.
 [DNLM: 1. Dietetics—Handbooks.   WB 39 Q5 2006]
RM217.2.Q53 2006
615.8′54—dc22   2005017235

6048

Production Credits
Publisher: Michael Brown
Associate Editor: Kylah Goodfellow McNeill
Production Director: Amy Rose
Associate Production Editor: Kate Hennessy
Associate Marketing Manager: Wendy Thayer
Manufacturing and Inventory Coordinator: Amy Bacus
Cover Design: Kristin E. Ohlin
Composition: ATLIS Graphics and Design
Printing and Binding: Malloy, Inc.
Cover Printing: Malloy, Inc.

Printed in the United States of America
 10 09 08 07 06   10 9 8 7 6 5 4 3 2 1

This book was written in memory of my dad—
my best friend, my mentor—Walter H. Lysen,
the publisher of 14 suburban Chicago newspapers for 52 years
who always found time for his family . . .

Who blessed me with the fruits of his labor,
the tenacity to pursue my dreams,
and his gift of the "power of the pen".

Born January 1, 1918–Died December 28, 2003

And to my mom—Margaret D. Lysen,
my pillar of continued strength,
who has dedicated her life to her family,
and to keeping our legacy alive . . .

Who continues to share her wisdom and intellect,
her amazing courage,
and—always—her unconditional love.

Table of Contents

Contributors

Pamela L. Amann, RD
Wellness Dietitian
Tacoma, Washington

Lucille Beseler, MS, RD, LD
President
Family Nutrition Center of South Florida
Margate, Florida

Chris Biesemeier, MS, RD, FADA
Assistant Director, Nutrition Services
Vanderbilt University Medical Center
Nashville, Tennessee

Regine Birkenhauer, MS, RD, CNSD
Nutrition Program Director
Virginia Commonwealth University Health
    System
Richmond, Virginia

Abby S. Bloch, PhD, RD, FADA
Vice President, Programs and Research
The Dr. Robert C. Atkins Foundation
New York, New York

Pamela Charney, MS, RD, CNS
PhD Candidate
Clinical Nutrition Management Consultant
Mercer Island, Washington

Ronni Chernoff, PhD, RD, FADA
Associate Director, Geriatrics Research,
    Education and Clinical Center
Central Arkansas Veterans Healthcare System
Little Rock, Arkansas

Kimberly Dong, RD, LDN
Research Dietitian
Tufts University School of Medicine
Nutrition/Infection Unit
Boston, Massachusetts

Jül L. Gerrior, RD, LDN
Research Dietitian
Tufts University School of Medicine
Boston, Massachusetts

**Michele M. Gottschlich, PhD, RD, LD,
    CNSD**
Director, Nutrition Services
Shriners Hospital for Children
Adjunct Associate Professor, Department of
    Dietetics and Nutrition Education
College of Allied Health Sciences
University of Cincinnati
Cincinnati, Ohio

**Carol Frankmann, MS, RD, LD,
    CNSD**
Director of Clinical Nutrition
The University of Texas M.D. Anderson
    Cancer Center
Houston, Texas

**Kathy Hammond, MS, RD, LD,
    CNSD, RN**
Coordinator, Continuing Education
Chartwell Diversified Company
Adjunct Assistant Professor
Department of Foods and Nutrition
University of Georgia
Athens, Georgia

**Jeanette M. Hasse, PhD, RD, FADA,
    CNSD**
Transplant Nutrition Specialist
Transplant Services
Baylor University Medical Center
Dallas, Texas

Edward A. Hatchigian, MD
Medical Director
Bariatric Surgery Program
Departments of Medicine and Surgery
Beth Israel Deaconess Medical Center
Harvard Medical School
Boston, Massachusetts

Kristy Hendricks, RD, DSc
Associate Professor
Tufts University School of Medicine
Boston, Massachusetts

Carol S. Ireton-Jones, PhD, RD/LD, CNSD
Director, Nutrition Services
Coram Healthcare
Carrollton, Texas

Donald F. Kirby, MD, FACP, FACN, FACG, CNSP
Professor of Medicine
Gastroenterology/Nutrition
Medical College of Virginia
Chief, Section of Nutrition
Virginia Commonwealth University Health System
Richmond, Virginia

Sarah Harding Laidlaw, MS, RD, MPA
Nutrition Services Director
Mesa View Regional Hospital
Mesquite, Nevada

Elizabeth A. Lennon, MS, RD, LD, CNSD, PA-S
Metabolic Support Clinician
Nutrition Support and Vascular Access Department
The Cleveland Clinical Foundation
Cleveland, Ohio

Lucinda K. Lysen, RD, LD, RN, BSN
Registered Dietitian and Registered Nurse Consultant
Chicago, Illinois
and
Medical Editor and Assistant Publisher
Southwest Messenger Press Newspapers
Midlothian, Illinois

Karen Masino, MS, RD, RN, CNP, OCN, ONP, CNSD
Clinical Dietitian/Oncology Nurse Practitioner
Northwestern Memorial Hospital
Hematopoietic Stem Cell Transplant Unit
Chicago, Illinois

Laura E. Matarese, MS, RD
Director of Nutrition
Thomas E. Starzl Transplant Institute
University of Pittsburgh Medical Center
Pittsburgh, Pennsylvania

Jo Ann McCrae, MS, RD
Nutrition Support Home Care Specialist
Hospital of the University of Pennsylvania
Philadelphia, Pennsylvania

Anne McNamara, RN
Clinical Research Nurse
Beth Israel Deaconess Medical Center
Boston, Massachusetts

P.K. Newby, ScD, MPH, MS
Scientist III
Jean Mayer USDA Human Nutrition Research Center on Aging
Tufts University
Boston, Massachusetts

Neha Parekh, RD
Metabolic Support Clinician
The Cleveland Clinic Foundation
Cleveland, Ohio

Janice S. Raymond, MS, RD, CNSD
Regional Nutrition Manager
Apria Healthcare
Redmond, Washington

Susan Roberts, MS, RD, LD, CNSD
Transplant Nutrition Specialist
Transplant Services
Baylor University Medical Center
Dallas, Texas

Michelle Romano, RD, LD, CNSD
Clinical Dietitian
Assistant Professor of Nutrition
St. Luke's Hospital
Jacksonville, Florida

Denise Baird Schwartz, MS, RD, FADA, CNSD
Nutrition Support Coordinator
Providence Health System
San Fernando Valley
Burbank, California

James S. Scolapio, MD
Director of Nutrition
Associate Professor of Medicine
Mayo Clinic
Jacksonville, Florida

Barry Sears, PhD
President, Inflammation Research
    Foundation
Zone Laboratories
Danvers, Massachusetts

Deborah Silverman, MS, RD, CNSD, FADA
Assistant Professor, School of Health Sciences
Eastern Michigan University
Ypsilanti, Michigan

Linda Veglia, MA, RD, LDN, RN
Bariatric Nutritionist
Beth Israel Deaconess Medical Center
Boston, Massachusetts

Christine A. Wanke, MD
Associate Professor
Tufts University School of Medicine
Boston, Massachusetts

Marion F. Winkler, MS, RD, LDN, CNSD
Surgical Nutrition Specialist
Rhode Island Hospital
Providence, Rhode Island

Introduction

In this second edition of *Quick Reference to Clinical Dietetics,* Ms. Lysen again offers busy practitioners an easy-to-read, well-organized guide to managing the nutritional needs of their patients. Each month, hundreds of journal articles are published on nutrition, and it is impossible for someone involved in patient care to keep up with the latest trends and practices. Ms. Lysen has enlisted the help of leading nutrition experts to author the chapters in the book, giving a concise synthesis of the developments in his or her field. Many of the authors have written authoritative textbooks on nutrition practice: Gottschlich, Matarese, Chernoff, and Sears. Others have published cutting-edge articles on the same subject as the chapter they wrote: Bloch, Hendricks, Wanke, Hasse, and Newby. Still others in the past have written guidelines for providing nutritional care that were ultimately adopted by such pre-eminent organizations as the American Dietetics Association: Ireton-Jones, McCrae, Schwartz, and Charney.

The result of this collaboration is the most concise and sound guide to giving patients the best nutritional care that we've seen. Anyone responsible for the nutritional management of patients—dietitians, pharmacists, nurses, and physicians—will benefit from the pearls contained in this book. And although one may end up only using the chapters that are applicable to the patients they counsel, the diversity of authors makes it tempting to glance at the other short chapters just to gain a few new ideas from the experts.

One of the greatest benefits we found as readers was that the pithy chapters made information clear and accessible—a vast improvement over wading through the pages of a giant nutrition tome to learn about a technique for unclogging a feeding tube, or managing acid/base balance, or conducting a nutritional assessment of a patient with HIV infection. Moreover, Chapter 7, Meal Planning, is a gem. As most readers of this book undoubtedly know, each department of dietetics has its own manual for feeding the patient. But none is likely to be as current or to contain the opinions of so many practitioners, as the section in this book.

Last but not least, a real plus is the book's extensive appendices. They are chock full of charts and tables that you'll actually use. And if you aren't using them, the chapters may end up convincing you to update your practice and incorporate a few of them into your daily recommendations.

We think that you will find the second edition of *Quick Reference to Clinical Dietetics* a valuable tool that will help you give the best patient care possible. The book is a "must" for every clinician in America.

Stacey J. Bell, DSc, RD
Research and Development
IdeaSphere Inc.
Grand Rapids, MI

George L. Blackburn, MD, PhD
S. Daniel Abraham Associate
Professor of Nutrition
Harvard Medical School/
Beth Israel Deaconess Medical School
Boston, MA

CHAPTER 1

Screening and Assessment

- Nutrition Screening
- Nutrition Assessment
- Physical Assessment

Nutrition Screening

Lucinda K. Lysen, RD, LD, RN, BSN

DESCRIPTION

Nutrition screening is vital for any patient in the hospital, receiving home care, or at an extended-care facility. Screening identifies the patient at nutritional risk and the steps required for nutrition consultation and assessment. An ongoing nutrition screening will alert the health care practitioner to changes in patient condition that will ultimately affect nutrition status. The objective of nutrition screening is to identify risk factors that can lead to nutrition compromise.

INITIAL SCREENING

Initial screening with the patient and/or significant other should cover the following areas:

- physical ability to ingest food
- food tolerance and/or intolerance
- previous diet history and/or dietary modifications
- change in weight/weight history
- alcohol use/abuse
- polypharmacy
- possible food/drug interactions

REVIEW OF MEDICAL HISTORY

A review of medical history should cover the following areas:

- Past and current diagnoses and/or problem list that may alter nutrition status of the patient
  1. changes in requirements for certain nutrients due to respiratory, cardiac, gastrointestinal, and other diseases
  2. any interference with the ability to ingest or digest food, absorb nutrients, or excrete waste
- Objective evidence of nutrition status
  1. weight history
     - weight at admission
     - height
     - usual body weight
     - percentage of weight change
  2. laboratory data
     - serum albumin level
     - hemoglobin and hematocrit
     - disease-specific blood work
  3. physical assessment (see Physical Assessment later in this chapter)
     - edema/skin turgor

      –cachexia/muscle wasting
      –obesity
      –presence of lesions/wounds/pressure sores
      –skin color
- Medical treatments that may affect nutritional status
  1. drug/nutrient interactions
  2. chemotherapy
  3. radiation therapy
  4. dialysis
  5. surgery
- Type of diet patient is ingesting
  1. number of days NPO
  2. oral supplementation
  3. enteral tube feeding
  4. parenteral nutrition

RISK IDENTIFICATION

Nutritional risk is based upon results of nutritional screening. Patients identified as being at nutritional risk need nutrition assessment. Patients not at nutritional risk are periodically reevaluated on the basis of criteria established by the individual institution.

Specialized nutrition support may be required in the following instances:

- poor nutrient intake—inability to meet nutrient and food requirements for greater than 5 days
- weight loss
  a. unintentional weight loss of 10% of usual weight in 6 months, or
  b. involuntary weight loss of greater than 5 lb in 1 month
- serum albumin level of less than 3.5 g/dL

Nutrition Assessment

Lucinda K. Lysen, RD, LD, RN, BSN

DESCRIPTION

The purpose of nutrition assessment is to investigate the nutrition status of the patient when screening indicates the need for comprehensive nutrition consultation. Nutrition assessment enables one to determine the safest, most convenient, and most economical means by which nutrient intake can be provided to the patient. It also enables one to manage the nutritionally compromised patient for the best nutritional outcome.

Areas of nutrition assessment follow.

COMPREHENSIVE INTERVIEW WITH THE PATIENT AND/OR SIGNIFICANT OTHER

- Extent and duration of physical factors affecting food ingestion
- Exploration of food tolerances and intolerances
  1. appetite changes
  2. anorexia
  3. difficulty swallowing
  4. gastrointestinal compromise, such as vomiting, nausea, diarrhea, or malabsorption
  5. food allergies or aversions

- Previous diet history, including the use of nutrition supplements and prior use of enteral and parenteral support
- Estimation of nutrient intake based on diet history
- Weight history
  1. usual body weight
  2. history of weight loss or gain and time frame

REVIEW OF MEDICAL MANAGEMENT OF THE PATIENT

- Medical diagnoses and/or problem list
  1. indications for medical nutrition therapy
  2. disease-specific problems requiring adjustments in nutrient intake
  3. indications for enteral nutrition support, such as cancer of the head or neck, chewing disorders, difficulty swallowing, tooth or jaw injuries, or benign obstructions of the upper gastrointestinal tract
- Metabolic gastrointestinal tract dysfunction, such as pancreatitis, radiation enteritis, or chemotherapy that would impair the ability to digest some nutrients
- Increased metabolism, causing an increase in nutrient needs beyond the level that can be achieved by regular oral means
- Respiratory failure
- Anorexia
- Psychiatric disorders
- Neurologic disorders
- Cardiac and/or pulmonary disorders/cachexia

REVIEW OF CONTRAINDICATIONS TO ORAL OR ENTERAL NUTRITION

- Intractable vomiting
- Upper gastrointestinal hemorrhage
- Severe intractable diarrhea
- Intestinal obstruction
- Upper gastrointestinal high-output fistula
- Pertinent laboratory data
  1. blood glucose level
  2. blood urea nitrogen (BUN) level/creatinine level

  3. electrolyte abnormalities
  4. serum albumin level
  5. hemoglobin and hematocrit levels

CRITERIA TO EVALUATE

- Review of systems
  1. cardiac
  2. pulmonary
  3. renal
  4. hepatic
  5. gastrointestinal
  6. endocrine
- Enteral nutrition risk profile
  1. aspiration
  2. dehydration
  3. diarrhea
- Anthropometric evaluation
  1. weight on admission, usual body weight, desirable body weight, ideal body weight
  2. height
  3. Body Mass Index (see Body Mass Index in Appendix 6)
- Physical assessment
  1. cachexia/muscle wasting
  2. obesity
  3. edema/skin turgor
  4. ascites
  5. dehydration
  6. skin lesions and/or pressure sores
  7. signs of vitamin and or mineral deficiencies

Refer to the section on Physical Assessment later in Chapter 1 for more specific details.

REFERENCES

Charney P, Marian M. Nutrition Screening and Risk Assessment. In: Charney P, Malone A, eds. *ADA Pocket Guide to Nutrition Assessment.* Chicago, IL: American Dietetic Association; 2004:1–22.

Marian M. Nutrition and Laboratory Assessment. In: Kalista-Richards M, Marian M, eds. *Sharpening Your Skills as a Nutrition Support Dietitian.* Chicago, IL: Dietitians in Nutrition Support Dietetic Practice Group, American Dietetic Association; 2003:245–254.

Matarese L, Gottschlich M, eds. *Contemporary Nutrition Support Practice: A Clinical Guide.* St. Louis, MO: Elsevier Science; 2005:1–9.

Shopbell J, Hopkins B, Shronts E. Nutrition Screening and Assessment. In: Gottschlich M, Fuhrman P, Hammond K, Holcombe B, Seidner D, eds. *The Science and Practice of Nutrition and Support: A Case-Based Core Cur-* *riculum.* Dubuque, IA: Kendall-Hunt Publishing Co; 2001:107–140.

Winkler MF, Lysen LK. *Suggested Guidelines for Nutrition and Metabolic Management of Adult Patients Receiving Nutrition Support.* Chicago, IL: American Dietetic Association; 1993:2–5.

Physical Assessment

Kathy Hammond, MS, RD, LD, CNSD, RN

DESCRIPTION

Physical examination is part of a comprehensive approach to the assessment of nutritional status. Key information is gathered through interviewing, observation, and hands-on examination techniques and measurements. Physical examination is necessary not only to assess physical features of nutritional deficiency but also to assess other related dynamics of nutritional status including one's ability to care for oneself, procure food, prepare food, and eat food.

EXAMINATION TECHNIQUES

Inspection

- Critical observation to assess color, shape, texture, and size
- Most frequently used technique
- Uses the senses of smell, sight, and hearing

Palpation

- Touching to assess texture, temperature, size, and mobility of a body part
- Two types:
  1. light—uses the fingertips for maximum sensitivity
  2. deep—uses the hand for heavier pressure

Percussion

- Tapping fingers and hands quickly and sharply against body surfaces
- Produces sounds to locate the border, shape, and position of organs
- Determines if an organ is solid or filled with fluid or gas
- Two types:
  1. Direct—tapping the fingertips or hand directly against the body surfaces
  2. Indirect—using the nondominant hand as the stationary hand while hyperextending the middle finger and placing the distal portion against the skin; the middle finger of the dominant hand is used to strike against the hyperextended middle finger

Auscultation

- Last technique to be used in assessment (except when assessing the abdomen, in which it is perfomed after inspection)
- The stethoscope is used to listen to different sounds produced by the lungs, heart, liver, and intestines

INSTRUMENTS

- Thermometer
- Stethoscope

- Sphygmomanometer
- Penlight
- Wooden tongue depressor
- Tape measure/ruler
- Scales
- Skin calipers
- Reflex hammer
- Nasoscope
- Otoscope
- Cotton balls
- Magnifying glass

PREPARATION

- Gather all needed equipment
- Provide privacy for the client
- Expose only the area being examined
- Explain purposes and each process as the examination progresses
- Recognize cultural aspects of care

ASSESSMENT

General Survey

- Reflects overall nutritional status
- Note general state of health including orientation, speech, body type, and mobility
- Note mental status
- Note energy status
- Notes signs of nutritional depletion, such as skeletal muscle wasting, especially in the quadriceps and deltoids; subcutaneous fat wasting in the face, triceps, thighs, and waist; and overall weight loss
- Note any complaints of pain that affect sleep, appetite, and/or physical and emotional well-being

Anthropometric Measurements (see also Appendix 3)

- Height
- Weight, including usual, ideal, and current. Usual body weight is more useful than ideal weight in ill populations. Percent deviation from usual weight assists in determining the degree of malnutrition.

- Knee-height calipers can be used to estimate height and weight measurements for nonambulatory patients, especially in the home, where weights may be difficult to impossible to obtain
- Body mass index (BMI): determined by weight in kilograms divided by the height in meters squared (see BMI chart in Appendix 6)
- Waist-hip ratio: a measure that correlates with risk for diabetes mellitus, stroke, coronary artery disease, and early mortality if over 0.8 for women or over 1.0 for men
- Subcutaneous fat measurements (triceps, biceps, subscapular, and suprailiac skinfolds): a measure of somatic fat stores
- Midarm muscle circumference: a measure of skeletal protein mass

Vital Signs

- Temperature
- Pulse
- Respiration
- Blood pressure

Skin

- Inspect/palpate for the following: color changes, pigmentation, lesions, and bruises. Also assess texture, moisture, temperature, and turgor. Assess wounds and ulcers for size, color, drainage, smell, and warmth.
- Skin should be warm, dry, and smooth to the touch, and without color changes, lesions, bruises, or rashes. Skin is the first line of defense.

Nails

- Inspect/palpate the nails for the following: color, shape, contour, angle, lesions, and circulation
- The nail plate is pink in the white population and bluish in the dark-skinned population.
- The nail surface should be smooth with a translucent plate. The surface may be flat or slightly curved. When squeezed, the nail should appear white and then return to its pinkish color when released.

Hair

- Inspect/palpate for the following: color, shine, quantity, and texture.
- Hair should be consistent in color, quantity, and texture. Natural shine should be present.

Face

- Inspect/palpate for the following: color, lesions, texture, and moisture.
- Face should be consistent in color, warm, dry, smooth, and without lesions.
- Assessment of cranial nerve V (trigeminal) is performed by having the patient clench teeth and noting muscle contraction. Cranial nerve VII (facial) is tested by having the patient show upper and lower teeth. These nerves are important in the eating process.

Eyes

- Inspect/palpate for the following: moisture; color of surrounding skin; condition of conjunctiva, cornea, and sclera.
- The skin surrounding the eye should be warm, dry, and consistent in color. The conjunctiva should be red and without drainage. The sclera is normally white, and the cornea is clear without opacities.
- Vision check should be completed.

Ears

- If trained in using otoscope examine ear according to adult or pediatric standards.
- Inspect color of inner and outer ear, color of inner ear, drainage, fluid, wax build-up.
- Hearing test if appropriate.

Nose: Internal and External

- Inspect/palpate for the following: shape, discharge, patency, septum deviation, and condition of mucous membranes.
- Note any discharge from the nose, including color and consistency
- Do internal inspection by tilting the head slightly back and assessing nasal passages for patency; lack of patency may influence the passage of enteral feeding devices.

- Use different items to test smell—cinnamon, lemon, fragance
- Mucous membranes should be pink.

Jaws

- Inspect/palpate for the following: opening and closing of the jaw, movement from side to side, and condition of the parotid gland.
- The upper and lower front teeth should align, and the jaw should be able to move from side to side without making a "popping" sound. This is important in assessing chewing ability. Also assess the parotid gland, located anterior to the ear lobes, for enlargement.

Lips

- Inspect/palpate for the following: color, symmetry, and lesions.
- The lips should be pink, symmetrical, and without lesions.

Tongue

- Inspect/palpate for the following: symmetry, color, moisture, and texture.
- Inspection is performed by having the patient protrude his tongue. Symmetry can then be noted if the tongue protrudes in midline without deviations or tremors. The tongue should be pink and should appear moist. The tongue is slightly rough in texture from taste buds present.
- Using a tongue blade look under the tongue and surrounding areas.
- Note taste sensations—sweet, sour, bitter, and salt

Buccal Mucosa

- Inspect/palpate for the following: color, moisture, and lesions.
- The oral mucosa should have a pink or red undertone in white populations and may have a bluish undertone in dark-skinned populations. The mucosa should appear moist and smooth without lesions.

- Assess the gag reflex by touching the back of the pharynx with a tongue blade to elicit a response.

Teeth

- Inspect/palpate for the following: color, state of repair, absence, and inflammation.
- The teeth should be same shade of white and in a state of good repair without mottling or patches noted. No inflammation should be present.
- Dentures should be removed to assess surrounding gums and mucosa.

Gums

- Inspect/palpate for the following: color, moisture, and lesions.
- The gums should be pink and moist, without lesions or sponginess noted.

Neck

- Inspect/palpate for the following: neck vein distention, condition of the thyroid gland, parotid gland, and presence of feeding devices.
- The neck veins should be flat and nondistended. Assess the thyroid gland by standing behind the patient, placing the right fingers between the trachea and sternomastoid muscle, and while slightly retracting the muscle, asking the patient to swallow. Repeat for the left side. The thyroid should move slightly up. No hardened nodules or growths should be present.
- Feeding devices should be noted.

Thorax/Respiratory

- Inspect/palpate for the following: muscle development and respiratory rate, depth, and rhythm.
- Auscultate for breath sounds. Breath sounds should be clear with high quality.
- Assess the thorax for adequate muscle and fat stores. Respiratory rate should be within a normal range (adults= ~16–20 breaths/minute). Depth should be even and rhythm regular.

- When auscultated, the breath sounds should be clear with a high quality.

Heart

- Inspect for the following: muscle and fat wasting and the presence and condition of vascular access and surrounding skin.
- Adequate muscle and fat stores should be noted in the general assessment, including the supraclavicular and temporal areas of the body.
- Auscultate heart sounds for presence of normal and abnormal sounds and evaluation of rate and rhythm.

Abdomen

- Inspect for the following: color, warmth, moisture, symmetry, contour, shape, and muscle development; placement and inversion of umbilicus; movements and presence of any feeding devices and/or ostomies. The abdomen should be pink, warm, and dry. The abdomen should be symmetrical bilaterally; contour may range from flat to rounded, depending upon nutritional status, gas, and the presence of fluid. The umbilicus should be midline and inverted. Feeding devices and/or ostomies should be noted, including condition of device, drainage, inflammation, or swelling.
- Auscultate for bowel sounds, using a stethoscope. Dividing the abdomen in four quadrants, begin to listen for bowel sounds in the right lower quadrant where the ileocecal valve is located. Proceed in a clockwise position around the abdomen. Normal bowel sounds occur 5–34 times per minute and are high pitched, with gurgling sounds occurring at irregular intervals. Bowel function including diarrhea or constipation should be assessed.
- Percuss the four quadrants to assess the density of abdominal contents. Tympany is present over the intestines, indicating the presence of air over the stomach, since a gastric air bubble is present. Solid organs and masses produce a dull sound.

- Palpate all four quadrants lastly to determine the size and location of specific organs and the presence of tenderness or pain. Perform light palpation in all four quadrants, using circular motions. The liver may be palpated if necessary. No masses or tenderness should be present.

Renal

- Inspect urine for color and turbidity.
- Urine is normally yellow to amber-yellow in color and clear in appearance.

Musculoskeletal

- Inspect/palpate for fat stores, muscle mass, range of motion, and joint changes, swelling, pain, and tenderness. Also assess motor skills.
- Adequate fat and muscle stores should be present. Triceps skinfold measurements and midarm muscle circumference measurements can assist in this determination. In addition, examination of the gastrocnemius muscle for muscle mass is appropriate along with examination of the deltoid muscle. Degree of mobility of the fingers, wrist, hand, elbow, and shoulder can indicate the need for adaptive equipment to assist with eating.
- No pain, swelling, or tenderness should be present.

Neurologic

- Inspect for the following: mental alertness, orientation, motor status, coordination, weakness, and reflexes.
- Observation during general conversation will reveal alertness and orientation. Assess motor status by observing gait and performance with utensils. Hand-to-mouth coordination can easily be observed during mealtime. Any weakness should be noted.
- Assess reflexes to note central nervous system functioning. A reflex hammer may be used. Reflexes to assess include the biceps, brachioradialis, and patella. Reflexes are graded from 0 to 4, where 2+ is normal response, 0 is absence of response, and 4+ is hyperactivity.

PROBLEMS

General Survey

- Loss of weight, muscle mass, and fat stores
- Mental status (e.g., confusion, depression) can affect food preparation, desire to eat, confusion as to whether meal was eaten or when to eat—resultant weight loss and associated nutritional deficiencies
- Excess fat stores in obesity
- Anemia and fatigue
- Pain affects appetite and ability to prepare food

Skin

- Poor wound healing, pressure ulcers
- Red, swollen, and/or with lesions
- Rash, pellagrous dermatitis
- Bleeding, poor skin turgor
- Xerosis (dry, shedding skin) and follicular hyperkeratosis (spinelike plaques that feel like sandpaper on the buttocks, thighs, elbows, and knees)
- Lesions with irregular borders, asymmetry, or unusual size, color, and/or diameter (usually non-nutritional related)

Nails

- Koilonychia (spoon-shaped, concave nails): be sure to rule out any cardiopulmonary disease
- Dull and lackluster appearance, with transverse ridging across the nail plate
- Bruising and bleeding
- Pallor, poor blanching, irregular shape

Hair

- Lack of shine, luster, thin and sparse distribution with wide gaps between hairs; alopecia
- Dyspigmentation (R/O bleaching)
- Easily plucked hair
- Alternating bands of light and dark hair (Flag sign)
- Corkscrew hair

Face

- Diffuse pigmentation
- Swelling
- Moon face
- Paresthesia
- Temporal wasting
- Maxillary wasting

Eyes

- Visual changes including macular degeneration
- Bitot's spots
- Conjunctival xerosis (inner lids and whites are dull and dry in appearance)
- Keratomalacia (softening of the cornea)
- Pale conjunctiva
- Angular palpebritis (cracked corners of the eye)
- Corneal arcus (grayish-white ring of arc surrounding cornea due to lipid deposition)
- Xanthelsasma (soft, raised yellow plaques on the eyelids)

Ears

- Vestibular disorder (inner ear balance disorders caused by an imbalance of volume and concentration of inner ear fluid).
- Signs/symptoms of vestibular disorder may include vertigo, dizziness, spinning, imbalance, nausea, falls, motion sickness.

Nose

- Seborrhea
- Obstruction; deviated septum
- Inflamed mucous membranes
- Decreased ability to distinguish smells

Jaws

- Malocclusion
- Enlarged parotid gland (bilateral)

Lips

- Cheilosis (vertical cracks, red, swollen)
- Angular stomatitis (cracks and redness at corners of mouth)

Tongue

- Asymmetry
- Atrophic filiform papillae
- Glossitis (beefy red, atrophied tongue)
- Magenta or scarlet color
- Fissures

Mucous Membranes

- Pallor
- Lesions
- Texture

Teeth

- Mottling
- Decay
- Missing teeth; poor repair of teeth
- Inflammation

Gums

- Sponginess
- Receding gumline
- Bleeding
- Lesions

Neck

- Distended veins
- Enlarged thyroid

Thorax/Respiratory

- Depressed muscle mass
- Decreased muscle strength
- Shortness of breath
- Fatigue
- Decline in pulmonary function

Cardiac

- Heart failure, irritability, other disease
- Volume overload
- Hyperlipidemia
- Gastrointestinal
- Anorexia, nausea
- Vomiting
- Diarrhea
- Constipation

- Absent bowel sounds
- Sluggish bowel sounds
- Hyperactive bowel sounds
- Poor wound healing
- Scaphoid abdomen (loss of subcutaneous fat)
- Protuberant abdomen (obesity, gaseous distention)
- Ascites
- Pain

Urinary

- Dark, concentrated urine
- Light, dilute urine
- Presence of blood in urine

Musculoskeletal

- Rickets
- Craniotabes (softening of back and sides of skull in infants less than 1 year of age)
- Enlargement of epiphyses
- Osteomalacia
- Osteoporosis
- Muscle wasting
- Fat store depletion
- Painful, swollen joints
- Limited range of motion

Neurologic

- Listlessness, apathy
- Confusion
- Dementia
- Paresthesia in hands and feet
- Lack of coordination
- Tetany
- Hyperactive reflexes
- Hypoactive reflexes

TREATMENT MANAGEMENT
(see Appendix 4, Assessment of Vitamin Nutriture Tables)

General Survey

- Adequate protein and calories to ensure adequate protein and fat stores
- Avoidance of overfeeding

- Adequate iron intake to prevent microcytic hypochromic anemia and fatigue
- Schedule meals when comfortable and desired
- High-calorie and protein supplements may be beneficial when reduced appetite is present

Skin

- Adequate protein, vitamin C, and zinc to assist with wound healing and prevention of decubitus ulcers
- Adequate B vitamins, especially niacin, to prevent swollen, red skin
- Adequate biotin and zinc to prevent rashes
- Adequate niacin to assist with prevention of pellagrous dermatitis
- Adequate vitamin A and essential fatty acids to assist with maintaining skin
- Vitamins K and C to prevent excessive bleeding, petechiae, and purpura
- Adequate fluid intake to prevent dehydration

Nails

- Adequate iron to prevent koilonychias
- Adequate protein and calories for nails to have a healthy shine and smoothness
- Vitamins A and C to prevent mottling, irregularities, and poor blanching

Hair

- Adequate protein to prevent dull, dry hair, and thinning
- Adequate calories and protein to assist with preventing alopecia that is not related to disease or treatment
- Protein and copper to prevent dyspigmentation and to prevent hair from being easily plucked
- Copper to maintain texture

Face

- Adequate calories and protein to prevent temporal and maxillary wasting

- Protein to maintain color and to prevent dyspigmentation and swelling
- Calcium to prevent paresthesia

Eyes

- Vitamin A for various disorders, including visual changes, Bitot's xerosis, and keratomalacia
- Iron, folate, and B_{12} to prevent potential for anemias
- Niacin, riboflavin, and pyridoxine for angular palpebritis
- Prevention and/or control of hyperlipidemia
- Vision changes should be corrected so safety is maintained while cooking and preparing meals

Ears

- Medical nutrition therapy for vestibular disorders can help alleviate some of the symptoms.
- Foods high in salt and sugar may influence fluid balance of inner ear
- Monitor intake of sugar, salt, alcohol, and caffeine

Nose

- Adequate B vitamins (riboflavin, niacin, pyridoxine) for seborrhea
- Obstructions for deviated septum will influence decision of feeding tube placement
- Smell deficit can have effect on intake—monitor

Jaws

- Malocclusion will influence feeding (textures and types of food)
- Enlarged parotid gland may signal eating disorders, such as bulimia from vomiting

Lips

- Adequate niacin and riboflavin to prevent cheilosis
- Adequate riboflavin, pyridoxine, niacin, and iron to prevent angular stomatitis

Tongue

- Zinc for taste atrophy
- B vitamins such as riboflavin, folic acid, B_6, iron, and B_{12} for glossitis
- Niacin for scarlet tongue
- Mucous membranes
- Iron and B_6 for microcytic anemia
- Folate for macrocytic anemia
- B_{12} for megaloblastic anemia

Teeth

- Adequate fluoride
- Avoidance of excess simple sugars

Gums

- Adequate vitamin C to maintain healthy tissues

Neck

- Adequate iodine to prevent thyroid enlargement
- Maintenance of appropriate fluid status

Thorax/Respiratory

- Adequate protein to maintain muscle mass and strength
- Adequate calories and phosphorus to provide necessary energy
- High-calorie formulas when necessary to decrease amount of energy expended on eating and chewing

Cardiac

- Adequate protein, calories, thiamin, phosphorus, selenium, potassium, calcium, and magnesium for cardiac muscle
- Maintenance of fluid balance
- Avoidance of excess fat intake

Gastrointestinal/Hepatic

- Adequate magnesium and B_{12} for anorexia
- Adequate fluid and fiber for bowel function

- Appropriate access for feeding; small-bowel options for feeding in many cases of gastric paresis, vomiting, early postoperative feeding
- Protein, calories, zinc, and vitamin C to promote wound healing
- Maintenance of appropriate fluid status and sodium and chloride balance with ascites

Urinary

- Giving adequate fluid for age and disease state to prevent dark, concentrated urine
- Avoiding excess fluid intake to prevent light, dilute urine

Musculoskeletal

- Adequate vitamin D and calcium to ensure proper bone development and prevention of rickets, osteomalacia, and osteoporosis
- Adequate vitamin C for joints
- Adequate protein for growth
- Assistance with increasing strength in order to shop, prepare food, and for general well-being

Nervous System

- Protein to maintain alertness and prevent listlessness, apathy, and confusion
- Pantothenic acid, biotin, and folate for lethargy
- Thiamin to assist with mental confusion, weakness, and peripheral neuropathy (beriberi)
- B_6 to treat polyneuritis
- Niacin and B_{12} to assist in prevention of dementia
- Calcium and magnesium to prevent tetany, tremors, and some behavioral disturbances
- Coordination assistance if needed to promote proper hand-to-mouth coordination, chewing, and swallowing ability

REFERENCES

Bates B, Bickley LS, Hoekelman RA, eds. *A Guide to Physical Examination and History Taking.* 6th ed. Philadelphia, PA: JB Lippincott Co; 1995.

Cecere C, McCash K. Health history and physical examination. In: *Medical–Surgical Nursing.* St. Louis, MO: CV Mosby; 1992:29–49.

Curtas S, Chapman G, Meguid NM. Evaluation of nutritional status. *Nurs Clin North Am.* 1989;24:301–313.

Flory C. Skin assessment. *RN.* June 1992;22–26.

Freis SB. Medical nutrition therapy and vestibular disorders. *Today's Dietitian.* 2003;5(10):38–40.

Fuller J, Schaller-Ayers J, eds. *Health Assessment: A Nursing Approach.* 2nd ed. Philadelphia, PA: JB Lippincott Co; 1994:115–184.

Grant A. *Nutrition Assessment Guidelines.* Seattle, WA: Northgate Station; 1979.

Hammond K. Dietary and clinical assessment. In: Mahan LK, Escott-Stump SK, eds. *Krause's Food, Nutrition, and Diet Therapy.* Philadelphia, PA: WB Saunders Co; 2004.

Herbert J. Health history and physical assessment. In: Bausbaum BS, Mauro E, Norris CG, eds. *Illustrated Manual of Nursing Practice.* 2nd ed. Springhouse, PA: Springhouse; 1994:48–75.

Heineken J, McCoy N. Establishing a bond with clients of different cultures. *Home Healthc Nurse.* 2000;18(1):45.

Hopkins B. Assessment of nutritional status. In: Gottschlich MM, Matarese LE, Shronts EP, eds. *Nutrition Support Dietetics Core Curriculum.* 2nd ed. Silver Spring, MD: American Society for Parenteral and Enteral Nutrition; 1993:15–70.

Jarvis C. *Physical Examination and Health Assessment.* Philadelphia, PA: WB Saunders Co; 1992.

Konstanstinides N. Nutritional care. In: Bauxbaum BS, Mauro E, Norris CG, eds. *Illustrated Manual of Nursing Practice.* 2nd ed. Springhouse, PA: Springhouse; 1994:789–835.

Owen G. Physical examination as an assessment tool. In: Simko MD, Cowell C, Gilgride JA, eds. *Nutrition Assessment: A Comprehensive Guide for Planning Intervention.* 2nd ed. Gaithersburg, MD: Aspen Publishers, Inc; 1995:85–90.

Poncor PJ. Who has time for a head to toe assessment? *Nursing.* 1995;25:59.

Sherman JL, Fields SK. *Guide to Patient Evaluation.* Garden City, NY: Medical Examination; 1982.

Vogelzang JL. Making nutrition sense from OASIS. *Home Healthc Nurse.* 2003;21(9):592–600.

Weisner RI, Morgan SL, eds. *Fundamentals of Clinical Nutrition.* St. Louis, MO: CV Mosby; 1993.

Zulkowski K, Albrecht D. How dental status affects healing in older adults. *Nursing.* 2003;33(10):22.

CHAPTER 2

Indirect Calorimetry

Carol S. Ireton-Jones, PhD, RD/LD, CNSD

INTRODUCTION TO INDIRECT CALORIMETRY

- *Definition:* Indirect calorimetry is the determination of heat production (energy expenditure) by measuring the oxygen consumption and carbon dioxide production during respiratory gas exchange.
- The technique of indirect calorimetry is based on the premise that all energy is derived from the oxidation of protein, carbohydrate, and fat and that the amount of oxygen consumed and carbon dioxide produced are characteristic and constant for each fuel.
- Measurement of energy expenditure by indirect calorimetry provides an assessment of an individual's energy expenditure and therefore energy requirements.
- Use of indirect calorimetric measurements enables the clinician to assess more accurately a patient's energy requirements and ability to utilize nutrient substrates.
- Indirect calorimetry measures actual energy expenditure as opposed to that estimated by energy expenditure formulae, and therefore provides important information to adjust the patient's intake accordingly.

COMPONENTS OF TOTAL DAILY ENERGY EXPENDITURE

- *Basal energy expenditure or basal metabolic rate (BMR)* is the approximate energy cost of maintaining basic physiologic activities including heartbeat, respiration, kidney function, osmotic balance, brain activity, and body temperature. Determined twelve to fourteen hours after the ingestion of food and with the individual at complete rest.
- *Resting metabolic rate (RMR)* includes the BMR and any increases that occur following awakening and with minimal activity.
- *Diet-induced thermogenesis* (the "thermic effect" of food) accounts for a 5%–8% increase above RMR in daily energy expenditure. It includes an obligatory process due to the inevitable energy costs of digestion, absorption, and processing or storage of substrates and a component which involves stimulation of the sympathetic nervous system.
- *Shivering* and *nonshivering thermogenesis,* or "cold-induced thermogenesis," play a minor role in everyday life. Nonshivering thermogenesis is difficult to demonstrate in adult individuals and therefore is considered to be of little or no consequence in overall daily energy expenditure.
- *Physical activity:* the energy costs of many activities have been measured and it has been found that the amount of energy expended is proportionate to the rate of sustained muscle contraction.
- *Disease, stress, and other factors:* the energy costs of stress from injury or illness caused by specific diseases such as cancer, by fever, or by the therapeutic interventions of pharmacotherapy and chemotherapy.

13

PHYSIOLOGY OF ENERGY EXPENDITURE

- The maintenance of body functions is dependent on a constant amount of voluntary and involuntary energy expenditure and varies among individuals.
- Energy expenditure is proportionate to the body surface area and to the percentage of lean body mass.
- Males typically have higher metabolic rates than do females.
- Energy expenditure is generally depressed during starvation and in chronic dieters and anorexics.
- Energy expenditure increases in people residing in cold climates as compared to those in warmer climates, in the obese, in smokers, and under conditions of stress and disease.

METHODS OF PERFORMING INDIRECT CALORIMETRY (MEASURING RESTING METABOLIC RATE [MRMR])

- *Open-circuit method:* The subject is permitted to breathe air from the environment, while his expired air is collected for volumetric measurement. The gas volume is then corrected for standard conditions and is analyzed for its oxygen and carbon dioxide content, with a subsequent calculation being done to determine oxygen consumption and carbon dioxide production. This method is employed by most of the indirect calorimeters on the market today.
- *Closed-circuit method:* The subject is isolated from outside air and breathes from a reservoir containing pure oxygen. The decrease in the gas volume in the closed method is related to the rate of the oxygen consumption, from which the metabolic rate is then calculated.
- The Weir Equation is used to calculate energy expenditure from the minute volume of oxygen consumed and carbon dioxide produced as measured by indirect calorimetry.
- Adults, children, and neonates can be measured using indirect calorimetry. When measuring pediatric patients or neonates using a metabolic measurement cart, appropriate technique and equipment must be used to account for lower ventilatory volumes.

EQUIPMENT TO PERFORM INDIRECT CALORIMETRY

- Indirect calorimeters, usually called Metabolic Measurement Carts
  Two types of indirect calorimeters to measure RMR:
  1. Provides measurement of VO_2 and VCO_2
     –*Advantages:* Ease of use, accurate among various operators, reproducible results, instantaneous results, can be used with a variety of patients in many settings if patient interfaces are available.
     –*Disadvantages:* Expensive
  2. Provides measurement of VO_2 only
     –*Advantages:* Ease of use, application to spontaneously breathing patients specifically; usually less expensive
     –*Disadvantages:* Respiratory quotient (RQ) cannot be measured and therefore a standard RQ of 0.85 is most often used; accuracy may be diminished, although not significantly
- Douglas bags/pulmonary physiology lab
  –*Advantages:* Considered by some to be the "gold standard" for performing indirect calorimetry.
  –*Disadvantages:* Cumbersome, accuracy relies on the operator's skills in obtaining and analyzing the data, results are not usually available quickly, not often used in the hospital or home care settings.
- Ventilators which are able to perform indirect calorimetry
  –*Advantages:* Patient can be measured 24 hours per day without additional equipment.
  –*Disadvantages:* Single use because only the patient using the ventilator can be measured—indirect calorimetry is part of the ventilator; expensive.

CONDITIONS FOR PERFORMING INDIRECT CALORIMETRY

- Energy expenditure can be accurately determined under standard conditions
- Patients should be measured when they are awake and two hours after a meal unless they are on continuous nutritional support.
- Measurements should be taken at least sixty minutes following strenuous activity such as a dressing change, chest physiotherapy, or physical therapy.

PROCEDURE FOR COMPLETING AN MRMR USING INDIRECT CALORIMETRY

- Patient is connected to the metabolic cart according to the specifications for spontaneously breathing or ventilator-dependent patient.
- Measurement is initiated and continued until a "steady state" has been achieved. This is indicated by 3 to 5 consecutive minute measurements in which the MRMRs are within 10% of each other and the corresponding RQs are within 5% of each other, or until the resting state has been maintained for 10–15 minutes.
- Long-term measurements of greater than 2 hours and up to 24 hours can be done with most metabolic carts depending on the patient's medical status and cooperation.
- See sample indirect calorimetry procedure (see Exhibit 2–1)

TYPES OF PATIENTS FOR WHOM INDIRECT CALORIMETRY IS USEFUL

Hospital

- All patients receiving intensive nutritional support (parenteral or enteral nutrition) should have their energy expenditure measured (MRMR) using indirect calorimetry as a part of the initial nutritional assessment.
- Patient prioritization for indirect calorimetry:
  1. all intensive care unit (ICU) patients receiving nutrition support
  2. patients receiving parenteral nutrition other than those in the ICU
  3. all other patients
- MRMR should be done weekly for ICU patients; all other patients should have their energy expenditures reassessed biweekly unless otherwise indicated. Any patient's energy expenditure should be reassessed when a significant change occurs affecting the condition, such as changing the route of nutritional support from parenteral to enteral or the method of ventilation from mechanical ventilator support to spontaneous breathing.
- Reassessment of MRMR should be done following each major surgical procedure, change in medical status, or by a standard protocol.

Home

- Because the type and complexity of patients seen at home is increasing, the use of indirect calorimetry in the home can be an important part of initial and follow-up assessments for people receiving nutrition support.
- Patients on home TPN may be inadequately nourished when the Harris-Benedict equations are used to estimate energy requirements. The Harris-Benedict equations were developed from MRMRs of adult normal subjects, not acutely ill or chronically ill people.
- Most indirect calorimeters are too cumbersome and are not portable enough to take into the patient's home. A new indirect calorimeter is small and easily portable and can be used to measure VO_2 and RMR of individuals not on a ventilator in the home or alternate site care setting (MedGem, HealtheTech, Golden, CO).

Other

- There are uses for indirect calorimetry other than for patients receiving intensive nutritional support, such as patients whose energy requirements are difficult to assess (obese patients, children).
- Inpatient and outpatient centers dealing with eating disorders will find the assessment of energy expenditure a useful adjunct to therapy.

Exhibit 2–1 Sample Indirect Calorimetry Protocol

WHO

Any patient receiving nutrition support or who is at nutritional risk. Must have MD order to see patient. Hospitalized patients as per MD order.

WHEN

Measured resting metabolic rate (MRMR) must be calculated under the following standard conditions:

1. MRMR is done two hours after a meal or calorie-containing fluid is ingested and/or two hours after discharged home on TPN or tube feeding (TF). If on TPN or TF continuously, then feeding is not discharged for test.
2. Patient must be at rest for one hour prior to the test (i.e., the patient can shower and dress but cannot exercise, such as a walk or workout).
3. Water or noncaloric beverage is acceptable intake before a test.

METHODOLOGY

SPONTANEOUSLY-BREATHING PATIENTS are connected to the metabolic cart using a canopy. VENTILATOR-DEPENDENT PATIENTS are connected to the metabolic cart using a single-piloted exhalation valve to collect expired gas. Inspired gas is sampled on the "dry side" of the ventilator humidifier.

INTERPRETATION

Measurements of oxygen consumption and carbon dioxide production are made in one-minute intervals until a steady state is achieved. MRMR and respiratory quotient (RQ) are calculated. A steady-state is achieved when three consecutive one-minute measurements of MRMR are within 10% of each other and the corresponding RQs are within 5% of each other.

RESULTS

1. Minute measurements of MRMR and RQ are averaged to determine the patient's energy expenditure.
2. Results are provided to the physician so that modification of the nutrition support regimen can be made in a timely manner.

- Study protocols may be devised to examine segments of the patient population in conjunction with specific diseases or injury.
- Indirect calorimetry may be integrated as a component of other programs, such as wellness programs.

RESPIRATORY QUOTIENT (RQ)

- RQ is calculated from the ratio of carbon dioxide produced (VCO_2) to oxygen consumed (VO_2) and reflects net substrate utilization (VCO_2/VO_2).
- Oxidation of each major nutrient class occurs at a known RQ, ranging from 0.7 for fat oxi-

dation to 1.0 for glucose oxidation. Net fat synthesis is demonstrated by the occurrence of an RQ greater than 1.0.

RQ (Respiratory Quotient) (specific fuel utilization)	
Substrate	*RQ*
Fat	0.70
Protein	0.80
Carbohydrate	0.95–1.00
Mixed diet	0.85
Net fat synthesis	>1.00

INTERPRETATION OF THE RESULTS OF INDIRECT CALORIMETRY MEASUREMENTS

- The indirect calorimetric measurement represents the patient's MRMR and may need to be modified to account for daily energy requirements.
- Suggested factors to add to the MRMR are:
  1. Light activity, inactive disease state: MRMR $\times$ 1.1–1.2
  2. Light activity, active disease state: MRMR $\times$ 1.2–1.5
  3. High activity, inactive disease state: MRMR $\times$ 1.5
- The MRMR is evaluated taking into account the results of the nutrition assessment. This information should be provided to the physician in a timely manner so that the nutrition support regimen can be modified accordingly.

BENEFITS OF USING INDIRECT CALORIMETRY TO MEASURE ENERGY EXPENDITURE

- Provides accurate assessment of energy expenditure—overfeeding of patients may be as harmful as underfeeding
- When VO_2 and VCO_2 are measured, RQ can be determined. Overfeeding and fat synthesis can be identified by an RQ > 1.0. Fat synthesis may lead to hepatic steatosis. Also, extra carbon dioxide and fluid loads produced as a result of excess nutrient intake exert deleterious effects in patients with impaired ventilator function.

LIMITATIONS OF INDIRECT CALORIMETRY

- Patients who are ventilator-dependent receiving pressure support, high-frequency ventilation, or levels of F_{IO_2} greater than 60% often cannot be accurately measured.
- In some cases, isolation techniques will prevent the use of the measurement equipment.

- For spontaneously breathing patients, cooperation is necessary for connection to the metabolic cart.
- Presence of an incompetent tracheal cuff will invalidate the measurement data because of the potential for dilution by room air or other sources of air.
- Patients receiving dialysis should not be measured during treatment.
- Patients with leaking chest tubes should not be measured.
- When indirect calorimetry is not available, appropriate energy equations should be used to predict the energy expenditures of hospitalized and home care patients. (Refer to other chapters which may include specific recommendations for energy expenditure estimation.)
- When a steady state is not achieved or there is wide variability in minute measurements of MRMR and RQ, this is indicative of an inaccurate indirect calorimetric measurement and the resulting MRMR and RQ data should not be used.

CHARACTERISTICS TO CONSIDER IN THE ACQUISITION OF A METABOLIC MEASUREMENT CART

- The population the metabolic cart will be applied to: ventilator-dependent and spontaneously breathing adult and/or pediatric patients.
- The type of measuring technique the metabolic cart uses (mixing chamber or breath by breath).
- The type and ease of connections to ventilator-dependent patients.
- The type and ease of connections to spontaneously breathing patients (mask, canopy).
- Special considerations such as ease of movement, warranty, training, and support services, both technical and scientific.

REFERENCES

Amato P, Keating KP, Quercia RA, et al. Formulaic methods of estimating calorie requirements in mechanically ventilated obese patients: A reappraisal. *Nutr Clin Pract.* 1995;10:229–232.

Frankenfield D, Muth ER, Rowe WA. The Harris-Benedict studies of human basal metabolism: History and limitations. *JADA.* 1998;98:439–445.

Frankenfield DC, Rowe WA, Smith JS, et al. Validation of several established equations for resting metabolic rate in obese and non-obese people. *JADA.* 2003:103(9): 1152–1159.

Ireton-Jones CS, Borman KR, Turner WW. Nutrition considerations in the management of ventilator-dependent patients. *Nutr Clin Pract.* 1993;8(2);60–64.

Ireton-Jones CS, Long A, Garritson B. The use of indirect calorimetry in the assessment of energy expenditure in patients receiving home nutrition support. *JADA.* 1994; 94(9); suppl;A30.

Ireton-Jones CS, Turner WW. The use of respiratory quotient to determine the efficacy of nutritional support regimens. *JADA.* 1987;87(2):180–183.

Ireton-Jones CS, Turner WW, Liepa GU, et al. Equations for the estimation of energy expenditures in patients with burns with special reference to ventilatory status. *J Burn Care Rehabil.* 1992;13(3):330–333.

Jequier E. Measurement of energy expenditure in clinical nutritional assessment. *JPEN.* 1987;11(5):86S–89S.

Kinney JM. Indirect calorimetry in malnutrition: nutritional assessment or therapeutic reference? *JPEN.* 1987;11(5): 90S–94S.

Makk LJ, McClave SA, Creech PW, et al. Clinical application of the metabolic cart to the delivery of total parenteral nutrition. *Crit Care Med.* 1990;18(12);1320–1327.

McClave SA, Snider HL. Use of indirect calorimetry in clinical nutrition. *NCP.* 1992;7:202–221.

McClave SA, Snider HL, Greene L, et al. Effective utilization of indirect calorimetry during critical care. *Intern Care World.* 1992;9:194–200.

McClave S, Snider HL, Ireton-Jones C. Can we justify continued interest in indirect calorimetry? *NCP Bull.* 2002;17(3):133–136.

Porter C, Cohen NH. Indirect calorimetry in critically ill patients: Role of the clinical dietitian in interpreting results. *JADA.* 1996;96(1):49–57.

Sedlet KL, Ireton-Jones CS. Energy expenditure and the abnormal eating pattern of a bulimic: A case report. *JADA.* 1989;89(1):74–77.

Weissman CW, Sadar A, Kemper MA. In vitro evaluation of a compact metabolic measurement instrument. *JPEN.* 1990;12:216–221.

CHAPTER 3

Nutrition Management for Specific Medical Conditions

- The Burn Patient
- Cardiovascular Disorders
- Cancer
- Nutrition Support in the Critically Ill Patient
- Diabetes Mellitus
- Gastrointestinal Disorders
- Geriatric Nutrition

- Hematopoietic Cell Transplantation
- Otolaryngology
- HIV/AIDS
- Obesity
- Pediatric Conditions
- Pulmonary Conditions
- Renal Conditions
- Solid Organ Transplantations

The Burn Patient

Michele M. Gottschlich, PhD, RD, CNSD

DESCRIPTION

Burns, as commonly defined, represent tissue destruction resulting in circulatory and metabolic alterations that characterize the compensatory response to injury (Table 3–1). These events have important effects on nutritional status.

CAUSE

The causes of burn wounds include excessive exposure to thermal (heat or cold), chemical (acids or alkalis), electrical, or radioactive agents.

ASSESSMENT

Classification

Burns are usually classified according to depth of skin involvement:

- First-degree burns: Limited involvement of outer epidermal layers only.

- Second-degree burns: Damage extends through the epidermis into varying depths of the dermis.
- Third-degree burns: Full-thickness injury with destruction of all epithelial elements.

Initial Assessment of Nutritional Status

Obtain diet/medical history to determine if the patient presents with significant risk factors that may further compromise nutritional status (e.g., inadequate intake prior to burn, > 20% burns, concomitant injury, sepsis, recent weight loss > 10%).

Estimation of Nutritional Requirements

Energy

- Alterations in metabolism
  1. The increased energy expenditure of burns exceeds that of any other injury.
  2. Oxygen consumption is near normal during resuscitation, then rises and peaks

Table 3–1 Metabolic Alterations Following Burns

	Ebb Response	Flow Response	
		Acute Phase	Adaptive Phase
Dominant factors	Loss of plasma volume	Heightened total body blood flow	Stress hormone response subsiding
	Poor tissue perfusion	Elevated catecholamines	Convalescence
	Shock	Elevated glucagon	
	Low plasma insulin levels	Elevated glucocorticoids	
		Normal or elevated serum insulin	
		High glucagon-insulin ratio	
Metabolic and clinical characteristics	Decreased oxygen consumption	Catabolism	Anabolism
	Depressed resting energy expenditure	Hyperglycemia	Normoglycemia
	Decreased blood pressure	Increased respiratory rate	Energy expenditure diminished
	Cardiac output below normal	Increased oxygen consumption and hypermetabolism	Nutrient requirements approaching preinjury needs
	Decreased body temperature	Increased carbon dioxide production	
		Increased body temperature	
		Redistribution of polyvalent cations such as zinc and iron	
		Increased urinary excretion of nitrogen, sulphur, magnesium, phosphorus, potassium, and creatinine	
		Accelerated gluconeogenesis	
		Fat mobilization	
		Increased use of amino acids as oxidative fuels	

Source: Gottschlich MM, Alexander JW, Bower RH. Enteral nutrition in patients with burns or trauma. In: Rombeau JL and Caldwell MD, eds. *Enteral and Tube Feeding.* Philadelphia, PA: WB Saunders Co; 1990:307.

around postburn day 10, with a maximum level 2 to 2.5 times greater than the normal metabolic rate.

3. Chronic elevation of catecholamines seems to be the dominant stimulus for increased oxygen consumption and enhanced energy needs.
4. The greater percentage of body surface area burned, the more pronounced the hypermetabolic response; other factors also affect the response (i.e., fever, sepsis, surgery, nutrient intake, environmental temperature, body composition, physical activity, drugs).
5. Metabolic rate returns to normal after wound coverage is achieved.

• Guidelines for estimating caloric needs
1. Many mathematical equations exist for estimating energy expenditure.
   –*Curreri formula* for children > 3 years old and adults: (25 × kg weight) + 40 × % burn)
   –*Polk formula* for children < 3 years old: (60 × kg weight) + (35 × % burn)
   –*Harris-Benedict equation* to derive basal energy expenditure (BEE): BEE × (activity factor) × (injury factor) will estimate total caloric needs.
   Activity factor
   Confined to bed = 1.2
   Out of bed = 1.3
   Injury factor
   Burns = 2.1
2. Indirect calorimetry permits a more accurate, individualized measure of energy – expenditure.
   –Multiply resting energy expenditure by activity factor 1.2 – 1.3 to estimate daily needs. Reassess at least twice weekly.
   –If respiratory quotient (RQ) is > 1.00, reduce total caloric intake and/or reduce carbohydrate/lipid ratio; if < 0.80, increase total caloric intake.

Protein

• Alterations in metabolism
1. Protein may be the most important nutrient compromised by a burn injury.

2. Protein provides the amino acid building blocks for healing.
3. Increased gluconeogenesis from alanine and other gluconeogenic amino acids exists during the acute phase.
4. The plasma concentration of arginine decreases, whereas plasma phenylalanine and leucine are frequently elevated.
5. Extensive nitrogen losses occur in exudate and urine.
6. Protein catabolism, like energy expenditure, is related to the size of the injury; aberrations normalize after the wound is covered.

• Guidelines for intake
1. Considerable evidence supports the use of high-protein regimens (20% to 23% of caloric needs), which inherently contain a low calorie–nitrogen ratio.
2. The protein source should be of high biologic value.
3. Intact protein is superior to predigested/elemental amino acids in enteral nutrition.
4. Arginine enrichment improves cell-mediated immunity and wound healing and decreases morbidity and mortality in burns; glutamine is a key fuel for the intestinal mucosa and therefore should be included in nonvolitional feeding regimens for burns; branched-chain amino acid supplementation has not shown beneficial effects.

Carbohydrate

• Alterations in metabolism
1. Increased glucose production from gluconeogenesis occurs in response to the altered hormonal environment.
2. There is little evidence to suggest impaired glucose oxidation occurs.
3. The burn wound metabolizes large quantities of glucose, largely to lactic acid, a pathway apparently favored by healing wounds.
4. During the acute phase following major thermal injury and during periods of infection, the tendency for hyperglycemia has

resulted in terms such as *stress diabetes* and *diabetes of injury.*
- Guidelines for intake
  1. Carbohydrate has beneficial effects as a nutritional substrate.
     –Stimulates insulin release, a key anabolic hormone.
     –Protein is best utilized when abundant carbohydrate is present.
  2. Potential side effects of excessive carbohydrate intake are
     –Hyperglycemia.
     –Osmotic diuresis, resulting in dehydration and hypovolemia.
     –Excess CO_2 production with potential respiratory insufficiency.

Fat

- Alterations in metabolism
  1. Reduced lipolysis during the acute phase with preferential oxidation of lean body mass for fuel.
  2. Elevated levels of serum free fatty acids
  3. Increased serum triglycerides
  4. Decreased levels of serum cholesterol
- Guidelines for intake
  1. Conservative ingestion of fat is beneficial; diets containing 15% to 20% of nonprotein calories as fat seem to be optimal.
  2. Supplementation with fatty acids of the omega-3 family (e.g., fish oil) has been correlated with improved immunocompetence and tube-feeding tolerance; this may be due to their inhibitory effect in the omega-6 fatty acid conversion to the 2-series of prostaglandins or an unrecognized omega-3 dietary requirement.
  3. Complications related to excessive fat intake are
     –Hepatomegaly
     –Fat overload syndrome
     –Impaired clotting
     –Impaired host defense
     –Decreased resistance to infection
     –Increased incidence of diarrhea

Micronutrients

- Protein and energy cannot be efficiently utilized if micronutrient intake is inadequate.
- Current knowledge supports daily multivitamin supplementation.
- Further enrichment with vitamins A and C along with zinc is also important.
  1. Vitamin A
     –Important for maintenance of immunologic response and epithelialization.
     –Dietary guidelines should approximate 5000 IU of vitamin A per 1000 kcal of enteral nutrition.
  2. Ascorbic acid
     –Important coenzyme involved in collagen synthesis and immune function.
     –Ingestion of 1 g of ascorbic acid per day (500 mg twice daily) should be routine protocol.
  3. Zinc
     –Cofactor in energy metabolism, protein synthesis.
     –Supplementation with 220 mg of zinc sulfate daily is recommended.

PROBLEMS

- Underfeeding has a direct negative impact on wound healing, immunocompetence, and mortality.
- Overfeeding can cause complications such as hyperglycemia, fatty liver, and elevated CO_2 production (respiratory insufficiency).

TREATMENT/MANAGEMENT

Enteral Nutrition

- Adequate oral intake is probable with burns ≤ 20% surface area.
- Feeding tubes should usually be inserted for patients with burn area exceeding 20% or patients presenting with significant nutritional risk factors.
- Begin enteral nutrition as soon as possible postburn.

Table 3–2 Nutrition Parameters to Monitor in Burn Patients

Parameter	Frequency	Comments
Diet history	On admission	Look for evidence of preinjury malnutrition, food allergies, intolerances that could put a critically ill patient at heightened risk.
Indirect calorimetry	Biweekly	Valuable indicator of severity of hypermetabolism. Nutrition support is inadequate when REE $\times$ 1.3 exceeds caloric intake or when RQ is less than 0.83.
Weight	3 times weekly	Weight loss in excess of 10% of preinjury weight represents a nutritional emergency. A weight change greater than 1 lb/day indicates fluid imbalances and will skew interpretation of visceral proteins. Corrections must be made for amputations, supportive apparatus, occlusive dressings, and major escharotomies.
Triceps skinfold, midarm muscle circumference	Weekly	Detect long-term changes in lean body mass and fat stores. In the absence of physical therapy, the immobile patient patient will lose somatic protein even with aggressive nutritional suport.
Nitrogen balance	Daily	Amount of urine urea nitrogen excreted/24 hours is a valuable index of severity of hypercatabolism. Nitrogen balance indicates whether nitrogen intake is exceeding body mass breakdown. Nutrition support is considered inadequate if nitrogen balance is negative.
Serum albumin, transferrin, prealbumin, retinol-binding protein levels	Weekly	Indicative of extent of depletion of visceral proteins. Delivery of a large quantity of blood products or the long half-life of certain secretory proteins can complicate interpretation.
Delayed hypersensitivity skin testing, total lymphocyte count, C3, IgG	Optional	Suboptimal nutritional status can cause deficits in immune function and infection can cause derangements in nutrition parameters.
Serum glucose	Daily until stable, then twice weekly	Some patients with previously normal glucose tolerance prior to injury may require sliding-scale insulin therapy during aggressive nutritional support.
Fluid status, blood urea nitrogen, and serum creatinine	Daily until stable, then twice weekly	Need to be monitored for all patients receiving high-protein regimens because of high renal solute load. If azotemia develops, increase the delivery of free water, decrease the protein content of nutrient substrate, or both.
Nutrient intake from all sources (oral, tube feeding, parenteral)	Daily	Immediate modification in nutrition support should be made if deviation of actual intake from goal is detected. The use of a computer can greatly improve speed and sophistication of nutrient analysis (e.g., vitamin intake).

continues

Table 3–2 continued

Parameter	Frequency	Comments
Follow reports of skin graft adherence, healing process, or percent open wound	Weekly	Poor wound healing may suggest inadequate consumption of protein and/or micronutrients. Reassess needs/intake and supplement as indicated.

REE = resting energy expenditure; RQ = respiratory quotient.
Source: Adapted with permission from Gottschlich MM, Alexander JW, Bower RH. Enteral nutrition in patients with burns or trauma. In: Rombeau JL and Caldwell MD, eds. *Enteral and Tube Feeding,* Philadelphia, PA: WB Saunders Co.; 1990:318.

1. Delayed enteral feeding is associated with loss of gastrointestinal mucosal mass, decreased tube-feeding tolerance, elevated catabolic hormones, increased metabolic rate, and increased risk of postburn malnutrition.
2. Tube feeding bypassing the stomach into the small intestine makes enteral nutrition possible during times of gastric ileus.
3. Selection of enteral feeding products must consider the unique energy, protein, fat, and micronutrient needs of burn patients; many commercial tube-feeding products are unacceptable for burns.
4. A moderately low-fat, high-protein diet therapy program is recommended.
5. Since digestive and absorptive capabilities are intact in burns (assuming enteric feeding is implemented early), hydrolyzed products are not warranted.
- Enteral nutrition is favored over parenteral because of specific advantages derived from alimentation by the enteral route.
  1. Decreased incidence of complications such as pneumothorax, bleeding, infection
  2. Lower cost
  3. Maintenance of optimal intestinal anatomy and function

Parenteral Nutrition (PN)

- If calorie requirements cannot be entirely met by enteral feedings, PN can save burn

patients from the morbidity and mortality of malnutrition.
- However, PN implemented during the first 10 days postburn has no positive effect on immune function or survival.
- Conservative administration of intravenous fat is recommended in view of its hyperlipidemic and immunosuppressive tendencies.
  1. Intravenous lipids are unnecessary if enteral support containing fat is delivered simultaneously.
  2. When PN is the sole source of nutrition, 500 mL of 10% fat emulsion three times weekly is adequate.

Monitoring

Monitoring the feeding regimen to determine tolerance and effectiveness of the diet therapy program is important. Table 3–2 outlines suggested clinical and laboratory parameters that should be continuously monitored.

REFERENCES

Alexander JW, MacMillan BG, Stinnett JD, Ogle CK, Bozian RD, Fischer JE, et al. Beneficial effects of aggressive protein feeding in severely burned children. *Ann Surg.* 1980;192:505–517.

Alexander JW, Saito H, Trocki O, Ogle CK. The importance of lipid type in the diet after burn injury. *Ann Surg.* 1986;204:1–8.

Bell SJ, Molnar JA, Krasker WS, Burke JF. Prediction of total urinary nitrogen from urea nitrogen for burned patients. *J Am Diet Assoc.* 1985;85:1100–1104.

Gottschlich MM. Assessment and nutrition management of the patient with burns. In: Winkler MF and Lysen LK, eds. *Suggested Guidelines for Nutrition and Metabolic Management of Adult Patients Receiving Nutrition Support.* Chicago, IL: The American Dietetic Association; 1993:64–70.

Gottschlich MM. Nutrition in the burned pediatric patient. In: Queen P and Lang C, eds. *Handbook of Pediatric Nutrition.* Gaithersburg, MD: Aspen Publishers, Inc; 1999:493–512.

Gottschlich MM, Jenkins ME, Mayes T, Khoury J, Warden GD. An evaluation of the safety and effects of early versus delayed enteral support and effects on clinical, nutritional and endocrine outcomes following burns. Awarded the American Burn Association's Clinical Research Award. *J Burn Care Rehabil.* 2002;23:401–415.

Gottschlich MM, Jenkins M, Warden GD, Baumer T, Havens P, Snook JT, et al. Differential effects of three enteral regimens on selected outcome variables in burn patients. *JPEN.* 1990;14:225–236.

Gottschlich MM, Mayes T, Khoury J, Warden GD. Significance of obesity on nutritional, immunological, hormonal and clinical outcome parameters in burns. *J Am Diet Assoc.* 1993;93:1261–1268.

Gottschlich MM, Mayes T, Khoury J, Warden GD. Hypovitaminosis D in pediatric burn patients. *J Am Diet Assoc.* In press.

Gottschlich MM, Warden GD, Michel MA, Havens P, Kopcha R, Jenkins M, et al. Diarrhea in tube-fed burn patients: Incidence etiology, nutritional impact, and prevention. *JPEN.* 1988;12:338–345.

Gotschlich MM, Warden GD. Vitamin supplementation in the burn patient. *J Burn Care Rehabil.* 1990;11:275–279.

Gottschlich MM, Warden GD. Parenteral nutrition in the burned patient. In: Fischer E, ed. *Total Parenteral Nutrition.* Boston, MA: Little, Brown and Co; 1991:270–298.

Hart DW, Wolf SE, Herndon DN, Chinkes DL, Lal SO, Obeng MK, Beauford RB, Mlcak RP. Energy expenditure and caloric balance after burn. Increased feeding leads to fat rather than lean mass accretion. *Ann Surg.* 2002;235:152–161.

Herndon DN, Stein MD, Rutan TC, Abston S, Linares H. Failure of TPN supplementation to improve liver function, immunity, and mortality in thermally injured patients. *J Trauma.* 1987;27:195–204.

Hildreth M, Gottschlich MM. Nutritional support of the burned patient. In: Herndon DN, ed. *Total Burn Care.* Philadelphia, PA: WB Saunders Co; 1996:237–254.

Ireton CS, Hunt JL, Liepa GU, Turner WW. Evaluation of energy requirements in thermally injured patients. *JPEN J Parenter Enteral Nutr.* 1982;6:577.

Ireton-Jones C, Gottschlich MM. The evolution of nutrition support in burns. *J Burn Care Rehabil.* 1993;14:272–280.

Jenkins M, Gottschlich M, Baumer T, Khoury J, Warden GD. Enteral feeding during operative procedures. *J Burn Care Rehabil.* 1994;15:199–205.

Mayes T, Gottschlich MM. Burns and wound healing. In: Gottschlich MM, ed. *The Science and Practice of Nutrition Support: A Case-based Core Curriculum.* Dubuque, IA: Kendall/Hunt Publishing Co; 2001:391–419.

Mayes T, Gottschlich MM. Burns. In: Matarese L and Gottschlich M, eds. *Contemporary Nutrition Support Practice.* Philadelphia, PA: WB Saunders Co; 2003: 595–615.

Mayes T, Gottschlich MM, Khoury J, Warden GD. An evaluation of predicted and measured energy. *J Am Diet Assoc.* 1996;96:24–29.

Mayes T, Gottschlich MM, Warden GD. Nutrition intervention in thermally injured pediatric patients requiring laparotomy. *J Burn Care Rehabil.* 2000;21:451–456.

Mochizuki H, Trocki O, Dominioni L, Alexander JW. Reduction of postburn hypermetabolism by early enteral feeding. *Curr Probl Surg.* 1985;42:121–125.

Morath MA, Miller SF, Finley RK, Jones LM. Interpretation of nutritional parameters in burn patients. *J Burn Care Rehabil.* 1983;4:361–366.

Saffle JR. Practice guidelines for burn care. Initial nutritional support of burn patients. *J Burn Care Rehabil.* 2001;22:59S–66S.

Saffle JR, Medina E, Raymond J, Westenskow D, Kravitz M, Warden GD. Use of indirect calorimetry in the nutritional management of burned patients. *J Trauma.* 1985;25:32–39.

Waxman K, Rebello T, Pinderski L, O'Neal K, Khan N, Tourangeau S, et al. Protein loss across burn wounds. *J Trauma.* 1987;27:136–140.

Wilmore DW, Long JM, Mason AD, Skreen RW, Pruitt BA. Catecholamines: Mediator of the hypermetabolic response to thermal injury. *Ann Surg.* 1974;180:653–669.

Wray C, Mayes T, Khoury J, Warden G, Gottschlich M. Metabolic effects of vitamin D on serum calcium, magnesium and phosphorus in pediatric burn patients. Awarded the American Burn Association's Moyer Research Award. *J Burn Care Rehabil.* 2002;23:416–423.

Zhou YP, Jiang ZM, Sun YH, Wang XR, Ma EL, Wilmore D. The effect of supplemental enteral glutamine on plasma levels, gut function, and outcome in severe burns: A randomized double-blind, controlled clinical trial. *JPEN.* 2003;27:241–245.

Cardiovascular Disorders

Janice Raymond, MS, RD, CNSD and Pam Amann, RD

INTRODUCTION

Despite mountains of data from thousands of studies and an ever-increasing arsenal of drugs, cardiovascular disease (CVD) remains the leading cause of death in the United States. The importance of nutrition in the prevention and treatment of CVD is now doctrine. For the most part the dietary regimen recommended for prevention is also used for treatment.

CORONARY ARTERY DISEASE

Coronary artery disease (CAD) is any disorder of the coronary arteries that leads to an interference in blood supply to the myocardium. In the past, CAD was believed to be caused by the attachment of fatty plaques to the inner arterial wall, thus altering the lumen size and functional capacity of the coronary artery. We now know that these plaques actually arise in the vessel walls themselves and that inflammation plays a key role. The process of plaque formation has been described as that of a cut; an injury is followed by inflammation and the formation of a blood clot. When one of the plaques ruptures it can cut off blood flow and result in a myocardial infarction, a stroke, or a pulmonary embolus, depending on the location of the obstruction. An excess of low-density lipoprotein

(LDL) in the blood is apparently part of the inflammation initiation.

The diet for prevention and treatment of CAD is now focused on decreasing LDL cholesterol and decreasing the inflammation.

HYPERTENSION

Approximately 50 million—one in four—adult Americans have high blood pressure or hypertension. As the population ages, the prevalence of hypertension will increase further. Studies suggest that individuals who are normotensive at age 55 have a 90 percent lifetime risk for developing hypertension. The relationship between blood pressure (BP) and risk of CVD is consistent and independent of other risk factors. The higher the BP, the greater the chance of myocardial infarction, heart failure, stroke, and kidney disease. For individuals aged 40 to 70 years, each increment of 20 mm Hg in systolic BP or 10 mm Hg in diastolic BP doubles the risk of CVD across the entire BP range from 115/75 to 185/115 mm Hg.

A new classification, prehypertension, was introduced as a strategy to involve patients and professionals in prevention of hypertension. At the same time, the definitions of hypertension were changed. (See Table 3–3.)

Table 3–3 Classification of Blood Pressure (BP)

Category	Systolic Blood Pressure mm Hg		Diastolic Blood Pressure mm Hg
Normal	< 120	and	< 80
Prehypertension	120–139	or	80–89
Hypertension, Stage 1	140–159	or	90–99
Hypertension, Stage 2	≥ 160	or	≥ 100

HEART HEALTHY EATING

The Heart Healthy Food Pyramid (Figure 3–1), developed at MultiCare Health System, incorporates the most up-to-date recommendations from the American Heart Association (AHA), the National Cholesterol Education Panel (NCEP), the Dietary Approaches to Stop Hypertension (DASH) studies, and the Mediterranean Diet Pyramid.

The American Heart Association recommends consuming a balanced diet to include a variety of fruits and vegetables, grains, low-fat and nonfat dairy products, fish, legumes, poultry, and lean meats. The AHA guidelines also include information on consuming appropriate energy levels to maintain or achieve a healthy body weight.

The Executive Summary of the Third Report of the National Cholesterol Education Program (NCEP) Expert Panel on Detection, Evaluation and Treatment of High Blood Cholesterol in Adults (Adult Treatment Panel III [ATP III]) provides a set of evidence-based guidelines on cholesterol management that includes therapeutic lifestyle changes. In addition to recommending physicians refer patients

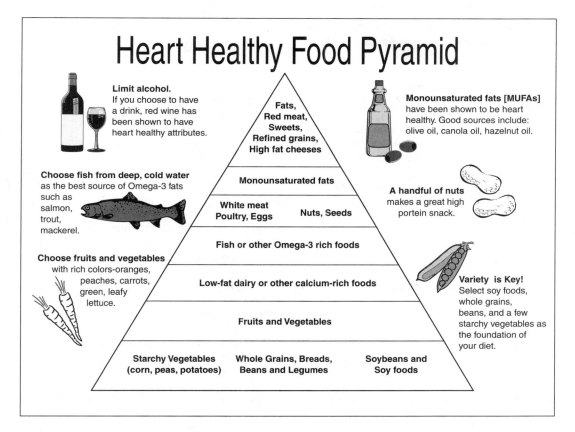

Figure 3–1 Heart Healthy Food Pyramid. Reprinted courtesy of Multicare Health System, Tacoma, Washington.

to see a registered dietitian, this set of guidelines includes: reduction in saturated fat and cholesterol, inclusion of stanols/sterols and soluble fibers, and increased activity along with weight management.

The Dietary Approaches to Stop Hypertension (DASH) eating plan is based on the research findings from two studies supported by the National Heart, Lung, and Blood Institute (NHLBI). The key findings of these studies showed that not only is the re-duction of sodium important in controlling blood pressure, but a diet rich in potassium, calcium, magnesium, protein, and fiber is also important. The DASH eating plan focuses on fruits and vegetables and low-fat dairy foods. It also includes whole grains, fish, poultry, and nuts, yet is limited in red meats, sweets, and beverages that contain sugar.

The Mediterranean Diet came out of the Seven Countries Study. This study showed that, despite a high intake of fat, certain Mediterranean

Table 3–4 The Heart Healthy Food Pyramid Is a Teaching Tool Meant to Accompany the Specific Recommendations for Dietary Changes

Fiber	30 grams daily	
Fat	• 20%–35% of total calories • < 7% of total calories from saturated fats • Avoid trans fatty acids	• Focus on monounsaturated fats such as olive oil, canola oil, and most nut oils • Include adequate omega-3 fats • No daily value for trans fatty acids has been established
Cholesterol		
Soy	25 grams of soy protein per day	In 1999, the Food and Drug Administration approved a health claim that can be used on labels of soy-based foods that meet the qualifying guidelines. The health claim reads: "Diets low in saturated fat and cholesterol that include 25 grams of soy protein a day may reduce the risk of heart disease."
Calcium	1200 mg per day	Sources: • Low-fat or nonfat dairy foods • Fortified calcium foods such as soy milk, tofu, whole-grain cereals, or orange juice • Nondairy sources of calcium such as broccoli, some leafy green vegetables or legumes, and sesame seeds
Fruits and vegetables	8–10 servings per day	• Highlight a variety of colorful fruits and vegetables • Phytochemicals produce the color in fruits and vegetables; the more color, the more nutrients
Sodium	2400 mg per day or less	• Most Americans consume 4–5 grams of sodium per day • 1 teaspoon of table salt contains 2400 mg of sodium • Foods, as they come from nature, are low in sodium; sodium is added in the processing and flavoring

populations had a very low incidence of CAD. However, the fat consumed was different than the typical American diet. Fat sources are primarily monounsaturated found in olive oil, nuts and seeds, and some omega-3 fat from fish with small amounts of saturated fat from poultry. There was very little consumption of red meat. The Mediterranean style of eating also includes an abundance of plant food (fruits, vegetables, whole-grain cereals, nuts, and legumes), and a moderate consumption of wine, normally with meals.

The Heart Healthy Food Pyramid visually depicts how to build a healthy diet, with the foods that should be consumed in the greatest quantity toward the bottom of the pyramid and the foods that should be eaten in limited quantities at the top. (See Figure 3–1 and Tables 3–4 through 3–8.)

HEART FAILURE

Heart failure (HF) is a complex clinical syndrome that can result from any cardiac disorder that impairs the ability of the ventricle to eject blood. Heart failure afflicts about 5 million people in the United States with 400,000 to 700,000 new cases diagnosed each year. This represents about 2% of the population. Heart failure is the only major cardiovascular disorder that is increasing in incidence and prevalence and is the leading cause of hospitalization in people age 65 and older. Annual direct expenditures for HF in the United States have been estimated at $20 to $40 billion. The cost of hospitalization for HF is twice that for all forms of cancer.

HF is a complex clinical syndrome that can result from any structural or functional cardiac disorder that impairs the ability of the ventricle to fill with or eject blood. The cardinal symptoms are shortness of breath, fatigue, and fluid retention.

Coronary artery disease is the cause of HF in about two-thirds of patients with left ventricular function. The remainder have nonischemic causes of systolic dysfunction such as hypertension, valvular disease, Beriberi, or myocarditis.

When no specific cause is identified it is known as idiopathic dilated cardiomyopathy.

Evaluation of Patients with Heart Failure

- The functional status of patients with heart failure is most commonly assessed using the New York Heart Association classification. Patients are assigned to 1 of 4 classes, depending on the degree of effort needed to elicit symptoms. Patients may have symptoms of HF at rest (Class IV); on less than ordinary exertion (Class III); on ordinary exertion (Class II); or only at levels that would produce symptoms in normal individuals (Class I). (See Table 3–9.)
- The single most important measurement in the patient with HF is the assessment of left ventricular ejection fraction. This is generally done with an echocardiogram coupled with Doppler flow studies; however, new noninvasive technology (Impedence Cardiography) has recently become available and may be used more frequently in the future.
- Measurement of circulating levels of brain natriuretic peptide (BNP). While this biochemical marker cannot distinguish diastolic dysfunction from those with systolic dysfunction, it does identify patients with elevated left ventricular filling pressure (ventricle stretch). *Note:* The synthetic form of BNP is known as nestiritide and is used as treatment for HF. It must be given intravenously.
- Assessment of fluid status is what determines the use of diuretics.

Management of Heart Failure

In heart failure, the inability to meet the body's metabolic needs is based on hemodynamic derangement and suboptimal oxygen-carrying capacity of the blood itself. Current pharmacologic therapy attempts to improve survival and reduce symptoms by optimizing hemodynamics and to increase oxygen delivery and oxygen-carrying capacity. Patients with HF are generally on multiple medications, many with negative effects on dietary intake and nutritional status. (See Table 3–10.)

Table 3–5 The NCEP Adult Treatment Panel (ATP) III Guidelines and Implication of Recent Clinical Trials

For high-risk patients—Individuals who have coronary heart disease (CHD) or disease of the blood vessels to the brain or extremities, or diabetes, or multiple (2 or more) risk factors that give them a greater than 20% chance of having a heart attack within 10 years.

ATP III	The treatment goal for high risk patients is an LDL less than 100 mg/dL	Update	The overall goal for high-risk patients is still an LDL less than 100 mg/dL. There is a therapeutic option to set the goal at an LDL less than 70 mg/dL for very high-risk patients—those who have had a recent heart attack, or those who have cardiovascular disease combined with either diabetes, or severe or poorly controlled risk factors (such as continued smoking), or metabolic syndrome (a cluster of risk factors associated with obesity that includes high triglycerides and low HDL cholesterol).
ATP III	Recommended consideration of cholesterol-lowering drug treatment in addition to lifestyle therapy for LDL cholesterol levels 130 mg/dL or higher in high-risk patients. Characterized drug treatment for LDL levels 100–129 mg/dL as optional, and not needed for LDL less than 100 mg/dL.	Update	Recommends consideration of drug treatment in addition to lifestyle therapy for LDL levels 100 mg/dL or higher in high-risk patients, and characterizes drug treatment as optional for LDL less than 100 mg/dL.

For moderately high-risk patients—Individuals who have multiple (2 or more) CHD risk factors together with a 10–20% risk for a heart attack within 10 years.

ATP III	The treatment goal is an LDL less than 130 mg/dL, and drug treatment is recommended if LDL is 130 mg/dL or higher.	Update	The overall goal for moderately high-risk patients is still an LDL less than 130 mg/dL. There is a therapeutic option to set the treatment goal at an LDL less than 100 mg/dL, and to use drug treatment if LDL is 100–129 mg/dL.

For high risk and moderately high-risk patients.

ATP III	Did not explicitly emphasize achieving a certain percentage lowering of LDL cholesterol.	Update	Advises that the intensity of LDL-lowering drug treatment in high-risk and moderately high-risk patients be sufficient to achieve at least a 30% reduction in LDL levels.

For people who are at moderate risk—those with 2 or more risk factors, plus a less than 10% risk for heart attack within 10 years, or lower risk—those with 0–1 risk factor, the update does not modify the ATP III recommendations.

Table 3–6 Table of Definitions

Definitions	
Saturated fatty acids	Tend to raise serum cholesterol. Are solid at room temperature. Major sources of saturated fatty acids are the following: animal fats (dairy products such as butter, whole milk, ice cream, and cheese), beef, pork, poultry, and plant oils (coconut oil, palm kernel oil, palm oil, cocoa butter).
Trans fatty acids	Artificially created form of fat that occurs when an unsaturated fat is hydrogenated, a process that makes the fat solid and spreadable.
Monounsaturated fatty acids	Lower serum cholesterol when used as part of a low-saturated fat diet. They do not appear to lower HDL cholesterol. Major sources of monounsaturated fatty acids are the following: olive oil, canola oil, peanut oil, rice oil, hazelnut oil, and avocado.
Polyunsaturated fatty acids	Some are known to lower serum cholesterol but can tend to lower HDL cholesterol, too. Major sources of polyunsaturated fatty acids include omega-6 polyunsaturates (linoleic acid) of corn oil, safflower oil, sunflower oil, and soybean oil, and omega-3 polyunsaturated fish oils. An increased intake of omega-3 fatty acids is associated with a disruption of platelet aggregation, which may reduce the risk of coronary thrombosis. Omega-3 fatty acids appear to be more effective at lowering triglyceride levels than lowering serum cholesterol.
Soluble fiber	Is considered an adjunct to a cholesterol-lowering diet.

Table 3–7 Table of Terms Used in Labeling

Terms Used on Food Labels for Fat, Cholesterol, and Sodium	
Fat-free	< 0.5 grams of fat per serving
Low-fat	≤ 3 grams of fat per serving
Reduced or less fat	At least 25% less fat per serving than the regular or reference product (cannot be used if product meets definition for low-fat)
Lean	< 10 grams of fat, < 4 grams of saturated fat, and < 95 mg of cholesterol per serving
Extra lean	< 5 grams of fat, < 2 grams of saturated fat, and < 95 mg of cholesterol per serving
Low in saturated fat	≤ 1 gram saturated fat per serving and $\leq 15\%$ of calories from saturated fatty acids
Cholesterol free	< 2 mg of cholesterol and ≤ 2 grams of saturated fat per serving
Low cholesterol	≤ 20 mg of cholesterol and ≤ 2 grams of saturated fat per serving
Reduced cholesterol	At least 25% less cholesterol than the regular or reference product and ≤ 2 grams of saturated fat per serving (cannot be used if product meets definition for low cholesterol)
Sodium free (no sodium)	< 5 mg of sodium per serving and no sodium chloride in ingredients
Very low sodium	≤ 35 mg of sodium per serving
Low sodium	≤ 140 mg of sodium per serving
Reduced or less sodium	At least 25% less sodium per serving than the regular or reference product (cannot be used if product meets definition of low sodium)

Table 3–8 Common CVD Medications

Classes of Cholesterol Lowering Drugs	
Class	*Example*
HMG CoA reductase inhibitors (statins)	Lovastatin
Bile acid sequestrants	Cholestyramine
Nicotinic acid	Niacin
Fibric acids	Clofibrate

Nutrition Therapy for Patients with Heart Failure

1. Lessen demands on the heart
   –decrease blood volume through sodium and fluid restriction
   –eat smaller amounts at each meal/snack
2. Eliminate or reduce edema
   –sodium and fluid restriction
3. Avoid distention and elevation of diaphragm
   –eat smaller amounts
   –avoid difficult-to-digest foods
   –decrease fat in meals
4. Attain ideal body weight, replace lean body mass
5. Limit cardiac stimulants like caffeine
6. Prevent cardiac cachexia
   –gradual feeding of a cachetic patient is critical to prevent refeeding syndrome. Serum electrolytes, Mg, and PO_4 should be carefully monitored.
7. Correct nutrient deficits
   –the most commonly reported nutrient deficiency is thiamin due to excessive losses from diuretic therapy and should be supplemented
   –Potassium supplementation is integral to thiazide diuretic therapy due to excessive losses.
   –A multivitamin with minerals and CoQ10 (see discussion that follows) is recommended for most patients
8. Prevent pressure ulcers from reduced activity and poor circulation

Coenzyme Q10

Coenzyme Q10 (CoQ10) is an important cofactor in several metabolic pathways. It is most abundant in cellular mitochondria. CoQ10 is one of the cofactors involved in converting adenosine diphosphate to usable energy, adenosine triphosphate (ATP). CoQ10 is prevalent in humans, with high endogenous concentrations found in the heart, liver, kidney, and pancreas.

Table 3–9 Stages of Heart Failure and Recommended Therapy

Stage	*Description of Stage*	*Therapy*
Stage A	At risk for heart failure but without structural heart disease or symptoms of HF	• Treat hypertension • Encourage smoking cessation • Treat lipid disorders with diet and medication • Encourage regular exercise • Discourage alcohol intake and illicit drug use • Use of ACE inhibitors in appropriate patients
Stage B	Structural heart disease but without HF	• All measures under A • ACE inhibitors in appropriate patients • Beta-blockers in appropriate patients
Stage C	Structural heart disease with prior or current symptoms of HF	• All measures under A • Diuretics, ACE inhibitors, beta-blockers and digitalis • Dietary sodium restriction
Stage D	Refractory HF requiring specialized interventions	• All measures under A, B, and C • Mechanical assist devices • Heart transplantation • Continuous IV inotropic infusions for palliation • Hospice care

Table 3–10 Nutritional Implications of Common HF Medications

Drug Class	Implications
ACE inhibitors	• Decrease production of angiotensin and aldosterone • End in "pril," such as catopril, enalapril, and lisinopril • Can cause hyperkalemia, nausea, vomiting, and dizziness.
Diuretics	• Furosemide is the most commonly used diuretic and can cause potassium depletion, anorexia, nausea, and decreased glucose tolerance.
Anticoagulants	• Warfarin is used in nonambulatory patients to prevent blood clots and in patients with atrial fibrillation, a common concomitant cardiac disorder. • High vitamin K foods should be eaten in consistent amounts each day to prevent fluctuations in clotting time.
Beta-adrenergic blockers	• Reduce cardiac output in competing for available receptor sites • Decrease sympathetic stimulation of the heart • End in "-ol," such as propranolol and acebutolol
Arterial vasodilators	• Include hydralazine and minoxidil • Reduce cardiac workload and can cause nausea and vomiting
Erythropoietin (Epogen)	• Stimulates production of red blood cells and therefore increases oxygen-carrying capacity of the blood • Must be given in conjunction with iron and the combination can cause nausea and constipation.

Heart failure is characterized by fatigue and has been associated with low endogenous CoQ10 levels. The purported role of CoQ10 in the treatment of CHF relates to its increase in ATP synthesis and enhancement of myocardial contractility. Ten randomized, double-blind, controlled studies evaluating adjuvant therapy with CoQ10 showed varying benefits in patients with HF. Eight of 10 studies revealed favorable effects. An improvement in quality of life and statistically significant reduction in the number of patients requiring hospitalization for worsening HF were reported in two studies.

Many patients with HF are on statin drugs to lower cholesterol. There is significant evidence that people who use statin drugs have reduced endogenous levels of CoQ10 and it is hypothesized that low CoQ10 levels may lead to statin-induced myopathy.

Patients should not take more than 300 mg per day of CoQ10. CoQ10 can decrease the effectiveness of warfarin and may decrease insulin requirements in patients with diabetes.

Sodium and Heart Failure

It is recommended that patients with HF restrict fluid to no more than 2 liters per day and restrict sodium to no more than 2 grams per day. The average American eats 4 to 5 grams of sodium per day, so the sodium restriction can be a difficult change for patients to make.

Most of the sodium in the American diet comes from eating processed foods or from adding table salt or salty seasonings to food. The only food group with naturally occurring sodium is dairy. One cup of milk has about 125 mg of sodium. (See Table 3–11.)

Examples of High-Sodium Seasonings and Condiments

Celery, onion, or garlic salt
Packaged sauces, gravies, and marinades
Fish sauce
Plum sauce
Soy sauce AND lite soy sauce
Meat tenderizer

Table 3–11 Four Basic Steps to a Low-Sodium (2-gram) Diet

---

1. Stop adding salt to food
2. Stop using all salt-containing seasonings and condiments
3. Eat fresh foods that have not been processed
4. Read labels and do not eat foods with more than 100 mg sodium per serving or more than 600 mg sodium in an entire meal

---

MSG
Pickle relish
Steak sauce
Teriyaki or stir-fry sauce
Pesto taco sauce
Worcestershire sauce
Sea salt and kosher salt
Salad dressings
Mustard*
Ketchup*
Barbeque sauce*

*These can be included in a low sodium diet if they are eaten in small amounts; be sure to read labels

REFERENCES

ACC/AHA Guidelines for the evaluation and management of chronic heart failure in the adult: Executive summary. *Circulation.* 2001;104:2996–3007.

De Lorgeril M, Salen P, Martin J, Monjaud I, Delaye J, Mamelle N. Mediterranean diet, traditional risk factors, and the rate of cardiovascular complications after myocardial infaction: Final report of the lyon diet study. *Circulation.* 1999, 99(6):779–785.

DePinieux G, Chariot P, Ammi-Said M, et al. Lipid-lowering drugs and mitochondrial function: Effects of HMG CoA reductase inhibitors on serum ubiquinone and blood lactate/pyruvate ratio. *Br J Clin Pharmacol.* 1996;42:333–337.

Heart Failure Society of America. How to Follow a Low-Sodium Diet. Heart Failure Society of America, 2002. www.hfsa.org.

Henkel J. *Soy: Health Claims for Soy Protein, Questions About Other Components.* FDA Consumer, May–June 2000.

Jeejeebhoy KN. Nutritional aspects of congestive heart failure. *Nutrition and the MD.* 2002;28(11):1–5.

Krauss RM, Eckel RH, Howard B, et al. AHA dietary guidelines: revision 2000: A statement for healthcare professionals from the Nutrition Committee of the American Heart Association. *Circulation.* 2000;102:2284–2299.

McBride BF and White M. Anemia management in heart failure: A thick review of thin data. *Pharmacotherapy.* 2004;24(6):757–767.

Mongthuong TT, Mitchell TM, Kennedy DT, Giles JT. Role of coenzyme Q10 in chronic heart failure, angina, and hypertension. *Pharmacotherapy.* 2001;21(7):797–806.

Packer M, Cohn J, eds. Consensus recommendations for the management of chronic heart failure. *Am J Cardiol.* 1999;83(2A):1A–38A.

Suter PM, Hany A, Vetter, W. Diuretic use: A risk factor for subclinical thiamine deficiency in elderly patients. *J Nutr Health Aging.* 2000;4(2):69–71.

Suter PM, Vetter W. Diuretics and vitamin B1: Are diuretics a risk factor for thiamin malnutrition? *Nutr Rev.* 1999;58(10):319–323.

U.S. Department of Health and Human Services. Third Report of the National Cholesterol Education Program (NCEP) Expert Panel on Detection, Evaluation, and Treatment of High Blood Cholesterol in Adults (Adult Treatment Panel III) Executive Summary. U.S. Department of Health and Human Services, National Heart, Lung, and Blood Institute. May 2001.

U.S. Department of Health and Human Services. Facts about the DASH Eating Plan. U.S. Department of Health and Human Services. National Heart, Lung, and Blood Institute. October 2003.

U.S. Department of Health and Human Services. Reference Card From the Seventh Report of the Joint National Committee on Prevention, Detection, Evaluation, and Treatment of High Blood Pressure (JNC 7). U.S. Department of Health and Human Services, National Heart, Lung, and Blood Institute. December 2003.

U.S. Department of Health and Human Services. The Seventh Report of the Joint National Committee on Prevention, Detection, Evaluation, and Treatment of High Blood Pressure. U.S. Department of Health and Human Services, National Heart, Lung, and Blood Institute. December 2003.

U.S. Department of Health and Human Services. Information about the Update of the Adult Treatment Panel III Guidelines. U.S. Department of Health and Human Services, National Heart, Lung, and Blood Institute www.nhlbi.nih.gov/guidelines/cholesterol/upd-info_prof.htm. January 2005.

U.S. Food and Drug Administration. How to Understand and Use the Nutrition Facts Label. www.cfsan.fda.gov/~dms/foodlab.html. November 2004.

Cancer

Abby S. Bloch, PhD, RD

DESCRIPTION

As the second leading cause of death in the United States, soon to surpass heart disease, cancer is of concern to both health professionals and the public. Studies have shown that 40%–80% of all patients who are diagnosed with cancer will develop clinical malnutrition. The clinical effects of poor nutrition may compromise the individual's ability to heal surgical wounds, maintain skin turgor, prevent breakdown or decubiti, prevent anastomotic leaks or dehiscence, maintain metabolic balance, and maintain effective immune activity; they may also increase morbidity and mortality. Therefore, feeding the cancer patient should be an integral aspect of care and management.

CAUSE

Cancer is caused by uncontrolled growth and spread of abnormal cells. Both external (chemicals, radiation, viruses, procarcinogens, and carcinogens ingested) and internal (hormones, immune conditions, inherited mutations) factors play a role in its development. Malnutrition in the cancer patient may be caused by any of the following:

- changes in dietary patterns, food intake, or appetite
- metabolic abnormalities caused by the disease process
- antineoplastic therapy (surgical resection of the gastrointestinal [GI] tract, chemotherapy, radiation therapy, hormones, or immunotherapy)
- functional status or logistical problems with food purchasing, preparing, and handling

ASSESSMENT

To determine the extent and depth of the nutritional problem, if any, a patient must be appropriately screened and assessed. The following are guidelines for performing a thorough, accurate assessment.

- Use the appropriate screening/assessment tool or measure to do the following:
  1. Establish risk category. (Table 3–12 provides a screening tool.)
  2. Flag nutritional deficits and problems.
  3. Develop a nutrition care plan and nutrient goals.
- Determine food intolerance, food aversions, and changes in taste perception or preferences.
- Assess the degree of decreased appetite, early satiety, head/neck or gastrointestinal discomfort, or symptoms affecting food intake or tolerance.
- Assess weight changes.
  1. Significant weight loss may be experienced by 45% or more of all adult hospitalized cancer patients.
  2. Assess pre-illness adult weight status, prior 6-month weight patterns, admission weight, and current weight.
  3. Consider influences such as edema, ascites, and hydration status.
- Assess medical status.
  1. Check for other clinical conditions such as diabetes, heart disease, hypertension, and renal disease.
  2. Obtain a list of all medications being taken.
  3. Obtain a history of previous therapy, treatments, or medical management.
- Evaluate nondietary factors affecting nutritional status:
  1. Age—if the individual is young or elderly, screening and assessment parameters should be age appropriate.

     Body composition, weight, and metabolic rate should be evaluated accordingly, using appropriate tables and algorithms.

Table 3–12 Memorial Sloan-Kettering Cancer Center Nutrition Care Process

Process	Low Risk	Moderate/High Nutritional Risk
MSKCC Patient Assessment Summary Nursing Review of Patient History and Data Base	Patient without weight loss or nutritional complications	Nurse Referral to Dietitian: 1. Weight status: Patient has a weight loss of 10 or more lbs in the last 3 months and/or 2. A 2- or more week history of food intake decreased from normal, nausea/vomiting, diarrhea, mouth sores, or difficulty chewing or swallowing.

Adult Oncology Screening Tool

	Low-Risk Criteria	Moderate Nutritional Risk Criteria	High Nutritional Risk Criteria
Dietitian's Evaluation of Nutrition Risk/ Intervention Plan	(patient does not meet nutritional risk criteria above; without weight loss/ nutritional complications): Rescreen on 6th day.	Nutritional Assessment completed within 24 hrs of referral. Reassessment within 5 days.	Nutritional Assessment completed within 24 hrs of referral. Reassessment within 3 days.
Diagnosis/ Complications	Nadir fever Comfort care Cancer of the: Prostate Bladder Ovary Renal cell Lung Liver	AIDS/HIV Ascites Emesis > 3 days Diarrhea > 3 days Diabetes Decubiti Stage II Edema Esophageal stricture GBM (Glioblastoma) Odynophagia Renal insufficiency Mucositis	Acute weight loss during hospitalization Chylous ascites/chylous leak Dysphagia GI (fistula, ileus, upper GI bleed, malabsorption, obstruction, short gut/ dumping syndromes) Graft vs. host disease Liver failure/Hepatic encephalopathy New-onset diabetes Pancreatitis Poor wound healing documented/Decubiti Stages III and IV Renal failure/dialysis

Adult Oncology Screening Tool

Dietitian's Evaluation of Nutrition Risk/ Intervention Plan	Low-Risk Criteria	Moderate Nutritional Risk Criteria	High Nutritional Risk Criteria
Treatment/Surgery	Biopsy Bronchoscopy One day chemotherapy Head and Neck Surgery (without complications) including: Partial Thyroidectomy, Neck Dissection, Parotidectomy, Craniofacial, Small Check, Oral Lesions, Nasal Polyps, Sinus Surgery, Biopsy, Tonsillectomy	Autologous Bone Marrow Transplant (BMT) Head & Neck Surgery: Craniotomy Total Thyroidectomy Free Flap, Skin Grafts, Bone Grafts, Palate Surgeries Base of Tongue, Floor of Mouth, Partial Glossectomy	Allogenic BMT Surgery for Esophageal Cancer Pancreatic Cancer Head & Neck Surgery: Commando Procedures, Mandibulectomy, Laryngectomy, Laryngopharyngoesophogastrectomy/ Gastric Pull-Up After Loading Catheters Head and Neck Brachytherapy
Weight status	(% UBW) > 90% UBW	(Loss) (1) 1%–2% UBW (over 1 wk) (2) < 5% UBW (over 1 mo) (3) < 10% UBW (over 6 mo)	(Loss) (1) > 2% UBW (over 1 wk) (2) > 5% UBW (over 1 mo) (3) > 10% UBW (over 6 mo) Enteral Nutrition TPN/PPN Dysphagia Diet Renal Diet NPO/Clear liquids ≥ 5 days (without nutrition support (Exceptions: nephrectomy, cystectomies, hemicolectomies)
Diet orders	Patient does not require diet instruction.	Patient requires diet instruction for diet modification or drug-nutrient interaction.	

Note: UBW = usual body weight.
Source: Courtesy of Memorial Sloan-Kettering Cancer Center, Food Service Department, New York, New York.

2. Functional status—mobility, dexterity, visual acuity, range of motion, mental status, pain status.
3. Determine whether adequate means are accessible to the patient to obtain, prepare, and ingest food.
4. Financial, psychological, and social conditions that may influence eating. Obtain laboratory parameters from the medical record that will provide insight on the clinical status of the patient.

• Assess the effect of the disease process on nutritional status.
1. Tumors within the GI tract may obstruct the passage of food.
2. Tumors outside the GI tract may press on or obstruct organs or parts of the GI tract.
3. Systemic effects of the tumor might lead to early satiety, or aversions to certain foods.

PROBLEMS

Metabolic Alterations Affecting Nutritional Status

• *Energy expenditure* may increase (sarcomas, leukemia, lymphomas, lung, head/neck, small-cell lung carcinoma, and gastric), decrease (pancreatic), or remain normal (colon). Resting energy expenditure cannot explain fully the cachexia seen in many cancer patients.
• *Carbohydrate metabolism* appears to be altered in the cancer patient, preventing adaptation to a starved state in which glycogen stores and ketone bodies can supply needed fuel to the brain, sparing glucose and muscle protein. Insulin resistance or impaired insulin sensitivity may be seen in wasting cancer patients.
• *Lipid metabolism* is altered in the malnourished cancer patient, as seen in the depletion of fat stores. Increased lipolysis and fatty acid oxidation may be related to the insulin resistance of the patient. Cancer patients do not suppress lipolysis after a glucose load is given, leading to body fat depletion of the cachectic cancer patient.

• *Protein metabolism* is also altered in the cancer patient. Malnourished cancer patients have protein metabolism similar to traumatized or infected noncancer patients. Most of these patients are in negative nitrogen balance that becomes more pronounced with the severity of the malignancy. Patients may have increased liver synthesis, decreased synthesis in the muscles causing muscle wasting, decreased serum protein levels, and increased whole-body protein turnover favoring the tumor over the host.

Treatments Affecting Nutritional Status

• *Chemotherapy* may cause nausea, vomiting, anorexia, diarrhea, mucositis, stomatitis, constipation, abdominal pain, pain on swallowing, generalized pain, altered taste, food aversions, cardionephrohepatotoxicity, and electrolyte and fluid abnormalities. (See Table 3–13 for emetogenic potential of specific chemotherapy agents.)
• *Radiation* may cause nausea, vomiting, anorexia, stenosis, radiation enteritis/malabsorption, decreased taste, decreased smell, problems with chewing/swallowing/mouth blindness, mucositis, dental caries, oral infections, inability to swallow, dry mouth, and mouth sores.
• *Surgery* may induce metabolic or nutritional compromise of the patient by altering or removing parts of the GI tract that play a role in digestion, absorption, or utilization of foodstuffs or nutrients. Surgical resection may compromise the physical capability of the patient, as in head/neck surgery, or create tolerance problems such as cramping, rapid transit, diarrhea, or fat malabsorption.

TREATMENT/MANAGEMENT

Nutritional Requirements

Calories

Caloric requirements should be established to ensure adequate energy and nutrients needed by the patient. To determine caloric levels, the following estimates are a quick guide that will

Table 3–13 Emetogenic Potential of Individual Chemotherapy Agents

High

Aldesleukin infusion (no dexamethasone)
Carboplatin
Carmustin
Cisplatin
Cyclophosphamide
Cytarabine
Dacarbazine
Dactinomycin
Daunorubicin
Doxorubicin
Epirubicin
Idarubicin

Ifosfamide
Lomustine
Mechlorethamine
Melphalan
Methotrexate
Oxaliplatin
Pentostatin
Procarbazine
Streptozocin
Thiotepa
Tirapazamine

Intermediate

Altretamine
Bleomycin
Doxorubicin, Liposomal
Gemcitabine
Hydroxyurea
Irinotecan

Mercaptopurine
Methotrexate
Mitomycin
Mitotane
Mitoxantrone
Topotecan

Low

Aldesleukin Sub-Q
Asparaginase
Busulfan
Chlorambucil
Cladribine
Docetaxel
Etoposide
Floxuridine
Fluorouracil
Fludarabine
Goserelin

Interferon
Leuprolide
Paclitaxel
Pegaspargase
Rituximab
Suramin
Thioguanine
Trastuzumab
Vincristine
Vinblastine
Vinorelbine

Disclaimer: The incidence of emesis with these and other agents varies greatly among individuals. Dose, schedule, concomitant therapy, other medical conditions, and psychological parameters may affect the incidence as well.

Note: Where dosage, onset, or duration information is not provided, the health professional working with a specific agent should fill in the blanks for that agent on the basis of clinical practice at his or her facility and personal experience of patients receiving the agent.

Source: Memorial Sloan-Kettering Cancer Center Classification of Antineoplastic-Based on the Emetogenic Potential, version 4.0 (2000). Memorial Sloan-Kettering Cancer Center Antiemetic Subcommittee, Pharmacy and Therapeutics Committee, New York, NY.

meet the needs of the majority of patients being managed:

- 25–30 kcal/kg body weight for nonambulatory or sedentary adults
- 30–35 kcal/kg body weight for slightly hypermetabolic patients, for weight gain, or for anabolic patients
- 35 kcal/kg body weight for hypermetabolic or severely stressed patients, or patients who have malabsorption

Protein

Adequate protein should be provided to meet protein synthesis and minimize protein degradation. Most malnourished cancer patients will be in negative nitrogen balance despite adequate nitrogen given.

- 0.6–0.75 g/kg body weight: Recommended Dietary Allowance (RDA) reference protein value
- 0.8–1.0 g/kg body weight: normal maintenance level
- 1.0–1.2 g/kg body weight: safe intake for a nonstressed cancer patient
- 1.5–2.5 g/kg body weight: intake if increased protein demands exist (e.g., protein-losing enteropathy, hypermetabolism, or extreme wasting)

Fluids

Fluid status should be considered in the overall dietary or nutrition plan. Hydration status may affect the clinical response of the patient and induce untoward clinical effects. The patient who is not at liberty to consume fluid ad libitum needs to have hydration status monitored closely to prevent hydration problems. Individuals with drainages or high output from fistulas, diarrhea, or other conditions that could dehydrate them should also be closely monitored.

Nutrition Support Modalities

Oral Intake

If the patient is struggling to meet nutritional and caloric needs, he or she may require modifi-cation in caloric density; modification in amounts, types, and volumes of food at each feeding; and supplements to augment total intake. Separation of fluids and solids may prevent early satiety or dumping symptoms if present. Pain and nausea should be managed by adequate medication at least 30 minutes prior to meals. (Exhibit 3–1 shows the antiemetic regimens recommended by the Memorial Sloan-Kettering Cancer Center.) This approach should be tried before alternative methods are used. However, the time period in which the patient attempts to meet nutritional needs with these techniques should not permit significant nutritional and weight deterioration before oral intake is abandoned for an alternative nutrition plan.

Enteral Management

This method of feeding is very safe, easy to administer, and cost-effective. Several types of enteral support may be chosen on the basis of the clinical and logistical needs of the patient.

- *Nasoenteric tube feeding*—for short-term management (i.e., if the patient will be able to eat adequately within 2–4 weeks). Placement is easily done at the bedside without equipment or special procedures involved. Placement should be verified before feedings begin.
- *Gastrostomy feeding tube*—for longer-term management of patients with a functional stomach. Several types of gastrostomy tubes are available:
  1. A percutaneous endoscopic gastrostomy (PEG) tube can be placed as an outpatient procedure.
  2. A surgically placed enterostomy tube can be placed at the time of a surgical procedure.
  3. A skin-level, low-profile feeding device (button) may replace a PEG tube after initial success with gastrostomy feeding is determined and when the patient will require such a tube for nutrition support in the future.
- *Jejunostomy feeding tube*—for longer-term management of patients who have compro-

Exhibit 3–1 Memorial Sloan-Kettering Cancer Center Adult Acute Antiemetic Regimens*

Recommended Antiemetic Regimens Based on the Emetic Potential of Specific Chemotherapy Programs
New Memorial Sloan-Kettering Cancer Center Guidelines: 2000

Emetic Potential	*Acute Antiemetic Regimen*
High	Granisetron 2 mg PO[1] + Dexamethasone 20 mg PO/IV
Intermediate	Dexamethasone 20 mg PO/IV
Low	PRN Antiemetics only

[1]The IV dose of Granisetron is 0.01 mg/kg.

Breakthrough Antiemetic Regimen:
If a patient requests additional antiemetic or vomits > 3 times, give: Metoclopramide 2 mg/kg IVPB ×
1 dose, and every 3–4 hours as needed + Diphenhydramine 50 mg IV every 30 minutes, PRN only, for
dystonic reactions.

Delayed Antiemetic Regimen:
To be given with: carboplatin, cisplatin, cyclophosphamide, dacarbazine, dactinomycin, daunorubicin,
doxorubicin, and idarubicin.
     To begin at 6 A.M. the day following chemotherapy: Dexamethasone 8 mg PO BID × 2 days; taper to
4 mg PO BID × 2 days + Metoclopramide PO × 2 days, 30 mg PO/IV QID × 2 days,
OR
     Dexamethasone 8 mg PO/IV × 2 days, then taper to 4 mg BID × 2 days, plus ondansetron 8 mg PO
BID × 2 days
     Diphenhydramine 50 mg PO every 4 hours PRN for dystonic reactions or restlessness.

PRN Antiemetics:
All patients receiving chemotherapy should have PRN antiemetics ordered
     Patients receiving Low Emetogenic chemotherapy regimens require PRN antiemetics ONLY.

- Lorazepam 1–2 mg PO/IV every 4–6 hours PRN nausea or anticipatory anxiety.
- Prochlorperazine 10 mg PO q6h PRN N/V or prochlorperazine spansule 15 mg PO BID PRN N/V
- Metoclopramide 30 mg PO/IV every 4 hours PRN N/V, plus diphenhydramine 50 mg PO PRN for
  dystonic reactions or restlessness.

CI–Continuous
Ondansetron 8 mg IVPB loading dose × 1 dose only, followed by ondansetron 1 mg/hour × 24 hours on
days of chemotherapy, plus dexamethasone 20 mg IVPB given each day of chemotherapy.

     NOTE: Patients should receive dexamethasone PO or IV concurrently with a serotonin antagonist where specified.
Dexamethasone is recommended for all patients at risk for delayed emesis. For leukemia, lymphoma, multiple
myeloma, and bone marrow transplant patients, refer to individual protocols for dexamethasone use. Patients may not
tolerate metoclopramide and/or prochlorperazine in delayed emesis regimens; however, dexamethasone should be used
if possible.
     Ondansetron 8 mg PO BID × 2 days can be substituted for metoclopramide in the delayed phase.
     *Antiemetic regimens are likely to change as new and more effective agents become available.
     Source: Memorial Sloan-Kettering Cancer Center Antiemetic Guidelines for Adults. Version 4.0, 2000.

mised gastric function. Two types of jejunostomy tubes, similar to gastrostomy tubes, are available: percutaneous endoscopic jejunostomy (PEJ) tubes and surgically placed tubes. A button may replace the initial tubes once the procedure is established.

Parenteral Nutrition

If the GI tract has been used unsuccessfully to maintain nutritional needs of the patient or the clinical indications of the patient preclude the use of the GI tract for feeding, then total parenteral nutrition (TPN) may be considered. In conjunction with an active plan of therapy, some appropriate indications for parenteral support are as follows:

- severe malnutrition unable to be corrected by enteral support
- chronic malabsorption, severe diarrhea
- short-bowel obstruction
- high-output fistula
- short-bowel secondary to bypass surgery
- radiation enteritis
- patient undergoing anticancer therapy that will be compromised if malnutrition interferes with treatment schedule
- patient NPO for 10 days or longer postsurgery and at risk for potential complications following surgery, such as wound dehiscence, anastomotic leak, infection, and compromised skin turgor

Nutrition Support Management

Feeding Options

- Oral intake
  1. Provide small, frequent feedings.
  2. Provide high-caloric density foods.
  3. Separate liquids and solids if appropriate.
  4. Make food consumption as easy, painless, and stress-free as possible.
- Enteral support
  1. Formula selection
     –General, intact formulas should be well tolerated. If the patient is lactose intolerant or if volume limitations or gastric dis-

comfort exists, appropriate modifications should be implemented.
     –Predigested or specialty formula is indicated if a metabolic abnormality exists or if the patient has a clinical condition such as short-bowel syndrome.
     –Most cancer patients have difficulty with adequate intake, so providing a feeding with adequate volume (enough calories) to meet nutritional needs is important.
     –If the cancer patient requires a higher protein content or a caloric density greater than 1 kcal/cc on the basis of determination of clinical status, then the appropriate formula should be selected.
     –A huge array of commercial formulas is available for specific medical needs and clinical requirements.
- Parenteral support
  1. Formula should contain adequate intravenous hypertonic glucose, protein, fat emulsion, vitamins, minerals, and electrolytes to meet the nutritional needs of the patient.
  2. Parenteral nutrition may be administered in the hospital or in an outpatient setting, including the home.
  3. If not contraindicated, oral intake should be encouraged for gut stimulation and the prevention of stasis, sludge, and gallstones.
  4. Delivery methods
     –The bolus method is the easiest, fastest, and physiologically closest to normal eating. If the patient has a normal-functioning stomach but has a mechanical limitation, anorexia, early satiety, or some other nonmetabolic reason for poor intake, then bolus feeding is recommended. The feedings may be scheduled 3–6 times daily, depending on the total daily volume needed to be consumed, the lifestyle of the patient, and availability of others for assistance, time constraints, and other logistical issues. Each feeding should be administered over a 10- to 20-minute period.
     –The gravity pump method is an option for the patient who cannot manipulate the sy-

ringe or tube during bolus administration or requires a little slower administration of each feeding. The patient may not be as mobile or active as the patient on bolus feeding; therefore, a gravity feeding may be more convenient. A feeding generally runs over an hour or so.

–Pump-assisted, continuous feeding over extended periods of time may be beneficial to patients who are fragile or very ill or who need the feeding in slow, controlled volumes, as in the case of patients with short-bowel syndrome or radiation enteritis. Patients who want to be free of the feeding during the day may prefer to receive their feeding at night while they sleep. Therefore, pump-assisted feedings may provide a controlled, regulated volume continuously throughout the night.

5. There are two delivery methods:

–The formula may be infused over a 24-hour period using a volumetric pump.

–The formula may be infused cyclically depending on lifestyle and clinical status of the patient.

Nutrition Support in the Home Setting

• A nutritional care plan should be developed and reviewed with the patient and/or caregiver prior to home management. Patients and/or caregivers should be thoroughly trained and knowledgeable in the management, care, potential complications, and outcome goals of enteral support. Ongoing monitoring of nutritional, clinical, and functional status of the patient should occur. When changes in the status of the patient are noted, adjustments should be implemented to meet the recent needs of the patient to prevent deterioration or complications from developing.

REFERENCES

Argiles JM, Lopez-Soriano FJ. New Mediators in cancer cachexia. In: Mason JB, Nitenberg G, eds. *Cancer & Nutrition: Prevention and Treatment.* Basel, Switzerland: Nestec Ltd, 2002.

ASPEN Board of Directors, and The Clinical Guidelines Task Force. Guidelines for the use of parenteral and enteral nutition in adult and pediatric patients. *JPEN.* 2002;26(1,Suppl):1SA–138SA.

Baracos VE, LeBricon T. Animal models for nutrition in cancer. In: Mason JB, Nitenberg G, eds. *Cancer & Nutrition: Prevention and Treatment.* Basel, Switzerland: Vevey/S. Karger AG, 2000:167–182.

Barber MD. Cancer cachexia and its treatment with fish-oil-enriched nutritional supplementation. *Nutrition.* 2001;17(9):751–755.

Barber MD, Fearon KC, McMillan DC, Slater C, Ross JA, Preston T. Liver export protein synthetic rates are increased by oral meal feeding in weight-losing cancer patients. *Am J Physiol Endocrinol Metab.* 2000;279(3): E707–E714.

Barber MD, Fearon KC, Tisdale MJ, McMillan DC, Ross JA. Effect of a fish oil-enriched nutritional supplement on metabolic mediators in patients with pancreatic cancer cachexia. *Nutr Cancer.* 2001;40(2):118–124.

Barber MD, Ross JA, Voss AC, Tisdale MJ, Fearon KC. The effect of an oral nutritional supplement enriched with fish oil on weight-loss in patients with pancreatic cancer. *Br J Cancer.* 1999;81(1):80–86.

Beutler B. Summary of the 5th International Congress on TNF and related cytokines: Scientific advances and their medical applications. *J Leukoc Biol.* 1995;57:11–12.

Bloch AS, Charuhas PM. Cancer and cancer therapy. In: Gottschlich MM, ed. *The Science and Practice of Nutrition Support: A Case-Based Core Curriculum.* Dubuque, IA: 2001: 643–661.

Bosaeus I, Daneryd P, Lundholm K. Dietary intake, resting energy expenditure, weight loss and survival in cancer patients. *J Nutr.* 2002;132(11 Suppl):3465S–3466S: 147–165.

Brady MJ, Cella DF, Mo F, Bonomi AE, Tulsky DS, Lloyd SR, et al. Reliability and validity of the Functional Assessment of Cancer Therapy-Breast quality-of-life instrument. *J Clin Oncol.* 1997;15(3):974–986.

Brown J, Byers T, Thompson K, et al. Nutrition during and after cancer treatment: A guide for informed choices by cancer survivors—American Cancer Society Workgroup on Nutrition and Physical Activity for Cancer Survivors. *CA Cancer J Clin.* 2001;51(3):153–187.

Cella DF, Bonomi AE, Lloyd SR, et al. Reliability and validity of the Functional Assessment of Cancer Therapy-Lung (FACT-L) quality-of-life instrument. *Lung Cancer.* 1995;12(3):199–220.

Chlebowski RT. Nutritional support of the medical oncology patient. *Hematol Oncol Clin North Am.* 1991;5:147–160.

Daly JM, Shinkwin M. Nutrition and the cancer patient. In: Murphy GP, Lawrence W, Lenhard RE, eds. *American Cancer Society Textbook of Clinical Oncology.* Atlanta, GA: American Cancer Society; 1995:580–596.

Eldridge B. Chemotherapy and nutrition implications. In: McCallum PD, Polisena CG, eds. *The Clinical Guide to Oncology Nutrition.* Chicago, IL: American Dietetic Association, 2001:61–69.

Espat NJ, Moldawer LL, Copeland EM 3rd. Cytokine-mediated alterations in host metabolism prevent nutritional repletion in cachectic cancer patients. *J Surg Oncol.* 1995;58(2):77–82.

Falconer JS, Fearon KC, Plester CE, et al. Cytokines, the acute-phase response, and resting energy expenditure in cachectic patients with pancreatic cancer. *Ann Surg.* 1994;219(4):325–331.

Fearon KC, Hansell DT, Preston T, et al. Influence of whole body protein turnover rate on resting energy expenditure in patients with cancer. *Cancer Res.* 1988;48:2590–2595.

Fleming ID. Basis for current major cancer therapies: Surgical therapy. In: Lenhard RE, Osteen RT, Gansler TG, eds. *The American Cancer Society's Clinical Oncology.* Atlanta, GA: American Cancer Society, 2001:160–165.

Fredrix EW, Soeters PB, Wouters EF, et al. Effect of different tumor types on resting energy expenditure. *Cancer Res.* 1991;51(22):6138–6141.

Garlick PJ, McNurlan MA. Protein metabolism in the cancer patient. *Biochimie.* 1994;76(8):713–717.

Gogos CA, Ginopoulos P, Salsa B, et al. Dietary omega-3 polyunsaturated fatty acids plus vitamin E restore immunodeficiency and prolong survival for severely ill patients with generalized malignancy: A randomized control trial. *Cancer.* 1998;82(2):395–402.

Hansell DT, Davies JW, Burns HJ. The relationship between resting energy expediture and weight loss in benign and malignant disease. *Ann Surg.* 1986;203:240–245.

Heber D, Byerley LO, Tchekmedyian NS. Hormonal and metabolic abnormalities in the malnourished cancer patient: Effects on host-tumor interactions. *JPEN.* 1992; 16(6):60s–64s.

Heber D, Chlebowski RT, Ishibashi DE, et al. Abnormalities in glucose and protein metabolism in noncachectic lung cancer patients. *Cancer Res.* Y1–1982 1996;42: 4815–4819.

Heber D, Tchekmedyian N. Cancer cachexia and anorexia. In: Heber D, Blackburn GL, Go VLW, eds. *Nutritional Oncology.* San Diego, CA: Academic Press, 1999: 537–546.

Herberman RB. Basis for current major cancer therapies: Immunotherapy. In: Lenhard RE, Osteen RT, Gansler TG, eds. *The American Cancer Society's Clinical Nutrition.* Atlanta, GA: The American Cancer Society, 2001: 215–223.

Herrington AM, Herrington JD, Church CA. Pharmacologic options for the treatment of cachexia. *Nutr Clin Pract.* 1997;12:101–113.

Inui A. Cancer anorexia-cachexia syndrome: Are neuropeptides the key? *Cancer Res.* 1999;59(18):4493–4501.

Kennedy LD. Common supportive drug therapies used with oncology patients. In: McCallum PD, Polisena CG, eds. *The Clinical Guide to Oncology Nutrition.* Chicago, IL: American Dietetic Association, 2000:168–181.

List MA, D'Antonio LL, Cella DF, et al. The performance status scale for head and neck cancer patients and the functional assessment of cancer therapy-head and neck scale. A study of utility and validity. *Cancer.* 1996; 77(11):2294–2301.

Lord L, Trumbore L, Zaloga G. *Enteral nutrition implementation and management. The A.S.P.E.N. nutrition support practice manual.* Silver Spring, MD: American Society for Parenteral and Enteral Nutrition, 1998:5-1–5-16.

Martin C. Calorie, Protein, fluid, and micronutrient requirements. In: McCallum PD, Polisena CG, eds. *The Clinical Guide to Oncology Nutrition.* Chicago, IL: The American Dietetic Association, 2000:45–52.

McCallum PD. Patient-generated subjective global assessment. In: McCallum PD, Polisena CG, eds. *The Clinical Guide to Oncology Nutrition.* Chicago, IL: American Dietetic Association, 2000:11–23.

McNamara MJ, Alexander HR, Norton JA. Cytokines and their role in the pathophysiology of cancer cachexia. *JPEN.* 1992;16:50s–55s

Moldawer LL, Copeland EM 3rd. Proinflammatory cytokines, nutritional support, and the cachexia syndrome. Interactions and therapeutic options. *Cancer.* 1997; 79:1828–1839.

Morita T, Tei Y, Tsunoda J, et al. Determinants of the sensation of thirst in terminally ill cancer patients. *Support Care Cancer.* 2001;9(3):177–186.

Murphy S, Von Roenn JH. Pharmacological management of anorexia and cachexia. In: McCallum PD, Polisena CG, eds. *The Clinical Guide to Oncology Nutrition.* Chicago, IL: American Dietetic Association, 2000:127–133.

Nelson KA. The cancer anorexia-cachexia syndrome. *Semin Oncol.* 2000;27(1):64–68.

Nixon DW, Kutner M, Heymsfield S, Foltz AT, Carty C, Seitz S, et al. Resting energy expenditure in lung and colon cancer. *Metabolism: Clinical & Experimental.* 1988;37:1059–1064.

Ottery FD. Cancer cachexia prevention, early diagnosis, and management. *Cancer Pract.* 1994;2(2):123–131.

Ottery FD. Supportive nutrition to prevent cachexia and improve quality of life. *Semin Oncol.* 1995;22:2(Suppl)3: 98–111.

Page RD, Oo AY, Russell GN, Pennefather SH. Intravenous hydration versus naso-jejunal enteral feeding after esophagectomy: A randomized study. *Eur J Cardiothorac Surg.* 2002;22(5):666–672.

Pisters PW, Pearlstone DB. Protein and amino acid metabolism in cancer cachexia: Investigative techniques and therapeutic interventions. *Crit Rev Clin Lab Sci.* 1993; 30:223–272.

Polisena CG. Nutrition concerns with the radiation therapy patient. In: McCallum PD, Polisena CG, eds. *The Clinical Guide to Oncology Nutrition.* Chicago, IL: The American Dietetic Association, 2000:70–78.

Roche AF, ed. The role of nutrients in cancer treatment: Report of the ninth Ross conference on medical research. Columbus, OH: Ross Laboratories, 1991.

Shaw JH, Wolfe RR. Whole body protein kinetics in patients with early and advanced gastrointestinal cancer: The response to glucose infusion and total parenteral nutrition. *Surgery.* 1988;103:148–155.

Shils ME, Shike M. Nutritional support of the cancer patient. In: Shils ME, Olson J, Shike M, Ross A, eds. *Modern Nutrition in Health and Disease.* Baltimore, MD: Williams & Wilkins, 1999:1297–1325.

Stratton RJ. Summary of a systematic review on oral nutritional supplement use in the community. *Proc Nutr Soc.* 2000;59(3):469–476.

Tayek JA. A review of cancer cachexia and abnormal glucose metabolism in humans with cancer. *J Am College Nutrn.* 1992;11:445–456.

Tayek JA. Nutritional and biochemical aspects of the cancer patient. In: Heber D, Blackburn GL, Go VLW, eds. *Nutritional Oncology.* San Diego: Academic Press, 1999:519–536.

Tchekmedyian N, Cella DF, Heber D. Nutritional support and quality of life. In: Heber D, Blackburn GL, Go VLW, eds. *Nutritional Oncology.* San Diego: Academic Press, 1999:587–593.

Tchekmedyian NS, Halpert C, Ashley J, Heber D. Nutrition in advanced cancer: Anorexia as an outcome variable and target of therapy. *JPEN.* 1992;88S–92S.

Tchekmedyian N, Zahyna D, Halpert C, Heber D. Assessment and maintenance of nutrition in older cancer patients. *Oncology (Suppl).* 1992;6:105–111.

Tisdale MJ. Wasting in cancer. *J Nutr.* 1999;129(1S Suppl):243S–246S.

Tisdale MJ. Catabolism of skeletal muscle proteins and its reversal in cancer cachexia. In: Mason JB, Nitenberg G, eds. *Cancer & Nutrition: Prevention and Treatment.* Basel, Switzerland: Vevey/S. Karger AG, 2000:135–146.

Tisdale MJ. Metabolic abnormalities in cachexia and anorexia. *Nutrition.* 2000;16(10):1013–1014

Tisdale MJ. Loss of skeletal muscle in cancer: Biochemical mechanisms. *Front Biosci.* 2001;6:D164–D174.

Ulander K, Jeppsson B, Grahn G. Postoperative energy intake in patients after colorectal cancer surgery. *Scand J Caring Sci.* 1998;12(3):131–138.

Wigmore SJ, Barber MD, Ross JA, et al. Effect of oral eicosapentaenoic acid on weight loss in patients with pancreatic cancer. *Nutr Cancer.* 2000;36(2):177–184.

Wigmore SJ, Todorov PT, Barber MD, et al. Characteristics of patients with pancreatic cancer expressing a novel cancer cachectic factor. *Br J Surg.* 2000;87(1):53–58.

Nutrition Support in the Critically Ill Patient

Janice L. Raymond, MS, RD, CNSD

DESCRIPTION

Patients with major trauma and burns, sepsis, or other conditions requiring intensive care present unique nutrition support challenges. These patients are difficult to assess due to the rapidly changing nature of critical illness. Standard nutritional assessment techniques are not applicable. Weight is more reflective of fluid status than energy status in the critically ill. Serum proteins such as albumin are difficult to evaluate when a patient has lost a lot of blood, was given blood products, or has been resuscitated with large volumes of fluid. Assessing and monitoring nutritional status in the critically ill

involves the use of more dynamic parameters and an understanding of the physiology of stress.

METABOLIC STRESS RESPONSE

The initial insult of trauma, injury, or infection/sepsis sets in motion a basic neuroendocrine response characterized by two phases. First is the "ebb" phase, that is characterized by decreased oxygen consumption, inadequate circulation, fluid and electrolyte imbalance, and decreased GI motility. This short period generally lasts only 24–48 hours and is commonly called "shock." It is characterized by hemodynamic instability. The "flow" phase is a state of hypermetabolism meaning increased oxygen consumption that peaks at 7–14 days dependent upon the degree of the stress.

Catecholamines, cortisol, and glucagon are released in response to stress and these stimulate catabolism of peripheral protein stores for gluconeogenesis. This process of accelerated gluconeogenesis results in nitrogen that must be excreted. Urinary nitrogen can be measured as an indicator of catabolism, but this requires an accurate 24-hour urine collection and is not generally practical in the clinical setting. When renal function is compromised the nitrogen cannot be excreted and remains in the blood, causing a rise in blood urea nitrogen (BUN).

EARLY ENTERAL FEEDING

Over the past decade early enteral feedings have been recognized as beneficial to the outcome of critically ill patients. It can blunt the catabolic response by providing energy to the cells. Enteral nutrition has been shown to prevent adverse structural and functional alterations of the gut barrier. Feeding the gut maintains mucosal integrity and decreases gut permeability, which in turn decreases the chance of bacterial translocation where organisms from the intestinal lumen enter the bloodstream. Additionally, enteral nutrition actually improves local and systemic immune responsiveness; there is an increase in immunoglobulin A secretion and increased trophic hormone secretion. Enteral nutrition stimulates gut blood flow in all layers, including the mucosa, submucosa, and muscularis.

There have been at least eight randomized controlled trials comparing early enteral nutrition versus delayed nutrient intake, with early being defined as 24 to 48 hours after resuscitation. When these studies were aggregated, early enteral nutrition was associated with a trend toward a reduction in infectious complications and mortality. While we now know that early enteral feeding can be beneficial, it can be diffi-

cult to establish due to altered GI function or difficulty with feeding tube placement.

GASTRIC VS. SMALL BOWEL FEEDING

Feeding via the stomach is easier in a critically ill patient because it is easier to place and to replace a tube if it becomes dislodged. This means feedings can be started sooner. Patients commonly have nasogastric tubes already in place for suction. They can sometimes be used for feeding. Larger bore feeding tubes can be used in the stomach, which generally means less clogging.

Patients Who Can Generally Be Fed via the Stomach Include:

- Trauma patients
- Non-GI surgery patients
- Patients with neurological conditions or diseases
- Patients with organic brain syndrome
- Patients who have had a CVA
- Patients with paralytic conditions

Patients Who Should Have Postpyloric Feeding Tubes Include:

- Patients on ventilators
- Patients with aspiration or significant gastroesophageal reflux
- Patients on significant pressor support
- Some GI surgery patients
- Patients with ileus
- Patients with pancreatitis*

Common Complications of Tube Feeding and Possible Solutions

High gastric residuals (defined as greater than 150–200 ml): May try a prokinetic agent or

---

*Patients with pancreatitis require tube feedings into the jejunum to prevent stimulation of pancreatic enzymes. The ligament of Treitz is used as a marker because this ligament is positioned at the duodenal-jejunal junction. Placement of these tubes often requires fluoroscopy.

advance the feeding tube past the pylorus. Feeding formulas that have whey as a protein source have been shown to empty the stomach faster than casein-based products. Fat and fiber delay gastric emptying and can contribute to high gastric residuals. Proper positioning of the patient is important. The head of the bed should be elevated to at least 30 degrees; 45 degrees is even better.

Abdominal distention: May try a motility agent (as above) and sometimes laxatives can help. Peptide-based formulas that are low in long-chain fat are often better tolerated. Advancing the feeding tube to the ligament of Treitz may help. A high-fat or a fiber-containing formula can contribute to the problem.

Diarrhea: Usually due to medications (talk to the pharmacist), underlying disease, or mucosal deterioration of the GI tract due to lack of use. Regeneration of the microstructure of the GI tract takes 2–3 days. The diarrhea should subside after this period of time. An elemental or semi-elemental formula may improve tolerance, since it does not require the same amount of digestive and absorptive capacity.

Hyperglycemia: Hyperglycemia is part of the physiological response to stress and can be present independent of tube feeding. It is now known that tight blood glucose control (80–110 mg/dl) can significantly improve the outcome of critically ill patients. Patients should be fed and treated aggressively with insulin to prevent hyperglycemia. Tube-feeding formulas marketed for hyperglycemia are high in fiber and high in fat (50%–62% of calories) and are therefore not usually well tolerated in this population of patients.

PARENTERAL NUTRITION

The American Society for Parenteral and Enteral Nutrition (ASPEN) has recommended the following guidelines for appropriate use of parenteral nutrition.

• Patient has failed EN trial with appropriate tube placement (postpyloric).

• Enteral nutrition is contraindicated or the intestinal tract has severely diminished function due to underlying disease or treatment. Specific applicable conditions are:
1. Paralytic ileus
2. Mesenteric ischemia
3. Small bowel obstruction
4. GI fistula except when enteral access may be placed distal to the fistula or volume of output (< 200 ml/day) supports a trial of enteral nutrition

There have been at least 13 major studies published comparing the efficacy of parenteral nutrition to enteral nutrition. When these results were aggregated statistically, enteral nutrition was associated with a significant reduction in infectious complications, when compared to parenteral nutrition.

METHODS FOR CALCULATING ENERGY EXPENDITURE IN CRITICALLY ILL PATIENTS

Harris-Benedict Equation

The Harris-Benedict Equation predicts basal energy expenditure (BEE):

BEE (female) = 655 + (9.6 × wt) + (1.8 × Ht) − (4.7 × age in yrs)

BEE (males) = 66 + (13.7 × wt) + (5 × ht) − (6.8 × age in yrs)

wt = Weight in kilograms

ht = Height in centimeters

Note: This equation was developed using a well, ambulatory population. It does not include energy needed for activity or stress. These factors account for great variability in how energy expenditure is calculated. In a recent study, Frankenfeld and colleagues measured energy expenditure using indirect calorimetry and compared it to several equations for predicting resting metabolic rate. They found a 33% difference between the Harris-Benedict calculation and the measured number. The difference was 74% in obese subjects.

Activity	Activity Factor
Confined to bed	1.2
Out of bed	1.3

Condition	Stress Factor
Elective surgery	1.0
Fracture	1.2
Skeletal trauma	1.3
Multiple trauma	1.4
SIRS/sepsis	1.5–1.8

Ireton-Jones Equations

Vented patients: 1784 − (11 × age in yrs) + (5 × wt in kg) + 244 if male + 239 for trauma

Spontaneously breathing patients: 629 − 11 (age in yrs) + 25 (wt in kg) − 609 if obese

Note: These equations were developed using a hospitalized population.

Formula for Hypocaloric Feeding for Obese Patients

< 20 Kcal/kg of Adjusted body weight with 2 g protein/kg IBW

Calculation for adjusted body weight = (current wt − IBW) × 0.25 + IBW

Note: This method of calculating energy needs in critically ill obese patients was used in a study by Dickerson and colleagues. They found that the patients fed according to the hypocaloric formula had shorter ICU stays and decreased duration of antibiotic therapy days. There was a statistical trend toward decreased ventilator days.

Indirect Calorimetry

Indirect calorimetry can be used to determine energy expenditure by measuring inspired oxygen and expired gases. When available, indirect calorimetry offers a more accurate method of assessing energy needs. However, indirect calorimetry requires expensive instrumentation, experienced technicians and strict adherence to manufacturer's guidelines in order to produce reliable results.

CALCULATING PROTEIN REQUIREMENTS IN THE CRITICALLY ILL

Mild stress/minor surgery: 1.2–1.5 g/kg
Major surgery and trauma: 1.5–1.75 g/kg
Multiple trauma, serious head injury, sepsis, major wound healing: 1.75–2.5 g/kg
Liver failure with encephalopathy: 0.6–0.8 g/kg to start and titrate up based on symptoms and ammonia level.
Renal failure: 1.5–2.0 g/kg—generally, protein should not be restricted in critically ill patients. They should be fed and dialyzed if necessary.
CVVH: 1.75–2.5 g/kg
Notes: There is no consensus of opinion on how to calculate protein needs in obese patients. Remember that recommended protein intake in the general population over 65 years is 1.0 g/kg. The recommended Kcal:N ratio decreases as age increases.

MONITORING NUTRITION THERAPY IN THE CRITICALLY ILL

Weight—does NOT reflect short-term response to nutrition but should be used to monitor fluid status.
Albumin—does NOT reflect short-term response to nutrition therapy due to its relatively long half-life of 17–21 days.
Prealbumin—has a shorter half-life and it is typically used to measure response to therapy. It is markedly decreased in SIRS, sepsis, and liver failure so it will not accurately measure nutrition repletion. Prealbumin is cleared through the kidneys and is therefore elevated in renal failure, which again limits its usefulness as a nutrition marker.
Transferrin—like prealbumin it has a short half-life, but because it is affected by iron status, it is not commonly used in critical care.
Note: All these serum proteins are affected by hydration, blood transfusion, liver function, and metabolic stress and must be used cautiously as nutrition parameters.

Common ICU Terminology

APACHE	Scoring system for severity of injury/illness
SIRS	Systemic Inflammatory Response Syndrome
DIC	Disseminated Intravascular Coagulation
HIT	Heparin Induced Thrombocytopenia
SVR	Systemic Vascular Resistance
PICC	Peripherally Inserted Central Catheter
BNP	Brain Natriuretic Peptide (measures stretch of the ventricle)
ICP	Intracranial pressure

Nutrition Support Practice Guidelines for the ICU

- Begin enteral feedings within 48 hours
- Unless contraindicated, start nasogastric feedings and start prokinetic agent such as metoclopramide.
- If gastric feedings are not tolerated place tube past pylorus. May need to be placed into the jejunum for tolerance.
- HOB 30 degrees or more.
- Begin formula at full strength 20–30 ml/hr and advance 10–20 ml every 8 hours to goal rate.
- Check gastric residuals every 4 hours. If residuals exceed 200 ml, hold feedings and recheck in 2 hours. Either restart or consider advancing tube.
- Check for abdominal distention and discomfort every 4 hours.
- If tolerance is not established despite advancing the tube, and elevating HOB, consider peptide formula and check medications for those that interfere with motility.
- Monitor blood glucose bid. If elevated increase frequency of blood glucose monitoring and start insulin therapy to maintain levels < 120 mg/dl.
- Obtain basic chemistry panel of electrolytes, BUN, creatinine, Mg, and PO_4.
- If feeding tube becomes clogged, instill one tablet Viokase and sodium bicarbonate (650-mg tablet) mixed with 5 ml water. Allow to sit for 30 minutes, then flush.

REFERENCES

Bozzetti F. Proceedings from Summit on Immune-Enhancing Enteral Therapy, *JPEN.* 2001;25(2):356–357.

Brantley S. Critical care nutrition support: An overview. *Support Line.* 2002;24(4):10–21.

Frankenfield D, Rowe WA, Smith JS, Cooney RN. Validation of several established equations for resting metabolic rate in obese and nonobese people. *JADA.* 2003; 103(9):1152–1159.

Halasa Esper, D. Metabolic response and nutrition management in patients with severe head injury. *Support Line.* 2004;26(2):9–13.

Heyland DK, Dhaliwal R, Drover JW, Gramlich L, Dodek P. Canadian clinical practice guidelines for nutrition support in mechanically ventilated, critically ill adult patients. *JPEN.* 2003;27(4):355–381

Rodriguez DF. Nutrition support in acute renal failure patients: Current perspectives. *Support Line.* 1997;19(7): 3–9.

The A.S.P.E.N. Nutrition Support Practice Manual, 1998.

The Science and Practice of Nutrition Support: A case based core curriculum for A.S.P.E.N. Edited by M. Gottschlich, Kendall/Hunt Publishers, Dubuque, IA, 2001.

Diabetes Mellitus

Pamela Charney, MS, RD, CNS

DESCRIPTION

Diabetes mellitus (DM) is the most common serious metabolic disease, affecting more than 13 million individuals in the United States alone. It is characterized by abnormal glucose metabolism due to relative or absolute insulin deficiency; protein and fat metabolism are also affected. DM is also characterized by pre- and postprandial hyperglycemia.

Serious long-term complications include retinopathy, neuropathy, and nephropathy. Life expectancy of individuals with DM is only two-thirds that of the general population. Complications of DM can be avoided by careful management of blood glucose levels and early treatment of symptoms.

Hormones involved with carbohydrate metabolism include the following:

- *Insulin* is secreted by the beta cells of the pancreas in response to elevated serum glucose and acts to lower blood glucose levels by facilitating entry into cells that are sensitive to insulin. Insulin also suppresses gluconeogenesis, and stimulates glycogen synthesis. An oral glucose load may lead to greater insulin release than an intravenous load, possibly due to an early secretion of insulin via action of gastrointestinal (GI) hormone release signaling the pancreas to secrete insulin.
- *Glucagon* is secreted by the alpha cells of the pancreas in response to a low serum glucose level (e.g., during a short fast). It acts to increase blood glucose levels by stimulating glycogenolysis and gluconeogenesis in the liver, thus ensuring available energy sources during the postabsorptive period. Glucagon acts only in the liver.
- The *catecholamines* (epinephrine and norepinephrine) are released in response to stress and act to increase blood glucose levels.
- *Cortisol* leads to relative insulin resistance and may increase glucose production.

Glucagon, cortisol, and the catecholamines are known as the counterregulatory hormones due to their known actions to raise blood glucose levels in opposition to insulin's effects to lower blood glucose levels.

Diabetes takes the following forms:

- Type 1 diabetes (formerly known as insulin-dependent diabetes)
  1. Patients require insulin for immediate survival
  2. Typical onset is at an early age (usually less than 40 years of age)
  3. Patients are prone to development of diabetic ketoacidosis
  4. Symptoms include polyuria, polydipsia, and polyphagia, often of acute onset, reflecting the inability of glucose to enter cells
  5. Condition may be diagnosed after development of diabetic ketoacidosis
- Type 2 diabetes (formerly known as non-insulin dependent diabetes)
  1. Insulin is not required for immediate survival
  2. Patient may require oral hypoglycemic agents and/or insulin for adequate blood glucose control
  3. Patient is often older and overweight at diagnosis, although diagnosis at a younger age is becoming more common
- Secondary diabetes
  1. Stress-induced hyperglycemia is often seen in acutely ill individuals who may or may not develop DM following their illness
  2. Gestational diabetes; impaired glucose tolerance with onset during pregnancy. It is thought that women with a history of gestational DM may be at higher risk for development of Type 2 DM later in life.
  3. Diabetes due to medications (steroids) or pancreatic disorders.

Normal Carbohydrate Metabolism

- Blood glucose levels normally maintained within a narrow range (70–110 mg/dL)
- Insulin levels increase after meals and promote entry of glucose into insulin sensitive cells. Insulin also promotes glycogen synthesis.
- During a short fast glucagon levels stimulate gluconeogenesis and glycogenolysis
- During stress or injury, counterregulatory hormones lead to increased gluconeogenesis and glycogenolysis as well as peripheral insulin resistance

CAUSE

Type 1 Diabetes Mellitus

- Type 1 DM may be genetic in some cases
- There is an autoimmune connection; Type 1 DM may be related to development of antibodies to beta cells of the pancreas
- Some trigger, such as viral illness, may be required for expression of diabetes

Type 2 Diabetes Mellitus

- There is insulin resistance at both hepatic and peripheral levels
- Pancreatic dysfunction leads to abnormal insulin secretion
- Consistently elevated blood glucose levels may lead to "exhaustion" of the beta cells that may be reversed with insulin therapy in some individuals
- Some overweight individuals may develop peripheral resistance to the actions of insulin; weight loss improves insulin resistance.

NUTRITION ASSESSMENT

- Nutrition assessment of patients with diabetes or abnormal blood glucose is similar to that of nondiabetic patients
- Monitor current weight and recent changes in weight
- Review medical and surgical history and current problems. Assess for complications of long-standing DM, including retinopathy, neuropathy, and nephropathy
- Medication history including timing and dosage of medications, including insulin and oral hypoglycemic agents
- Monitor laboratory data to include glucose levels and hemoglobin A1c (Hbg A1c) for long-term glucose control; other laboratory data as appropriate for the clinical condition
- Assess level of stress; adequate blood glucose control may be difficult in critically ill patients
- Nutrient requirements
  1. Various equations for estimating energy requirements are available. Avoid overfeeding in acutely ill patients. Indirect calorimetry allows for accurate measurement of energy requirements.
  2. Quick rule of thumb is to provide no more than 25–30 kcal/kg for normal weight individuals and no more than 20 kcal/kg actual weight for obese individuals.
  3. Provide 0.8–1.0 g protein/kg for nonstressed patients.
  4. Protein requirements may be as high as 1.5–1.75 g/kg body weight in metabolic stress.
  5. There is controversy over the need for protein restriction in renal failure. Many now suggest 0.6–0.8 g protein/kg body weight for stable patients not on dialysis. If protein restriction is desired, close monitoring is essential to prevent secondary malnutrition. Patients on maintenance dialysis need increased protein intake.

PROBLEMS

Effect of Stress and Illness on Glycemic Control

- Stress and illness increase levels of counterregulatory hormones
- Hepatic glucose production increases, while peripheral glucose uptake decreases
- Peripheral insulin resistance often complicates management, leading to hyperglycemia that is difficult to control

- Decreased or sporadic oral intake during illness contributes to suboptimal glycemic control

Diabetic Ketoacidosis

- Diabetic ketoacidosis (DKA) is a potentially life-threatening complication that is seen in Type 1 DM. It is probably related to insulin deficiency in the face of elevated counterregulatory hormones.
- Oxidation of fatty acids leads to increased levels of the ketone bodies (betahydroxybutyric acid and acetoacetic acid).
- Osmotic diuresis leads to dehydration, electrolyte abnormalities, and metabolic acidosis; if untreated, has adverse effects on renal and cardiovascular function.
- Treated with insulin and fluid and electrolyte replacement

Hyperosmolar, Hyperglycemic, Nonketotic Coma

- This is a complication seen in Type 2 DM, most often in those with a concurrent serious illness.
- Residual insulin secretion is thought to prevent the development of acidosis
- The condition is characterized by extreme hyperglycemia (> 600 mg/dL) and serum osmolarity > 330 mOsm/kg), mild acidosis, and serum bicarbonate > 20 mEq/L; patient may be obtunded
- Treatment is with insulin in addition to fluid and electrolyte replacement
- Prompt recognition and treatment are vital, as mortality may be as high as 50%

Hypoglycemia

- May occur as a result of overzealous insulin administration
- Other causes include missed meals after insulin administration
- Clinical signs (confusion, sleepiness) are difficult to recognize in intensive care unit patients so frequent blood glucose monitoring is important

- Repeated severe hypoglycemia may have adverse neurological effects.

Neuropathy

- Delayed gastric emptying or gastroparesis occurs in 45%–75% of individuals with DM
- Gastroparesis may be asymptomatic in some individuals. In others it may be characterized by acute exacerbations with symptom-free intervals.
- Pharmacologic treatment offers some relief
- Bowel rest and parenteral nutrition are rarely necessary; enteral feedings are usually possible with tube placement past the stomach.

Nephropathy

- Proteinuria is the first sign of diabetic nephropathy
- Protein-restricted diets (0.6–0.8 g of protein/kg body weight) are often recommended prior to the initiation of dialysis; patients should be monitored closely to prevent the onset of malnutrition.
- Patients receiving maintenance dialysis treatment require adequate protein intake (up to 1.5 g protein/kg body weight in patients on peritoneal dialysis).

Dyslipidemia

- The most common abnormality is elevated triglycerides along with low levels of high density lipoprotein (HDL) cholesterol
- Hypertriglyceridemia may improve with glycemic control
- Patients with triglyceride levels > 2000 mg/dL may be at risk for pancreatitis
- Treatment involves weight loss (if patient is overweight), exercise, and a low-fat, limited simple sugar diet.

TREATMENT/MANAGEMENT

- Treatment of DM involves diet, exercise, oral hypoglycemic agents, and insulin if needed. Patients with Type 1 DM will always require insulin for survival

- Exercise enhances weight loss and may improve metabolic control in some individuals
- Alcohol consumption is discouraged
- Results of the Diabetes Control and Complications Trial (DCCT) show that good control may prevent or delay onset of complications

Diet

- Improved insulin sensitivity with weight loss in obese individuals may lead to improvement in glycemic control as well as decreased reliance on pharmacologic therapy
- Increased fiber intake is often recommended, but glycemic response to fiber varies. Up to 50 g fiber per day has been recommended, but this level is difficult for many Americans to achieve.
- Approximately 10%–20% of total calories should come from protein
- Diet should also include less than 10% of calories from saturated fat
- The remaining calories should include complex carbohydrate sources and mono- and polyunsaturated fats.
- Moderate sucrose consumption is not contraindicated for individuals with good blood glucose control and as part of a well-balanced diet
- There has been much interest in the use of diets high in monounsaturated fats; more research is needed on the long-term effects.
- Consistency in timing of meals is important for patients on insulin therapy; however, intensive insulin therapy and home blood glucose monitoring allow for more flexibility. Meal planning must be accomplished according to the patient's lifestyle and food habits.
- The diabetic exchange system and carbohydrate counting systems are two methods often used to plan diets.
- Adherence to treatment regimens is enhanced through use of a multidisciplinary treatment team

Oral Hypoglycemic Agents

- Oral hypoglycemic agents are used in patients with Type 2 DM

- The actions of different medications vary and involve either enhancing residual insulin secretion, improving peripheral insulin resistance, and slowing absorption of carbohydrate from the GI tract
- The clinician should note the type of medication used and its metabolic effects
- Long-acting agents have been associated with the development of hypoglycemia and should not be used in the elderly or those at risk for hypoglycemia

Insulin

- In normal individuals, insulin is secreted as a bolus dose in response to a meal as well as at a constant basal level; most adults secrete approximately 30–40 units/day.
- Patients with Type 1 DM require exogenous insulin for survival; patients with Type 2 DM may require insulin for optimal blood glucose control.
- Currently beef, pork, and human insulin are available. The beef and pork insulins differ from human insulin by 1 and 3 amino acids.
- Short-acting (regular), intermediate (NPH), and long-acting (Lente) insulins are most commonly used. Shorter acting and longer acting insulins are also used. The longer acting insulin can be used to provide a basal insulin level without peaks. Shorter acting insulin can then be given at meal and snack times to optimize control.
- Currently there is no "ideal" recommended insulin regimen. Insulin therapy in Type 1 DM may be initiated with 0.6–0.8 units/kg body weight and adjusted according to blood glucose levels. Traditionally, patients have been managed using both morning and evening injections of a combination of short- and intermediate-acting insulins. More intensive therapy using multiple daily injections is showing good results in terms of blood glucose control and prevention of complications.
- Insulin pumps can provide insulin with the need for multiple injections and are being used more often. The pump is often discontinued during hospitalization

- Patient lifestyle, blood glucose levels, and desires must be considered when designing an insulin regimen
- Accurate home blood glucose monitoring is needed for optimal glycemic control.

NUTRITION SUPPORT IN PATIENTS WITH DIABETES MELLITUS

- Indications for nutrition support are the same as those for patients without diabetes
- Enteral feedings are preferred over parenteral feedings for several reasons: enteral feeding provides for a more physiological route of feeding, maintenance of the gut mucosal barrier, and fewer potentially serious complications.
- Glycemic control should be optimized prior to initiating enteral or parenteral feedings
- Insulin is the preferred pharmacologic agent for glycemic control; oral hypoglycemic agents are not recommended except for those patients who are stable on long-term enteral feedings.

Enteral Nutrition Support

- Small intestinal feedings are recommended for patients with a history of gastroparesis
- Balanced polymeric formulas are appropriate for most patients, including those with mild to moderate gastrointestinal impairment
- Disease-specific formulas are expensive and not well tested
- Feedings should not be diluted unless additional free water is desired
- For guidelines on insulin use in enteral nutrition see Exhibit 3–2

Parenteral Nutrition

- Parenteral nutrition is indicated in patients with a nonfunctional gastrointestinal tract
- Initiate total parenteral nutrition with 100–150 g of dextrose; advance dextrose to desired levels only after stable blood glucose levels are achieved.
- Approximately 30% of total calories given as lipid can assist with glycemic control and lessen the need for insulin in some patients

Exhibit 3–2 Insulin Use in Enteral Nutrition

If the patient has not previously been on insulin:

- Check blood glucose levels frequently (every 4–6 hours)
- Initiate sliding-scale, short-acting insulin as needed to keep blood glucose levels as close to normal as possible while avoiding hypoglycemia
- Add 1/4 to 1/2 of the previous day's sliding scale as NPH the following day
- Continue sliding-scale coverage with goal of eliminating sliding scale with daily insulin dose
- Split doses of NPH with regular insulin

If patient has been previously on insulin:

- Check blood glucose levels frequently (every 4–6 hours)
- Patient may require increased insulin with enteral feedings, particularly if critically ill
- Give 1/4 of usual NPH dose every 12 hours as continuous feedings are initiated. Closely monitor blood glucose levels and use sliding-scale or continuous insulin infusion to maintain near normal blood glucose levels.
- Add 1/4 to 1/2 of previous day's sliding-scale insulin to the next day as NPH (or continue with scheduled short-acting doses).
- Monitor insulin dose as well as enteral formula intake daily to prevent sudden fluctuations of insulin or formula intake and subsequent wide swings in blood glucose levels.

Exhibit 3–3 Insulin Use in Parenteral Nutrition

If the patient has not previously been on insulin:

- Do not give insulin in initial parenteral nutrition
- Check blood glucose levels frequently (every 4–6 hours)
- Give sliding-scale insulin to maintain blood glucose levels as close to normal as possible while avoiding hypoglycemia
- Add 1/4 to 1/2 previous day's sliding scale as regular

- Careful blood glucose monitoring is vital in all patients receiving nutrition support. Hyperglycemia has been associated with increased risk for complications, particularly infectious complications.
- Insulin can be added to parenteral nutrition solutions or given as a separate infusion in an ICU setting or as subcutaneous injections.
- There is no need for long tapering of parenteral nutrition if blood glucose levels are stable. Attention should be paid to last insulin dose and other sources of feeding during the tapering process to ensure adequate control.
- For guidelines on insulin use in parenteral nutrition see Exhibit 3–3.

REFERENCES

Bloomgarden ZT. (2002). Diabetes and nutrition. *Diabetes Care.* 25(10):1869–1875.

Boord JB et al. (2001). Practical management of diabetes in critically ill patients. *Am J Respir Crit Care Med.* 164:1763–1767.

Brown G, Dodek P. (2001). Intravenous insulin nomogram improves blood glucose control in the critically ill. *Crit Care Med.* 29(9):1714–1719.

Charney P. Diabetes mellitus. In *Contemporary nutrition support practice: A clinical guide.* LE Matarese and MM Gottschlich, Eds. (2003). Philadelphia: WB Saunders, 533–545.

Garg AX. (1998). High MUFA diets for patients with diabetes mellitus: A meta-analysis. *Am J Clin Nutr.* 67(suppl 3):577S–582S.

Granner DK. (2000). Hormones of the pancreas and gastrointestinal tract. In *Harper's biochemistry.* RK Murray et al., Eds. Stamford, CT: Appleton & Lange, 610–626.

Jenkins, DJA. (2002). High-complex carbohydrate or lente carbohydrate foods? *Am J Med.* 113(9B):30S–37S.

Koch KL. (1999). Diabetic gastropathy; gastric neuromuscular dysfunction in diabetes mellitus: A review of symptoms, pathophysiology and treatment. *Dig Dis Sci.* 44:1061–1075.

McMahon MM, Rizza RA. (1996). Nutrition support in hospitalized patients with diabetes mellitus. *Mayo Clin Proceedings.* 71:587–594.

The American Diabetes Association. (2003). Evidence-based nutrition principles and recommendations for the treatment and prevention of diabetes and related complications. *Diabetes Care.* 26(Suppl 1):S51–S61.

The American Diabetes Association. (2003). Translation of the diabetes nutrition recommendations for health care institutions. *Diabetes Care.* 26(Suppl 1):S70–S72.

The American Diabetes Association. (2004). Diabetes fact sheet. Accessed February 10, 2004. http://www.diabetes.org/diabetes-statistics/national-diabetes-fact-sheet.jsp.

Van Den Berghe G, et al. (2001). Intensive insulin therapy in critically ill patients. *New England J Med.* 345:1359–1367.

Gastrointestinal Disorders

Donald Kirby, MD, FACP, FACN, FACG, CNSP, CPNS and Regine S. Birkenhauer, MS, RD, CNSD

DESCRIPTION

The gastrointestinal tract is designed to convert ingested foods into a form that can be readily assimilated and used by the body. However, when the gastrointestinal tract becomes compromised as a result of gastrointestinal disorders, this assimilation may not be efficient and can lead to incomplete or inefficient digestion *(maldigestion)*. This can then result in the *malabsorption* of nutrients.

Diarrhea is a common manifestation of many gastrointestinal disorders. Nutritional consequences can ensue due to the loss of essential nutrients such as water, minerals, vitamins, electrolytes, and micronutrients. In its severest form, diarrhea can disrupt nutrient absorption to such an extent that malnutrition can occur.

ANATOMY AND PHYSIOLOGY

The gastrointestinal tract includes hollow organs that comprise the alimentary tract and solid organs, consisting of the pancreas, liver, and gallbladder that function in the digestive process.

- The upper gastrointestinal tract is composed of the
  1. mouth and pharynx (oral cavity)
  2. salivary glands
  3. esophagus
  4. secretory glands
  5. stomach
  6. duodenum
- The lower gastrointestinal tract is composed of the
  1. jejunum
  2. ileum, including the ileocecal valve
  3. colon, including the rectum and anus
  4. secretory glands
- The solid organs are composed of the
  1. liver
  2. gallbladder
  3. pancreas

The functions of different parts of the gastrointestinal tract are as follows:

- The *oral cavity* begins the digestive process with chewing, lubricating, digesting, and swallowing
- The *esophagus* is a muscular tube that helps propulse the food into the stomach
- The *stomach* mixes food with gastric juices and controls release into the small intestine for continued digestion and absorption. In addition, the acid secreting, parietal cells, also secrete intrinsic factor which is important for the absorption of vitamin B_{12}
- The *small intestine* (duodenum, jejunum, and ileum) continues the digestive process and absorbs most of the end products of digestion
- The *large intestine* (colon) absorbs water and sodium and secretes potassium and bicarbonate. The large intestine also absorbs short-chain fatty acids. As water is absorbed, waste material gradually becomes more solid for elimination. Bacteria in the colon create a significant portion of vitamin K which is absorbed and critical in the blood clotting cascade
- *Secretory glands,* which are distributed throughout the gastrointestinal tract, with the exception of the colon, release secretions into a duct *(exocrine)* or release secretions into the blood *(endocrine)*
- *Sphincters* are circular muscles located in the gastrointestinal tract. They assist in regulating the passage of contents from one segment of the tract to another.

Digestion

Table 3–14 summarizes the digestive process.

Absorption

Figure 3–2 shows sites of absorption for different nutrients.

Table 3–14 Summary of Digestive Processes

Source of Secretion and Stimulus for Secretion	*Enzyme(s)*	*Substrate(s)*	*End Products*
Salivary glands Saliva is produced in response to foods	Salivary amylase	Starch Glycogen	Maltose plus 1:6 glucosides plus maltotriose
Lingual glands	Lingual lipase	Primary ester link at sn-3 triacylglycerols	Fatty acids plus 1,2 diacylglycerols
Stomach glands	Pepsin A (fundus)		
	Pepsin B (pylorus)	Protein	Peptides
	Gastric lipase	As for lingual lipase	As for lingual lipase
	Rennin	Casein of milk	Coagulates milk
Pancreas	Trypsin	Protein Peptides	Polypeptides Dipeptides
Acid chyme from the stomach activates the duodenum to produce	Chymotrypsin	Protein Peptides	Same as trypsin More coagulating power for milk
• Secretin, which stimulates flow of pancreatic juice	Elastase	Protein Peptides	Polypeptides Dipeptides
• Cholecystokinin, which stimulates the production of enzymes	Carboxypeptidase	Polypeptides at the free carboxyl end of the chain	Small peptides Free amino acids
	Pancreatic amylase	Starch Glycogen	Maltose plus 1:6 glucosides (oligosaccharides) plus maltotriose
	Lipase	Primary ester linkages of triacylglycerol	Fatty acids, 2-monoacyl-glycerols, glycerol
	Bile	Triacylglycerol esters (cholesteryl ester, vitamin esters, lysophospholipids	Free fatty acids, vitamins, cholesterol
	Ribonuclease	Ribonucleic acid	Nucleotides
	Deoxyribonuclease	Deoxyribonucleic acids	Nucleotides
	Cholesteryl ester hydrolase	Cholesteryl esters	Free cholesterol plus fatty acids
	Phospholipase A_2	Phospholipids	Fatty acids, lysophospholipids
Liver and gallbladder Cholecystokinin, a hormone from the intestinal mucosa, and possibly gastrin and secretin, stimulate the gallbladder and secretion of bile by the liver	Bile salts and alkali	Fats—also neutralize acid chyme	Fatty acid-bile salt complexes and finely emulsified neutral fat-bile salt micelles and liposomes

continues

Table 3–14 continued

Source of Secretion and Stimulus for Secretion	Enzyme(s)	Substrate(s)	End Products
Small intestine	Aminopeptidase	Polypeptides at the free amino end of the chain	Small peptides, free amino acids
	Dipeptidases	Dipeptides	Amino acids
	Sucrase	Sucrose	Fructose, glucose
	Maltase	Maltose	Glucose
	Lactase	Lactose	Glucose, galactose
	Trehalase	Trehalose	Glucose
	Phosphatase	Organic phosphates	Free phosphate
	Isomaltase or 1:6 glucosidase	1:6 glucosides	Glucose
	Polynucleotidase	Nucleic acid	Nucleotides
	Nucleosidases (nucleoside phosphorylases	Purine or pyrimidine nucleosides	Purine or pyrimidine bases, pentose phosphate

Source: Adapted from Murray R, Granner D, Mayes P, Rodwell V. In: *Harper's Biochemistry,* 25th ed., pp. 668–669, © 2000, Appleton & Lange.

Secretion

- The GI tract handles approximately 9–12 liters of fluid per day. Approximately 2 liters of fluid is ingested, with the remaining 7–10 liters coming from endogenous secretions which include the following sources:
  1. salivary juice ~1500 mL
  2. gastric juice ~ 3000 mL
  3. pancreatic juice ~ 1500 mL
  4. bile ~ 500 mL
  5. intestinal ~ 1000 mL
- Fluids are absorbed throughout the GI tract
- Refer to Table 3–15 for a breakdown of the composition of different gastrointestinal fluids

Motility

- Many factors may alter the motility of the gastrointestinal tract
- Return of normal activity may precede the return of bowel sounds in postoperative patients

- The digestive organs resume normal activity postoperatively at different times
  1. Stomach: 48–72 hrs
  2. Small intestines: 12 hrs (therefore, the intestines is the best site for early postoperative enteral feeding)
  3. Colon: 72 hours (contractions that sustain the movement of gas and bowel contents)
- Factors that may prolong postoperative ileus include the following:
  1. sympathetic hyperactivity, usually due to pain
  2. abdominal distention
  3. intraperitoneal irritation
  4. the administration of autonomic, cardiac, or psychotrophic drugs
  5. electrolyte imbalances (in particular, potassium and magnesium)
  6. concomitant disease in the gastrointestinal tract
- The passage of flatus commonly indicates the end of a postoperative ileus

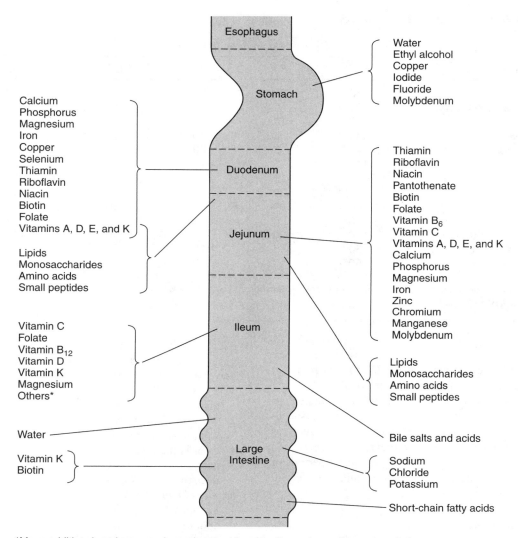

Esophagus

Stomach
- Water
- Ethyl alcohol
- Copper
- Iodide
- Fluoride
- Molybdenum

Calcium
Phosphorus
Magnesium
Iron
Copper
Selenium
Thiamin
Riboflavin
Niacin
Biotin
Folate
Vitamins A, D, E, and K

Lipids
Monosaccharides
Amino acids
Small peptides

Duodenum

Jejunum
- Thiamin
- Riboflavin
- Niacin
- Pantothenate
- Biotin
- Folate
- Vitamin B$_6$
- Vitamin C
- Vitamins A, D, E, and K
- Calcium
- Phosphorus
- Magnesium
- Iron
- Zinc
- Chromium
- Manganese
- Molybdenum

Vitamin C
Folate
Vitamin B$_{12}$
Vitamin D
Vitamin K
Magnesium
Others*

Ileum
- Lipids
- Monosaccharides
- Amino acids
- Small peptides

Water

Vitamin K
Biotin

Large
Intestine
- Bile salts and acids
- Sodium
- Chloride
- Potassium
- Short-chain fatty acids

*Many additional nutrients may be a absorbed from the ileum depending on transit time.

Figure 3–2 Sites of nutrient absorption in the gastrointestinal tract.
Source: Reprinted with permission Groff JL, Gropper S: Sites of nutrient absorption in the gastrointestinal tract. In: *Advanced Nutrition and Human Metabolism,* 3rd ed., 414, © 2000, Wadsworth, an imprint of the Wadsworth Group, a division of Thomson Learning.

Table 3–15 Electrolyte Composition of Various Body Fluids

Fluid	Electrolytes (mEq/L)				Volume (L/d)
	Na⁺	K⁺	Cl⁻	HCO₃⁻	

Fluid	Na^+	K^+	Cl^-	HCO_3^-	Volume (L/d)
Saliva	30	20	35	15	1–1.5
Gastric, pH < 4	60	10	90		2.5
Gastric, pH > 4	100	10	100		2.0
Bile	145	5	110	40	1.5
Duodenal	140	5	80	50	
Pancreatic	140	5	75	90	0.7–1.0
Ileal	130	10	110	30	3.5
Cecal	80	20	50	20	
Colon	60	30	40	20	0.5–2.0
Sweat	50	5	55		0–3.0
New ileostomy	130	20	110	30	0.5–2.0
Adapted ileostomy	50	5	30	25	0.4
Colostomy	50	10	40	20	0.3

Source: Reprinted with permission from Lyerly H, Gaynor J. *The Handbook of Surgical Intensive Care.* 3rd ed. p. 410. © 1992, Elsevier.

Adaptation

Maintenance of the trophic effects found in the mucosa of the gastrointestinal tract is best accomplished through provision of enteral nutrient sources. Provision of specific gastrointestinal tract-preferred fuel sources, such as glutamine for the enterocyte and short-chain fatty acids for the colonocyte during periods of growth following resection or injury, is helpful in promoting adaptation.

Immunologic Barrier

The mucosa of the gastrointestinal tract provides a protective barrier against bacterial translocation and potential toxins. Failure to maintain a normal mucosal barrier can lead to breakdown of barrier function and increase gastrointestinal tract permeability.

NUTRITIONAL IMPLICATIONS IN ASSESSMENT OF THE GASTROINTESTINAL TRACT

Assessment of an individual with a gastrointestinal disorder should cover the following areas:

- *Chief complaint:* If the patient presents with gastric pain, heartburn, vomiting, or altered bowel habits, ask questions about
  1. onset, duration, and severity of the complaint
  2. what precipitates symptoms
  3. what makes symptoms better or worse
  4. what is the location of the pain, if there is pain
  5. does the pain radiate to other locations
- *Medical history:* Ask about
  1. history of disorders of the mouth, throat, abdomen, and rectum
  2. long-term gastrointestinal conditions such as ulcerative colitis
  3. major disorders, including neurologic disorders that can impair movement of the tongue, mouth, and throat, gastric motility and/or disease states such as diabetes, hypothyroidism, and constipation
  4. allergies to foods
  5. medications, including over-the-counter products and herbal preparations that the patient is taking
  6. surgical history for procedures of the gastrointestinal tract, particularly resections
  7. ingestion of vitamins, mineral supplements, and laxatives

- *Family history:* Check for a history of inflammatory bowel disease, celiac disease, colon polyps or cancer, gallbladder disease, liver disease, alcoholism, or intestinal ulcers
- *Psychosocial history:* Investigate situations that might have emotional implications, including perception of self-image, a history of eating disorders, or current living situation issues that might impact on nutrition
- *Functional status/activities of daily living/ lifestyle changes:*
  1. nutrition history (detailed)
  2. appetite changes
  3. weight history
  4. ability to purchase and prepare food
  5. special dietary restrictions
  6. ability to exercise regularly
  7. smoking and drinking history
  8. dental history
- *Physical examination* for nutritional status:
  1. Obtain present height and weight, and weight history (determine if weight loss or gain is voluntary or involuntary, and if it is related to changes in eating habits or medical status/symptoms)
  2. Mouth: inspect the individual's mouth for dental caries and problems of the gums, tongue, lips, and general condition of teeth or presence of dentures
  3. Abdomen: use techniques of inspection, auscultation, percussion, and palpation to detect such signs as bowel sounds and location(s) of pain
- *Review of assessments/history/physical examinations by other health care professionals:* Ask about abnormal signs and/or symptoms such as:
  1. Symptoms: abdominal pain, constipation, diarrhea, dysphagia, nausea, vomiting
  2. Signs: distention and protrusion, abdominal pulsations related to intestinal obstruction, abnormal abdominal sounds (hyper- or hypoactive bowel), and/or ascites
- *Pertinent diagnostic tests*
  1. basic metabolic and/or comprehensive metabolic, CBC, liver function tests, including prothrombin time and ammonia levels, if indicated

  2. prealbumin
  3. hydration status indicators (patient may have a propensity to become dehydrated)
  4. stool analysis (common tests include stool for blood, white blood cells, stool cultures, *Clostridia difficile* toxin and presence of fat
  5. radiography: abdominal films, esophagram, upper gastrointestinal series, small-bowel series, barium enema, ultrasonography, computed tomography (CT) scan, magnetic resonance imaging (MRI)
  6. endoscopy (upper endoscopy, colonoscopy, endoscopic retrograde cholangiopancreatography (ERCP) and endoscopic ultrasound)

Optimally, to assess/determine problems of the gastrointestinal tract, one should have a solid knowledge of the normal processes of digestion, absorption, and metabolism.

If the individual is experiencing symptoms that do not appear to be normal, then the nutrition care plan should be based on achievement of an outcome as close to normal as possible.

SIGNIFICANT FACTORS THAT MAY AFFECT THE ABILITY TO DELIVER APPROPRIATE NUTRITION SUPPORT

- *Jejunal resection, intact ileum, intact colon.* Individuals rarely need aggressive nutrition support and can usually be fed immediately
- *Less than 100 cm of ileum resected; colon largely intact.* Individuals may have bile acid diarrhea but can usually be managed by controlled oral intake and medication therapy
- *100–200 cm of ileal resection with colon largely intact.* Individuals have both bile acid diarrhea and steatorrhea, but can usually be treated by diet modification and possibly medications will be required
- *More than 200 cm of small bowel resected or lesser resection with colostomy.* Individuals require a well-managed oral diet following a graduated regimen for adaptation
- *Less than 60 cm of small bowel remaining or only duodenum.* Individuals require parenteral nutrition support and may also receive adjunctive oral or tube feedings

- *Surgical removal of portions of the upper gastrointestinal system secondary to tumor, trauma, achalasia, or esophageal stricture.* Management will vary depending upon the extent of the surgical removal, the portion(s) of the upper gastrointestinal system removed, and the nature of possible postoperative therapy
- *Partial obstruction (e.g., secondary to tumor, stricture [scleroderma], or inflammation).* Individuals rarely need aggressive nutrition support and can be managed by controlled oral intake. Some require enteral access placement appropriate for the anatomical situation
- *Oral cavity abnormality, such as lesions or poor dentition.* Individuals rarely need aggressive nutrition support and can be managed by controlled oral intake
- *Gastroparesis as a result of diabetes mellitus, pancreatic cancer, a medication side effect, aging, neuromuscular disorders such as amyotrophic lateral sclerosis, chemotherapies such as vinblastine and vincristine, or uremia.* Individual management will vary depending on the etiology of the gastroparesis
- *Diseases that have a high risk for swallowing disorders, such as amyotrophic lateral sclerosis, Parkinson's disease, dementia, Alzheimer's disease, coma, cerebrovascular disease, multiple sclerosis, head trauma, or muscular dystrophies.* Individual management will vary depending on the etiology and extent of the swallowing disorder

SPECIFIC DISORDERS OF THE GASTROINTESTINAL TRACT: THE ORAL CAVITY AND ESOPHAGUS

Upon entering the mouth, food is chewed by the action of the jaw muscles and is made ready for swallowing by mixing with the secretions released from the salivary glands. The passage of food from the mouth through the pharynx into the esophagus constitutes *swallowing.* Swallowing is divided into four stages:

- Anticipatory
- Oral (or voluntary)
- Pharyngeal
- Esophageal

Swallowing is a reflex response initiated by a voluntary action and regulated by the swallowing center in the medulla of the brain. As the food passes through the pharynx, the swallowing center acts to inhibit the respiratory center, thereby preventing food from being aspirated into the larynx and lungs.

When food moves into the esophagus, both the striated muscles of the upper portion of the esophagus and the smooth muscles of the distal portion are stimulated by cholinergic (parasympathetic) nerves. The result is *peristalsis,* or a progressive wavelike motion that moves the food through the esophagus into the stomach.

At the lower end of the esophagus, just above the upper end of the stomach, lies the lower esophageal sphincter (LES). Normal LES pressure is higher than intragastric pressure. When swallowing is initiated, the LES pressure drops and relaxes the sphincter. Food passes from the esophagus into the stomach. Tonic pressure increases within the LES musculature to prevent gastroesophageal reflux.

Swallowing Difficulties/Dysphagia

Disruption of any phase of the swallowing process due to medical issues or medication side effects can result in dysphagia, either with or without aspiration. The interdisciplinary team should determine the best approach for management of the swallowing difficulties after weighing all relevant concerns and after identifying the underlying pathology.

If it is determined that further testing is needed via swallowing studies, then there are a variety of techniques available.

- *Videofluoroscopy* (also called Modified Barium Swallow): provides visualization of the structures, movement, and coordination of the swallow
- *Fiberoptic endoscopy:* visually assesses the function of the larynx and pharynx
- *Manometry:* monitors pressures within the esophagus, which can be used to determine motility disorders

If the team decides that a modified diet is appropriate, the prescribed diet should be individualized to a consistency that enables safe mastication and swallowing and yields adequate hydration and nutrition. The National Dysphagia Diet, from the task force of the American Dietetic Association, provides the first attempt to standardize dysphagia diets. Though it has not been peer reviewed, it defines common terminology that will enhance communication amongst professionals. (See the American Dietetic Association website: www.eatright.org.)

Reflux Esophagitis or Gastroesophageal Reflux Disease

Gastroesophageal reflux, often manifested as heartburn, results from LES incompetence (a decrease in pressure at the LES), which occurs when LES pressure is decreased or the LES is relaxed. Recurring reflux of caustic products, which can be acid or base, into the esophagus can damage the esophageal mucosa. Multiple mechanisms, including neural and hormonal, regulate LES pressure. Certain foods and/or food-related substances appear to increase, probably indirectly, the relaxation of the LES. Fat-containing foods increase relaxation by decreasing LES pressure and delaying gastric emptying. Other foods that can decrease LES pressure are chocolate, alcohol, and peppermint.

Nutritional management should be aimed at

- avoiding substances that can further lower LES pressure, which is already low due to the condition, or substances that may further irritate the esophagus, such as orange juice or tomato-based products
- avoiding substances that may promote the secretion of acid, which would then be present in higher concentrations than normal if refluxed
- Avoiding high-fat foods or meals with chocolate, coffee, alcohol, peppermint, and other plants with volatile oils
- Avoiding high-protein diets; the digestion of protein stimulates the release of gastrin, which increases LES pressure but is also a potent stimulator of hydrochloric acid secretion

- Consuming small meals and consuming fluids between meals to decrease gastric volume

Achalasia

Achalasia is a motility disorder of the esophagus associated with dysphagia or difficulty in swallowing. Classic achalasia is defined by a hypertensive LES which fails to properly relax associated with either diminished or absent peristalsis.

The main treatment of this disorder is the reduction on LES pressure by pneumatic dilatation, botox injection of the LES, or surgical treatment (Heller myotomy).

Other Esophageal Disorders

Esophageal Perforation

Esophageal perforation may be caused by blunt injury to the chest, abdominal trauma, spontaneously (Boerhaave's syndrome), endoscopic procedures, or a surgical procedure. Nutritional consequences include weight loss due to inability to ingest adequate oral nutrition and excessive protein loss because of catabolism and/or loss of protein-rich fluid.

In nutritional management:

- Enteral nutrition is the preferred modality, but the use of a nasogastric/enteric feeding route may need to be avoided so as not to increase esophageal irritation and reflux
- Percutaneous endoscopically placed feeding sites should also be avoided because the esophagus must be traversed for placement
- Gastrostomy or jejunostomy feedings may be appropriate

Esophageal Obstruction

The esophagus may be obstructed by cancer, congenital abnormalities, or strictures. Nutritional consequences include weight loss, dysphagia, and sepsis (aspiration pneumonia).

In nutritional management:

- Enteral nutrition is the preferred modality, if the GI tract can be accessed. Parenteral

nutrition is generally not indicated because the gastrointestinal tract is functional
- Use of endoscopically, radiologically or surgically placed feeding tubes (i.e., gastrostomy, jejunostomy feeding tubes) may be appropriate
- Polymeric formulas are generally well tolerated

Esophageal Varices

This is a condition resulting from elevated portal hypertension, which can have multiple etiologies. In its most severe form malnutrition can be seen, associated with the liver disease.

Nutritional management may include

- use of a soft diet, excluding high-roughage foods that can cause irritation
- use of enteral nutrition support may be appropriate, but is the physician's decision
- gastrostomy tubes may be placed, but usually in the absence of ascites

Esophageal Resection/Replacement

Esophageal resection or replacement may be required because of tumor, congenital abnormalities, or trauma. Nutritional consequences include swallowing difficulties due to differences in musculature and innervation between the colon/jejunum and the normal esophagus.

In nutritional management

- give small, frequent feedings of nutrient-dense foods to optimize intake
- an antidumping regimen may be indicated
- feeding jejunostomies may be placed at the time of the operative procedure
- oral daily intake may be augmented with nocturnal feedings

SPECIFIC DISEASES OF THE GASTROINTESTINAL TRACT: THE STOMACH

The bolus of swallowed food enters the stomach through the LES. The stomach is divided functionally and histologically into the following parts:

- Cardia
- Fundus
- Body
- Antrum
- Pylorus

The fundus and body contain most of the acid and pepsin-secreting cells; the antrum contains cells that secrete gastrin.

Blood supply arrives from the celiac trunk and the major branches that provide a very rich supply to the organ. Autonomic innervation is primarily parasympathetic through the vagus nerve and sympathetic through fibers that arise from T-6 to T-10.

The stomach has two curvatures, the lesser and the greater, with the lesser being shorter than the greater. The shape of the stomach allows it to serve as an excellent food reservoir.

One of the most important functions of the stomach is the production of hydrochloric acid and intrinsic factor for the absorption of vitamin B_{12}. The gastric mucosal barrier prevents hydrochloric ions from flowing back through the gastric mucosa, and mucus also lubricates the passage of solids and undigested food. It protects the epithelium from mechanical damage, delays the passage of chyme into the intestine so that the intestine is not overwhelmed, and enables food to be properly mixed for initial digestion. Hyper- and hypo-osmotic solutions, as well as fats, appear to delay emptying of the stomach, as a result of a reflux mechanism from receptors situated in the duodenum. Between meals, gastric motor function works to empty any residual of recently ingested food.

Peptic Ulcer Disease

Peptic ulcer disease is an ulceration of the gastrointestinal tract in areas that come in contact with gastric acid and pepsin. Treatment is directed at the reduction of gastric secretions and the buffering of gastric acid. Chronic antacid therapy, however, may affect nutritional status in the following ways:

- Excessive and prolonged use of calcium antacids products may induce hypercalcemia and development of renal calculi

- Phosphorus depletion may occur with use of magnesium hydroxide and aluminum hydroxide
- All acid-reducing drugs such as the following: H_2 receptor antagonists (i.e., cimetidine, famotidine, ranitidine, nizatidine) or Proton Pump Inhibitors (i.e., omeprazole, pantopraxole, rabeprazole, esomepraxole, lansoprazole) can decrease production of intrinsic factor and may decrease vitamin B_{12} absorption
- Pain, bleeding, hypermotility, and/or gastric outlet obstruction may occur
- Iron-deficiency anemia may develop secondary to poor intake, blood loss, impaired breakdown of iron-rich foods, and altered gastric pH
- Progression to oral intake and the variety of food items included is based on individual tolerance

Gastritis

Gastritis is the acute or chronic inflammation of the mucosal lining of the stomach. Etiologies vary but include alcohol abuse, ingestion of corrosives, bacterial, or viral infection (food poisoning), anemia, shock, and chronic drug use (especially nonsteroidal anti-inflammatory drugs such as aspirin, BC Powder, ibuprofen, and so forth)

The clinician should take into consideration the following implications for nutritional status:

- Pain on eating may prevent adequate oral intake
- Stimulation of gastric secretions should be reduced; modifications to the diet include avoidance of caffeine and excess liquids
- Reduced secretion of intrinsic factor may result from chronic gastritis, increasing the risk of inadequate vitamin B_{12} absorption

Vomiting

Aside from obvious impairment of intake, prolonged vomiting can lead to a metabolic alkalosis.

- Intractable vomiting may require parenteral support until oral intake or enteral support can be reestablished

- May be a part of an eating disorder and can lead to dental and nutritional ramifications

Hiatal Hernia

Hiatal hernia is herniation of a portion of the stomach through the hiatus of the diaphragm into the esophagus.

- Anatomical ramifications of this condition may complicate or contraindicate nasogastric or orogastric tube feedings
- Progression of oral feeds requires frequent small feedings, upright positioning during ingestion, avoiding food intake prior to retiring, and often elevation of the head of the bed to avoid regurgitation and aspiration

Gastric Outlet Obstruction

Gastric outlet obstruction is a disturbance in the normal emptying of the stomach. It may be

- *anatomical,* as in pyloric stenosis, stricture, or swelling near a pyloric or duodenal ulcer
- *functional* (occurring postvagotomy)

The patient may require parenteral support while diagnostic evaluation is in progress. If the disturbance is prolonged, the patient may require enteral feeding via jejunostomy.

GI Bleed

GI bleed may be accompanied by nausea and hematemesis.

- With resolution of hemorrhage, resume oral intake or enteral infusions as tolerated
- Chronic low-grade gastric bleeding or recurring gastrointestinal bleeds can induce iron deficiency anemia
- Endoscopic or surgical interventions may be indicated for continued bleeding or development of other complications

General Surgery

Gastric surgeries may be indicated in cases of tumor, ulcer disease, perforation, hemorrhage, Zollinger-Ellison syndrome (gastric acid hypersecretion due to excess gastrin from a tumor), gastric polyposis, and Menetrier's disease (large, tortuous gastric folds in the body and fundus of the stomach with hyperplasia that replaces most of the chief and parietal cells).

Vagotomy

Truncal vagotomy has the following effects:

- The resting tone of the stomach *(gastric stasis)* is altered, and the pyloric sphincter is widely patent
- Poor gastric emptying is the result of a disturbance in normal antral peristalsis
- Emptying of solids is slowed and emptying of liquids is accelerated
- Hypertonic fluids leave the stomach undiluted
- The grinding of solid foods and the sieving action of the pylorus are not normal, resulting in the emptying of larger masses of solid food into the small intestine
- The stomach is less able to perform the functions of storage, mixing, liquefying, digesting, and delivering the resulting chyme to the duodenum in a controlled fashion
- There is early satiety because of reduced storage capacity

Selective and parietal cell vagotomies have the following effects:

- There is minimal acceleration of liquid emptying
- Emptying of solids is not alerted
- There is early satiety because of reduced gastric capacity
- Vagotomy of the fundus will impair receptive relaxation
- Release of catecholamines or any means of sympathetic stimulation causes relaxation of fundic tone and occasionally gives rise to acute gastric dilatation *(adynamic ileus)*
- Once the process has resolved, all liquids are handled by the stomach in the same fashion, so the common practice of progression from a clear liquid to a full liquid to a soft diet in the postoperative period has no physiologic rationale

Pyloroplasty

- This surgery is commonly used to widen the opening of the pylorus
- Hypertonic fluids flow into the duodenum and can result in dumping syndrome

Total Gastrectomy

In cases of total gastrectomy (removal of the entire stomach), a reservoir may be created by using a section of the jejunum to form a pouch.

- The limitations of a reduced gastric pouch, however, dictate a need for small, frequent, nutrient-dense feedings limited in simple sugars
- Dumping syndrome is common due to the loss of the pyloric sphincter.
- Loss of cells that produce intrinsic factor, thus vitamin B_{12} must be provided to the patient

Subtotal or Partial Gastrectomy

This procedure removes a portion of the stomach (amount removed varies) accompanied by a reconstruction procedure. There are several variations of partial gastrectomy:

- *Antrectomy with gastroduodenostomy* (Billroth I) is the removal of the distal portion of the stomach and the pyloric sphincter. The stomach remnant is anastomosed to the duodenum
  1. dumping syndrome may occur
  2. some compromise of digestion may result as chyme rapidly mixes with duodenal, pancreatic, and biliary secretions
- *Antrectomy with gastrojejunostomy* (Billroth II) is the removal of the distal portion of the stomach, pyloric sphincter and part of the duodenum; the remnant of the stomach is anastomosed to the side of the jejunum, creating a blind loop
  1. dumping syndrome may occur
  2. some compromise of digestion, particularly fat, may occur as chyme mixes with duodenal, pancreatic, and biliary secretions in abnormal synchronization

- *Vertical banded gastroplasty* is a weight-loss surgical procedure that creates a stomach pouch that holds about 15–30 ml and drains through a 1-cm gastric channel reinforced by a band into the fundus of the stomach. It is a volume-restrictive surgery only, and does not deter the patient from consuming foods high in sugar and fat. Dumping syndrome does not occur as nutrient absorption proceeds normally
  1. average caloric intake ranges from 600–800 kcal per day during the weight loss phase
  2. foods low in simple sugars and fats are encouraged in order to prevent weight gain
  3. liquids are consumed between meals in an attempt to prevent overfilling of the pouch
  4. vitamin and mineral supplement is typically given due to the low caloric intake
- *Roux-en–Y gastric bypass or laparoscopic gastric bypass* are weight-loss surgical procedures that subdivide the stomach by rows of staples into two chambers. The ~ 30-ml proximal pouch is excluded from the fundus and antrum of the stomach, and is attached to the jejunum through a narrow anastomosis. Food enters into the pouch and empties into the jejunum, therefore bypassing the lower portion of the stomach and the duodenum
  1. average caloric intake ranges from 800–900 kcal per day
  2. protein intake of approximately 50–70 g per day is encouraged
  3. foods low in simple sugars and fats are encouraged in order to prevent weight gain
  4. liquids are consumed between meals to maintain hydration and to prevent overfilling of the pouch at mealtimes
  5. dumping syndrome may occur
  6. vitamin/mineral supplement, iron (for menstruating women), vitamin B_{12}, calcium are typically supplemented
  7. nausea, vomiting, constipation, gallstones, marginal ulcers, stomal stenosis, small bowel obstruction, and incisional hernias may occur, as well as other much less common complications

- *Lap-Band* is a weight-loss laparoscopic procedure whereby an adjustable band is placed around the top of the stomach creating a 60-ml pouch. Inserting or removing saline can adjust the diameter of the band. It is a volume-restrictive surgery. Typically, vitamin and mineral supplements are given due to low caloric intake.

Dumping Syndrome

This condition results from alteration, removal, or bypass of the pyloric sphincter.

- Approximately half of the gastric surgery patients develop dumping

The syndrome has two phases:

- *Early dumping* occurs 10 to 15 minutes after ingesting a meal (especially if the meal is high in simple carbohydrates)
- Symptoms include diaphoresis, nausea, vomiting, dizziness, palpitations, flushing, weakness, abdominal bloating, cramping, and diarrhea (within 1 hour after a meal)
- *Late dumping* occurs 1 to 2 hours after a meal
- Symptoms include perspiration, tachycardia, mental confusion, and syncope. This phase is thought to be the result of insulin-induced hypoglycemia
- The exact etiology of dumping syndrome is unknown but is thought to be related to extravascular fluid depletion resulting from rapid reflux of hypertonic gastric contents into the jejunum
- Release of intestinal hormones (serotonin, bradykinin, enteroglucagon, GIP, neurotensin)

Management of oral progression involves a low-carbohydrate, high-protein, modified-fat diet, limiting fluids to between meals.

- Meals served dry; liquids consumed 1 to 2 hours postprandially
- Avoidance of simple sugars to reduce osmolality of food contents directly entering the small bowel
- Increase in the concentration of complex carbohydrates

- Initially, lactose-containing foods may need to be limited and re-introduced as tolerance allows

Generally these dietary modifications are needed only for a short term, as most individuals can resume a general diet. However, some individuals may need to adhere to this diet indefinitely.

Dumping syndrome may be seen with initial enteral infusions following gastrectomy, gastroduodenostomy, or gastrojejunostomy. Enteral feeding requires attention to osmolality, related to small or predigested molecules of carbohydrate (sucrose), protein (amino acids), and fat medium-chain triglycerides (MCT). Introduction of enteral products as isotonic concentration or of hypertonic solution at low volume is recommended.

Bezoar Formation

This condition is the formation of masses from retained food and vegetable matter or hair in the stomach and intestine. It occurs because of reduced gastric motility, decreasing mixing and churning of the stomach, delayed gastric emptying, and reduction of gastric secretions. It is treated with efforts to improve motility, but may require endoscopic intervention to break up and remove the concretion or on rare occasions, surgical removal.

SPECIFIC DISORDERS OF THE GASTROINTESTINAL TRACT: THE INTESTINES

The adult has approximately 350 to 650 cm (11.5–21.5 feet) of small intestine, depending on the method and circumstances of the measurement.

The enterocyte is highly susceptible to injury, so provision of nutrients is essential for gastrointestinal function. The presence of food in the small intestine plays an integral part in the maintenance of normal villous structure and function.

During periods of stress, particularly critical illness, the mucosa of the gastrointestinal tract is susceptible to ulceration and bleeding.

The ileocecal valve protects the small intestine from a more rapid transit time of food and from the anaerobic bacterial flora of the colon. Loss of the valve permits bacterial reflux, which results in increased small intestinal colonization of highly anaerobic bacteria that can

- deconjugate bile salts, leading to diarrhea
- convert fatty acids to hydroxyl fatty acids that impair water absorption by the colon

Carbohydrate malabsorption may contribute to the diarrhea due to the increased osmotic concentration caused by breakdown of unabsorbed carbohydrate.

The severity of nutritional problems resulting from disorders of the intestines is multifactorial:

- Length and location of the remaining bowel
- Presence or absence of the ileocecal valve
- Concomitant colonic disease
- Mucosal integrity and function of the remaining gut
- Time since onset of the syndrome/disorder

Nutritional management of maldigestive/malabsorptive disorders is summarized in Table 3–16.

Disorders of Absorption

Disorders of absorption generally involve a defect in the mucosal absorptive mechanisms.

- A selective defect in specific transport systems of protein, lipid, or carbohydrate
- Disorders that invade the mucosa, such as intestinal lymphoma
- A marked decrease in absorptive surface area and a derangement in cellular maturation, genetic expression, and differentiation that results in an impairment in global absorptive function
- Bacterial overgrowth related to the stasis associated with motility disorders, multiple jejunal diverticula, blind loops, or surgical resection

Table 3–16 Nutritional Management of Maldigestive/Malabsorptive Disorders

Disorder	Nutritional Management
Acute malabsorption	Parenteral nutrition or hydrolyzed enteral nutrition
Disaccharidase deficiency	Lactase replacement with lactose; sucrose restriction
Bile salt diarrhea	Moderate to normal fat, medium chain triglycerides, cholestyramine
Primary pancreatic insufficiency	Low fat, medium chain triglycerides, pancreatic enzymes
Pancreatic insufficiency, secondary to rapid transit	Low fat, medium chain triglycerides, pancreatic enzymes, low osmolality, low lactose
Bacterial overgrowth	Antibiotics
Ileal impairment	Low fat, medium chain triglycerides, low osmolality
Mucosal alterations	Low fat, medium chain triglycerides, low lactose
Resection of < 100 cm of the ileum	Moderate to low fat, medium chain triglycerides, low oxalate, low osmolality
Resection of > 100 cm of the ileum	Low fat, medium chain triglycerides, low oxalate, low osmolality
Massive resection	Hydrolyzed enteral nutrition or parenteral nutrition

Source: Reprinted from *The Handbook of Surgical Intensive Care,* 3rd ed., Lyerly H et al, 1992, Mosby. With permission from Elsevier.

- *Celiac disease* is common genetic, autoimmune enteropathy that leads to intestinal mucosal damage
  1. Small bowel biopsy of the second portion of the duodenum is often used to determine presence of celiac disease. Other screening tests are available (e.g., anti-gliadin IgA and IgG, anti-endomysial (EMA) IgA and IgG, tissue transglutaminase IgA and IgG). However, they have a higher rate of false-negative and false-positive results. Genetically, celiac disease is associated with HLA alloantigens DQ2 and DQ8. An individual who has neither of these genes is unlikely to ever develop celiac disease. However, these are common HLA alloantigens in America, where up to 37% of the population may have one or both of these markers. Presence of one or both of these gene markers does not mean a person has the disease, but in the right setting may develop the disorder.
  2. Genetic, environmental, and immunological factors precipitate the development of celiac disease
  3. Gliadin in wheat, prolamins in rye and barley, oats, and gluten are known food factors that promote intestinal damage
  4. Common nutrient deficiencies: iron, folate, vitamin B_{12}, calcium, vitamin D, and other fat-soluble vitamins
  5. Treatment of celiac disease consists of nutrition counseling by a trained dietitian, lifelong elimination of gluten and other food intolerances, potential initial avoidance of lactose, and replacement of micronutrients as needed

Small Intestinal Obstruction

Small intestinal obstruction is a mechanical obstruction of the lumen resulting from adhesions, tumor, or hernia.

- Net absorption decreases in its early phase (≤ 12 hours), while net secretion remains constant
- The late phase begins after 12 hours, with net absorption decreasing further and net secretion increasing, thereby further exacerbating intestinal distention

- The resulting third-spacing of isosmolar fluid leads to an isosmolar volume contraction
- Intestinal distention, stasis, and accumulation of desquamated cells and debris allow intraluminal bacteria to flourish
- Partial or incomplete intestinal obstruction results from conditions that intermittently allow proximal intestinal content and gas to pass the point of obstruction
- The individual presents with crampy abdominal pain and intermittent diarrhea
- Nutritional management should proceed with caution. The individual should remain without enteral nutrition support until the nature and extent of the obstruction can be determined, and medical/surgical management is implemented. Advancement of nutrition support may use a transitional modality, with incorporation of parenteral nutrition support and enteral nutrition support individualized to the appropriate levels.

Lactase Deficiency/Lactose Intolerance

Lactase deficiency is the most common mucosal brush border enzyme deficiency. Nutritional consequences after lactose ingestion may include the following: abdominal pain, bloating, flatulence, and diarrhea. The amount of lactose tolerated by each individual can vary considerably in a range of < 3 g to as great as 15 g. Diagnosis can be confirmed by a lactose tolerance test or a hydrogen breath test.

Nutritional management must include a reduction of dietary lactose as the major aspect of treatment, with the amount of reduction adjusted to the individual's ability to tolerate lactose.

- The individual should be counseled on foods that contain lactose, how to read nutrition labels, how to watch for "hidden sources," and how to adjust ingestion of lactose to avoid symptoms
- Reduction of exposure by the mucosa to a quantity of lactose can be accomplished by dividing the total dose into smaller portions throughout the day

- Since a number of foods that contain lactose are also good sources of calcium, individuals should be counseled on how to incorporate other calcium-rich food sources into their dietary intake or advised to take a calcium supplement
- Tolerance to milk may be enhanced by adding lactase-enzymes to milk products per the manufacturer's recommendations, or using prepared low-lactose products such as Lactaid milk
- Yogurt that contains live bacteria cultures may be well tolerated by these individuals since the bacteria synthesize beta-galactosidase, which ferments lactose in the intestinal lumen

Inflammatory Bowel Disease

Inflammatory bowel disease (IBD) is an autoimmune disorder that can cause ulceration of the colonic mucosa (*ulcerative colitis*) or can affect both the large and/or small intestines (*Crohn's disease*).

Nutritional consequences include malnutrition, diarrhea, abdominal pain, bloody stools, steatorrhea, malabsorption, limited oral intake, anorexia, avoidance behavior, possibility of micronutrient deficiencies, and possible lactase deficiency.

- *Crohn's disease:* steatorrhea; loss of calcium, magnesium, and possibly zinc in the stool; excessive absorption of uncomplexed oxalate, hyperoxaluria, and increased risk of calcium oxalate kidney stones; small intestinal malabsorption; weight loss; and possible hypoalbuminemia, and low vitamins A and D levels
- *Ulcerative colitis:* loose stools, rectal urgency, bloody diarrhea, abdominal pain, fever, dehydration, weight loss, anemia, and possible development of colon cancer

Nutritional management of IBD varies depending upon individual severity of symptoms and the extent of mucosal involvement.

- The patient may have increased energy requirements. Adjust for degree of hypermetabolism and need for weight maintenance/repletion

- The patient may have increased protein needs secondary to enteric losses and/or use of corticosteroids in medical treatment modality. Required levels of intake may be 1.3 to 2.0 g/kg per body weight
- Bowel rest may alleviate some of the acute symptoms, with parenteral nutrition support used during these time periods to provide adequate nutritional intake
- When the disease is in remission, use of a standard oral diet, offered in small frequent feeding intervals, should be encouraged
- When enteral nutrition support is indicated, mild to moderate inflammation may benefit from use of polymeric diets, and moderate to severe inflammation may benefit from monomeric (defined or elemental) diets
- Avoidance of specific foods should be entirely dependent on the individual's needs and the food's influence on the severity of disease
- Other dietary modifications that may be efficacious include
  1. possible restriction of fiber in the diet to less than 30 g
  2. restriction of fat in the presence of steatorrhea, with the use of medium-chain triglycerides (MCT) to augment caloric intake and monitoring of individuals receiving MCT for nausea, vomiting, abdominal discomfort, and osmotic diarrhea
  3. lactose restriction if the individual is lactase deficient
  4. evaluation and treatment of vitamin and mineral deficiencies (common deficiencies are iron, folate, vitamin B_{12}, zinc, magnesium, calcium, and vitamin D)
  5. use of oral rehydration therapy solutions when individuals with malabsorption cannot maintain fluid and electrolyte homeostatis
  6. possible consideration of the "specific carbohydrate diet" (information available at www.scdiet.org). *Note:* There are no randomized trials of safety and efficacy, but many anecdotal reports of disease amelioration.

Short Bowel Syndrome

Short bowel syndrome is an array of metabolic and physiological consequences that occur as a result of massive surgical resection, bypass, or intrinsic disease of the bowel. It is generally defined as having less than 150 cm (about 60 inches) of small intestine remaining.

Nutritional Consequences

Nutritional consequences are entirely dependent upon the degree and location of resection, and the subsequent rehabilitation of the individual is dependent upon overall health status. Metabolic consequences include anemia, bile salt depletion, osteomalacia, cholelithiasis, dehydration, diarrhea, steatorrhea (particularly if the ileocecal valve is resected), bile salt diarrhea, hypocalcemia, hypomagnesemia, oxalate stones, trace mineral deficiencies, vitamin (A, D, E, K, B_{12}) deficiencies, and protein-energy malnutrition.

Nutritional Management

Nutritional management varies depending on site and extent of intestinal resection. Prior to initiation of nutritional therapy, assess the functional capacity of the remaining sections of the bowel, and note the stool pattern and volume. Resections of 70%–80% are associated with the most severe nutritional problems and necessitate aggressive nutritional support.

Management of any individual, independent of degree of resection, includes:

- Replacement of fluids and electrolytes
- Use of total parenteral nutrition in the initial postoperative phase
- Once diarrhea has stabilized, transition to an enteral route of nutrition support with gradual transition to enteral/oral feedings and parenteral nutrition tapered
  1. Use of continuous infusion of enteral nutrition may be better tolerated than bolus feedings.
  2. Monomeric diets may be efficacious in the early adaptive period, with consideration given to the osmotic concentration and the rate of feeding.

3. Polymeric diets have been demonstrated as efficacious, with attention paid to the content of fat (MCT may be useful).

- An oral diet consumption is low in fat and high in carbohydrates, except for individuals with osmotic diarrhea
- Estimation of energy requirements at 1.5–2.0 times the basal energy expenditure
- Estimation of protein requirements at levels that maintain nitrogen balance
- Individualized restriction of soluble fiber content and lactose in the oral diet
- For individuals with hyperoxaluria, possible restriction of high-oxalate foods such as chocolate, cola drinks, tea, carrots, celery, spinach, pepper, nuts, plums, figs, and strawberries

Long-term management for nutritional consequences should include monitoring of

- Electrolytes, fluid status, vitamin/mineral status (especially calcium, magnesium, sodium, potassium, zinc, phosphate, and iron), with replacement as necessary
- Weight status
- Tolerance to enteral feeding regimen, with adjustment as necessary
- Protein nutriture status, using appropriate biochemical markers such as prealbumin or albumin

REFERENCES

Allard JP, Jeejeebhoy KN. Nutritional support and therapy in the short bowel syndrome. *Gastroenterol Clin North Am.* 1989;18:589–601.

American Dietetic Association. *National Dysphagia Diet: Standardization of Optimal Care.* 2002.

American Gastroenterological Association. AGA technical review on Celiac Sprue. *Gastroenterology.* 2001; 120(6):1526–1540.

Bristol JB, Williamson RCN, Chir M. Nutrition, operations, and intestinal adaptation. *JPEN.* 1988;12:299–309.

Desao MB, Jeejeebhoy KN. Nutrition and diet in management of diseases of the gastrointestinal tract. In: Shils ME, Young VR, eds. *Modern Nutrition in Health and Disease.* Philadelphia, PA: Lea & Febiger; 1988:1092–1128.

Frankenfield DC, Beyer PL. Dietary fiber and bowel function in tube-fed patients. *J Am Diet Assoc.* 1991; 91:590–596.

Green PHR, et al. Characteristics of adult celiac disease in the USA: Results of a national survey. *Am J Gastroenterol.* 2001;96:126–131.

Klein S, Jeejeebhoy KN. Long-term nutritional management of patients with maldigestion and malabsorption. In: Sleisenger MH, Fordtran JS, eds. *Gastrointestinal Disease: Pathophysiology/Diagnosis/Management.* 5th ed. Philadelphia, PA: WB Saunders Co; 1993:2048–2061.

Lacey JM, Wilmore DW. Is glutamine a conditionally essential amino acid? *Nutri Rev.* 1990;8:48:297–309.

Messing B, Pigot F, Rongier M, et al. Intestinal absorption of free oral hyperalimentation in the very short bowel syndrome. *Surg Clin North Am.* 1987;67:551–571.

Picarelli A, diTola M, Sabbatella L, Mastracchio A, et al. Identification of a new celiac disease subgroup: Antiendomysial and antitransglutaminase antibodies of IgG class in the absence of selective IgA deficiency. *J Intern Med.* 2001;249(2):181–188.

Podolsky DK. Inflammatory bowel disease. *N Engl J Med.* 1991;325:928–937, 1008–1016.

Purdum PP, Kirby DF. Short-bowel syndrome: A review of the role of nutrition support. *JPEN.* 1991;15:93–101.

Geriatric Nutrition

Ronni Chernoff, PhD, RD, FADA

POPULATION DESCRIPTION

The geriatric population is defined as those people age 65 and older. Although this is an arbitrary designation, it has been used in common law to define retirement age, age of eligibility for federal and state entitlement programs, demographic categorizations, and for other purposes. In the over-65 population, there are stratifications for the "young-old" (65–74), "old" (75–84), and "very old" (85 and older). It is noteworthy that the most significant growth among the over-65 group has been among the very old.

The geriatric population as a percent of the American population is expanding more rapidly than any other group. It is expected to increase further when the oldest people of the "baby boom" generation, born between 1946–1964, reach the age of 65 in just a few years.

Through longitudinal studies, changes have been described that are part of the normal human aging process that impact the standard approaches to assessing nutritional status, defining nutrient requirements, selecting nutrition interventions, and providing nutrition support to older people. This chapter will briefly describe these issues.

PHYSIOLOGY OF HUMAN AGING

Humans are very heterogenous in genetic profile, predisposition to disease, health behaviors, cultural behaviors, and social and environmental factors, all of which contribute to the rate and manner in which individuals age. However, there are common physiological alterations that occur with age, although they may happen at a different rate among individuals. The following are the major changes that are associated with advancing age:

- decrease in body protein compartments
- decrease in total body water content
- loss of bone density
- increase in proportion of body fat

Decrease in Body Protein Compartments

The decrease in body protein compartments will contribute to the following potential effects:

- decrease in muscle mass with an associated reduction in muscle strength, coordination, and functional independence
- reduction in organ function, including cardiac, pulmonary, renal, epatic, gastrointestinal (including peristalsis), bladder, and urinary tract control
- decrease in basal metabolic rate and oxygen consumption, contributing to a decrease in need for dietary energy
- impairment of immune responses
- reduction in production of hormones, enzymes, metabolic substrates, and blood cell types
- decline in rate of physiological response to both internal and external events; recovery from illness, trauma, or surgery may be slower

Decrease in Total Body Water

In young adulthood, water is approximately 80% of body composition, but it may decrease to 60%–70% in older people. Water is an important compartment of the human body because it is involved in the:

- maintenance of cellular integrity
- regulation of body temperature
- transportation of nutrients
- dilution and transport of medications
- maintenance of normal body waste removal

Decrease in Bone Density

Loss of bone density occurs in males and females, although the primary focus has been on the pathologic loss of bone that may occur in women who are postmenopausal.

- Reduction in bone density can be minimized by a lifelong health plan that includes adequate dietary calcium, vitamin D, and weight-bearing exercise.
- In postmenopausal women, current therapy for avoiding excess bone loss includes menopausal hormone therapy which should be undertaken under the direction of a physician.
- Decreased bone density will contribute to the likelihood of fractures resulting from, or contributing to, falls.
- In advanced osteoporosis, collapse of the vertebrae contributes to a compression of the abdominal cavity with subsequent displacement and constriction of vital organs.

Increase in Proportion of Body Fat

Although the actual amount of body fat may not increase significantly, reductions in all the other major body compartments contribute to this change. There is also a shift in fat tissue deposition with more fat deposited in the abdominal area and an increase in the density of organ fat pads.

NUTRITIONAL REQUIREMENTS OF OLDER ADULTS

The physiological changes that occur with advancing age, changes in body composition, chronic disease, level of physical activity, medication use, and social and economic conditions all contribute to whether or not individuals meet their daily nutritional requirements. The need for specific nutrients is affected uniquely by age and generalizations cannot be made for most nutrients.

Energy

- Caloric needs are determined by the amount of energy needed for basal metabolic function, to sustain lean body mass, and to support physical activity.
- Energy needs tend to decrease with advancing age due to the reduction in total body protein and decreased physical activity.

- Energy needs increase when there is a demand for tissue synthesis to heal a wound, repair a bone fracture, or fight infection.

Protein

- Protein needs actually increase with advancing age.
- The RDA for adults (0.8 g/kg/body weight) will not achieve nitrogen equilibrium in healthy, ambulatory elderly people.
- One g/kg of body weight is a better base level for dietary protein intake.
- There may be greater demands for protein for tissue synthesis, bone repair, or infection resistance.

Carbohydrate

- There are no significant changes in carbohydrate requirements with age.
- Recommendations are the same for older adults as they are for younger adults: 55%–60% of calories from complex carbohydrates.
- Due to a decrease in bowel motility, emphasis should be placed on dietary intake of carbohydrates that are rich in fiber.
- Carbohydrate tolerance may decrease with advancing age.

Fat

- Dietary fat should be eaten in amounts adequate to provide needed energy, fat-soluble vitamins, and essential fatty acids.
- There is some controversy about restricting dietary fats, such as cholesterol, in elderly people.
- Risk factors for coronary heart disease change in the early 60s with systolic hypertension becoming a greater predictor than serum lipid profiles.

Water

- Thirst sensitivity decreases with advancing age and there is a risk of dehydration in older people.

- Requirements for free fluid are approximately 30 ml/kg body weight.
- Minimum fluid intake should approximate 1500 ml/day.

Vitamin B₁ (Thiamin)

- RDA for adults is 1.2 mg/day for men and 1.0 mg/day for women.
- There is no known decrease in absorption or alteration in metabolism of vitamin B_1 associated with age.
- Epidemiological studies reveal that approximately 50% of people over age 65 are ingesting less than two-thirds of the RDA for thiamin.
- The greatest risk factor for vitamin B_1 deficiency is alcoholism which interferes with intake, absorption, and utilization.

Vitamin B₂ (Riboflavin)

- RDA for adults is 1.4 mg/day for men and 1.2 mg/day for women.
- There is no known decrease in absorption or alteration in metabolism of vitamin B_2 associated with age.
- Inadequate dietary intake is the greatest risk factor for elderly due to decreased consumption of milk products, the primary source of riboflavin, associated with lactose intolerance.

Niacin

- RDA for niacin is 15 mg niacin equivalents (NE)/day for men and 13 mg NE/day for women, which appears to be adequate for older adults.

Vitamin B₆

- RDA for vitamin B_6 is 2 mg/day for men and 1.6 mg/day for women.
- Many studies have demonstrated an inadequate intake of vitamin B_6 among elderly people.
- There have been suggestions that vitamin B_6 requirements may be too low for elderly people because atrophic gastritis, which is more common among the elderly, may interfere with absorption, but this has yet to be supported by research.
- Alcoholism and liver disease are risk factors for vitamin B_6 deficiency among older adults.

Folate

- RDA for folate is 200 μg/day for men and 180 μg/day for women.
- There is no age-related impact on folate requirements.
- Alcoholism is a risk factor for folate deficiency in the elderly.
- Atrophic gastritis may contribute to malabsorption of folic acid in older adults.

Vitamin B₁₂

- RDA for vitamin B_{12} is 2 μg/day for both men and women.
- Atrophic gastritis and bacterial overgrowth may contribute to deficiency in older adults due to impaired absorption.
- There is some controversy over whether the RDA should be increased to the pre-1989 level of 3 μg/day for the elderly, but individuals at risk due to gastrointestinal problems should be monitored regularly.

Vitamin C

- RDA for vitamin C is 60 mg/day for both men and women.
- Elderly subjects have lower blood, plasma, and serum levels than do younger adults.
- Low blood levels of vitamin C can be corrected with supplementation, but when supplements are stopped, low levels return rapidly.
- There do not appear to be any age-related alterations in the absorption or utilization of vitamin C.
- Stress, smoking, and some medications may increase vitamin C requirements, so it is important to review dietary intake of vitamin C with individuals who may be at risk of inadequate intake.

Vitamin A

- RDA is 1000 mg/retinol equivalents (RE) for men and 800 mg/RE for women.
- It is rare to identify a vitamin A deficiency in older adults.
- Chronic hypervitaminosis may be a problem in elderly people who take large doses of supplementary vitamin A.
- High levels of vitamin supplementation have been associated with increased levels of circulating retinyl esters, which may indicate vitamin toxicity or liver damage.
- Low levels of vitamin A are associated with immune response impairment.
- Conversion of beta carotene to vitamin A is a well-regulated reaction that prevents hypervitaminosis with high level of beta carotene intake.
- Beta carotene supplementation has been promoted to quench free radicals; although this suggestion has not been fully investigated, large doses of beta carotene do not appear to be toxic.

Vitamin D

- RDA for vitamin D is 5 μg/day (200 IU) for both men and women over age 51.
- Vitamin D can be obtained from dietary sources or from sunlight exposure on the skin.
- Elderly people are at risk for vitamin D deficiency because of inadequate diets, lack of sun exposure, decreased 7-dehydrocholesterol levels in skin, and impaired conversion of vitamin D precursors in liver and kidney.
- Vitamin D is needed to facilitate calcium absorption.
- Vitamin D has an important role in immune function, and deficiency may contribute to increased susceptibility to communicable disease.
- Vitamin D supplementation at the RDA level should be considered for housebound or institutionalized elderly people.

Vitamin E

- RDA for vitamin E is 10 mg α-tocopherol equivalents for men and 8 mg α-tocopherol equivalents for women.

- There does not appear to be any age-related alteration in the absorption or metabolism of vitamin E.
- Vitamin E is a nutrient that is frequently taken as a supplement because of its antioxidant properties.
- Other claims made for the benefits of vitamin E in ischemic heart disease have yet to be scientifically confirmed.

Vitamin K

- RDA of 1 μg/kg body weight is considered sufficient.
- Vitamin K is derived from diet and synthesized by bacteria in the jejunum and ileum.
- Elderly persons at risk of developing a deficiency are those receiving sulfa drugs and anticoagulant therapy.
- People taking large supplements of vitamins A and E may develop an induced hemorrhagic condition associated with a vitamin K deficiency.

Calcium

- RDA for calcium is 800 mg/day for both men and women.
- This is controversial and suggestions have been made that the RDA for calcium be increased to 1000, 1200, or 1500 mg/day.
- The condition most closely associated with calcium metabolism in older adults is osteoporosis; this occurs in both males and females.
- Postmenopausal osteoporosis is currently treated with hormone replacement therapy, calcium, and vitamin D.
- Plasma calcium levels are not reflective of calcium status due to the close regulation of plasma calcium by several homeostatic mechanisms.
- Hypercalcemia in elderly people is usually indicative of malignant disease, hyperparathyroidism, overuse of thiazide therapy, or immobilization.

Sodium

- There is no RDA for sodium.
- Hyponatremia is a common finding among hospitalized and institutionalized elderly.

- Hypernatremia is often indicative of an acute disease process, but elderly individuals are prone to dehydration due to decreased thirst sensitivity.
- Sodium-restricted diets should be used with caution in older patients.

Potassium

- There is no RDA for potassium.
- Hypokalemia may occur in older adults who are on diuretic therapy.
- Hyperkalemia is most likely to occur in individuals with impaired renal function.
- There is some evidence that a diet rich in potassium may have a protective effect against cerebrovascular accidents.

Iron

- RDA for iron is 10 mg/day for men and women.
- Iron stores tend to increase with advancing age.
- Iron-deficiency anemia is most likely related to gastrointestinal blood loss from malignancies, peptic ulcer disease, or nonsteroidal anti-inflammatory drugs (aspirin, indomethacin).

Zinc

- RDA is 15 mg/day for both men and women.
- Evidence of zinc deficiency in elderly people is variable.
- Many elderly people have a decrease in taste sensitivity *(hypogeusia)* that has been associated with zinc deficiency, but the hypogeusia seen in elderly subjects is attributed to many factors other than zinc nutriture.
- Zinc requirements increase with a demand for tissue synthesis, but large doses for extended periods will interfere with absorption of other trace minerals (e.g., copper).

NUTRITIONAL ASSESSMENT OF THE ELDERLY

Assessing the nutritional status of older adults is often a challenge due to the physiological, physical, and disease-related changes that are associated with advanced age. An assessment that gathers as much information as possible, without making comparisons to standards that do not include equivalent populations, is an appropriate goal.

Physical Assessment

- Review condition of hair, skin, skin turgor, and signs of edema.
- Oral exam is important; the condition of the oral mucosa, tongue, gums, and teeth, and the presence of dentures or lesions all may be clues to nutritional status.
- Evaluation of physical disabilities should be part of a physical assessment.
- Obtain a history of past illnesses that might affect nutritional status.

Anthropometric Measures

- Weight for height is best evaluated by using a measure of body mass index: weight (kg)/height (m^2).
- Fluctuations in weight should be monitored closely; weight gain or loss may be an indication that physical conditions are changing.
- Height should be measured with the individual standing erect; if that is not possible, recumbent length, knee-to-heel, or segmental measurements should be used.
- Using measures that have standards derived from young adult populations are not reliable or valid in assessing nutritional status of older adults; these measurements can be used to gauge baseline data and track changes over time.
- Skinfold measures and midarm muscle circumference may not be reliable measures in older people because of the age-associated loss of lean body mass and loss of cutaneous elasticity.

Biochemical Assessment

- Serum albumin is the most reliable measure of visceral protein status in older adults; however, it is important to be aware of all the factors that may lower serum albumin that may not have any nutritional etiology.

- Transferrin is not reliable because older adults have increased iron stores and transferrin is more sensitive to iron nutriture than to protein status.
- When available, thyroxine-binding prealbumin and retinol-binding protein are the most sensitive indicators of protein status or response to nutrition intervention.

Hematological Measures

- Hematocrit, hemoglobin, and total lymphocyte count should be monitored regularly; these measures are not affected by advancing age.
- Anemia is common among elderly people, although its etiology is unknown.

Immunological Measures

- Immune system does not function as efficiently in older adults.
- The ability to respond to recall antigens diminishes with age as it does with chronic protein energy malnutrition; the only way to distinguish between age-related and malnutrition-related energy is to renourish the individual and retest with recall antigens.

Functional Assessment

There are many instruments that are available to assess functional status. The basic skills that they address include:

- *Bathing:* ability to manage personal hygiene
- *Dressing:* ability to dress oneself
- *Toileting:* ability to get to toilet without help
- *Transferring:* ability to transfer from a bed to a chair, and from a chair to an upright position
- *Continence:* ability to control bladder and bowel function
- *Feeding:* ability to feed oneself

These dimensions are measured on 3- or 4-point scales that allow the clinician to evaluate patient's skills at self-care. There is a strong correlation with the score on these activities of daily living and both serum albumin levels and the prediction of use of health resources, such as many hospitalizations or institutionalization.

There is a supplemental scale that assesses "instrumental" activities of daily living which include:

- using the telephone
- shopping
- preparing food
- housekeeping
- doing laundry
- transportation (i.e., driving)
- managing medications
- managing finances

These dimensions are also measured on a scale that assesses the ability of patients to live independently.

Medication Profile

Polypharmacy is a common problem in elderly people and must be considered as part of a comprehensive geriatric assessment. A medication profile should be kept on each patient.

- Medications, both prescription and over-the-counter, can have direct effects on the absorption, metabolism, and excretion of nutrients.
- Drugs can affect food intake by altering appetite, taste, or smell.
- Food can interfere with the absorption or utilization of medications.
- Drug–drug interactions may also impair nutritional intake.
- Drug–herb interactions may lead to deleterious outcomes.

Social History

- Socioeconomic status must be assessed, along with place and type of residence.
- Living situation, including with whom the patient is residing (spouse, adult children, relatives, friends, acquaintances, alone), must be assessed.
- Obtain a history of smoking and alcohol use.
- Determine whether the individual can afford to purchase adequate food or whether there is need for social intervention that provides access to senior meal programs, food stamps, food assistance programs, or home-delivered meals.

- Confirm that immunizations are recent.
- Confirm that screenings for cancer (prostate, breast, colon, skin) are up to date.

MODIFIED DIETS

It is well known that older people often have at least one, and frequently more than one, chronic condition that requires dietary modification. It is common for physicians to prescribe dietary modifications for many of these conditions (e.g., diabetes, coronary heart disease, hypertension, obesity). Additionally, some older adults assume responsibility for altering their own diets as a health promotion measure.

- Comprehension by the patient of the modifications required by the diet should be apparent to the counselor.
- Careful assessment of the value of dietary modification should be conducted, particularly if a medication(s) is also prescribed to manage the same condition.
- Some dietary modifications may affect the nutritional value of the individual's usual intake; if this occurs, appropriate supplements should be offered so that nutritional deficiencies do not add or compound existing health problems.
- For many older people, dietary modifications may contribute to chronic undernutrition.
- Serious consideration of restricting food selection must be given, particularly when older people are institutionalized, undernourished, or terminally ill.
- Flavor of food may be altered by dietary modifications.
- There should be a compelling medical indication to modify or restrict the diet of a frail elderly person.

CONSIDERATIONS IN FEEDING THE ELDERLY

Whenever possible, encouraging eating patterns close to usual for the individual is the best option when feeding elderly people. There are, however, many factors that must be reviewed when selecting the best route through which to feed someone.

Oral Feeding Considerations

- Is the person able to self-feed? Are modified utensils, plate slip guards, double-handled cups, nonspill glasses, or other devices needed to aid in independent feeding?
- Is impaired vision or neurological function a factor that demands the individual be helped with feeding or to be fed?
- Can the individual chew and swallow food? Is there a need for dental intervention? Is there a need for altering the consistency of food to accommodate any chewing or swallowing impairment?
- Are there religious or cultural dietary considerations? Are there medically related problems in digestion or absorption of food? Is there a requirement to modify the diet to address unique, disease-related needs?
- Is the individual eating a diet that meets nutrient requirements, or is a nutrient supplement needed? For diets that are nutritionally inadequate, a multivitamin/mineral supplement should be considered.
- If the individual cannot eat enough, a meal supplement may be a reasonable addition to the diet.
- Oral liquid feedings can supplement a diet by contributing protein, calories, vitamins, and minerals; they may be a viable option for between-meal feedings for individuals who have a limited capacity and experience early satiety at meals.
- For individuals who are unable to eat due to their medical conditions, another feeding route must be considered, such as enteral or parenteral feeding.

Enteral Feeding Considerations

- Determination of length of feeding should be part of feeding route selection. Short-term feeding can use nasal access; long-term feeding should consider placement of an indwelling tube (i.e., percutaneous endoscopic gastrostomy).

- Mental status should be evaluated because confused and agitated people resist tube placement and may pull out tubes and harm themselves.
- Gastrointestinal tract function must be evaluated to ensure best tube placement to maximize nutrient digestion and absorption.
- Formula selection depends on tolerance for volume, ability to digest and absorb nutrients, medical condition, nutritional requirements, and patient prognosis.
- Cost may be a factor in selecting enteral feeding; reimbursement for enteral feeding exists through a durable medical equipment (DME) component of Medicare. Enteral feeding is less expensive than parenteral nutrition interventions.
- Complications of enteral feeding must be minimized by regular, careful monitoring. Such complications may include
  1. Gastric retention
  2. Gastric reflux
  3. Mucosal ulceration
  4. Pulmonary infusion
  5. Pulmonary aspiration
  6. Hyperglycemia/dehydration
  7. Hypernatremia
  8. Hyperchloremia
  9. Azotemia
  10. Chronic undernutrition from inadequate feeding
  11. Bacterial contamination
  12. Interference with drug absorption
  13. Diarrhea
- Patency of feeding tube should be a high priority. Only enteral formula should be infused through the tube; flush tube regularly with water.

Parenteral Feeding Considerations

- Anticipated patient prognosis must be evaluated in the decision to provide parenteral nutrition support to an elderly patient.
- Venous access may present a problem in older adults.
- Parenteral solutions consist of hypertonic glucose solutions, aqueous protein solutions, lipid emulsions, vitamins, minerals, and trace elements.
- Elderly individuals are more likely to have glucose intolerance. Although it is an accepted practice to infuse insulin with hypertonic glucose solution, this technique would require very close monitoring in older patients.
- Lipid clearance rates should be assessed before infusing large volumes of lipid emulsions.
- Tolerance to large-volume fluid infusion must be judged because elderly adults are more sensitive to shifts in fluid compartments and volume expansion than are younger adults.
- Careful, close monitoring is necessary when supporting older patients on parenteral nutrition.

Home Nutritional Support

- Social circumstances must be carefully evaluated before sending an elderly patient home with either enteral or parenteral support.
- Finances, space for storage, caregiver support, and access to medical care all must be evaluated.
- When possible, options for home nutrition support should include visiting nurses, support from hospital personnel, support from family or close friends, or a home nutrition support company.
- Maintaining elderly patients who require nutrition support in their own homes is an acceptable and desirable option if all the requirements for safety, cleanliness, adequate storage (including refrigeration), and close medical supervision and monitoring are met.

REFERENCES

Baker MR, Peacock M, Nordin BEC. The decline in vitamin D status with age. *Age and Aging.* 1980:9:249–252.

Burns EA, Goodwin JS. Immunodeficiency of aging. *Drugs Aging.* 1997:11:374.

Campbell WW, et al. Increased protein requirements in elderly people: New data and retrospective reassessments. *Am J Clin Nutr.* 1996:60:501–509.

Chernoff R. Thirst and fluid requirements. *Nutr Reviews.* 1995:52:S3–S5.

Chernoff R. Nutrition monitoring and research studies: Nutrition screening initiative. In: Bernadier CD, ed. *Handbook of Nutrition and Food.* Boca Raton, FL: CRC Press, 2002.

Chernoff R. Nutritional rehabilitation and elderly individuals. In: Lewis CB, ed. *Aging: The Health Care Challenge,* 4th ed. Philadelphia, PA: FA Davis Company, 2002.

Food and Nutrition Board, National Research Council. *Recommended Dietary Allowances* 10th ed. Washington, DC: National Academy Press, 1989.

Fosmire GJ. Trace metal requirements. In: Chernoff R, ed. *Geriatric Nutrition: The Health Professional's Handbook,* 2nd ed. Gaithersburg, MD: Aspen Publishers, 1999.

Katz S. Assessing self maintenance: Activities of daily living, mobility, and instrumental activities of daily living. *J Am Geriatr Soc.* 1983:31:721–727.

Katz S, Akpom CA. A measure of primary sociologic functions. *Int J Health Services.* 1976:6:493–508.

Kohli M, Lipschitz DA, Chatta GS. Impact of nutrition on the age-related declines in hematopoiesis. In: Chernoff R, ed. *Geriatric Nutrition: The Health Professional's Handbook,* 2nd ed. Gaithersburg, MD: Aspen Publishers, 1999.

Krasinski SD, Russell RM, Ostradovec CL, et al. Relationship of vitamin A and vitamin E to fasting plasma retinol, retinol-binding protein, retinyl esters, carotene, α-tocopherol, and cholesterol among elderly people and young adults: Increased plasma retinyl esters among the vitamin A supplement users. *Am J Clin Nutr.* 1989: 49:112–120.

Lindeman RD, Beck AA. Mineral requirements. In: Chernoff R, ed. *Geriatric Nutrition: The Health Professional's Handbook,* 2nd ed. Gaithersburg, MD: Aspen Publishers, 1999.

Manolagas SC. Immunoregulatory properties of 1,25 $(OH)_2D_3$: Cellular requirements and mechanisms. In: Norman AW, Schaefer K, Grigoleit HG, et al., eds. *Vitamin D: Molecular, Cellular and Clinical Endocrinology.* New York: Walter de Gruyter & Co, 1988.

Mitchell CO, Chernoff R. Nutritional assessment of the elderly. In: Chernoff R, ed. *Geriatric Nutrition: The Health Professional's Handbook,* 2nd ed. Gaithersburg, MD: Aspen Publishers, 1999.

Ross AC, Stephenson CB. Vitamin A and retinoids in antiviral responses. *FASEB J.* 1996:10:979–985.

Shock NW, Greulich RC, Andres R, et al. *Normal Human Aging: Baltimore Longitudinal Study on Aging.* Washington, DC: NIH Publication No 84-2450; 1984.

Smith D. *The Older Population in the United States: March 2002.* Washington, DC: U.S. Census Bureau Current Population Reports, 20–546.

Sullivan DH. What do serum proteins tell us about our elderly patients? *J Gerontol: MED SCI.* 2001:56A(2): M71–M74.

Sullivan DH, Patch GA, Walls RC, et al. Impact of nutrition status on morbidity and mortality in a select population of geriatric rehabilitation patients. *Am J Clin Nutr.* 1990:51:749–758.

Suter PM. Vitamin status and requirements of the elderly. In: Chernoff R, ed. *Geriatric Nutrition: The Health Professional's Handbook,* 2nd ed. Gaithersburg, MD: Aspen Publishers, 1999.

Hematopoietic Cell Transplantation

Susan Roberts, MS, RD, LD, CNSD

DESCRIPTION

Hematopoietic cell transplantation (HCT) is utilized to restore marrow function in patients treated with intensive chemotherapy and total body irradiation (TBI) therapy for malignant and nonmalignant diseases. Table 3–17 describes the five key phases of HCT.

The types of HCT are:

- *Autologous:* Patient's own hematopoietic cells are infused.

- *Allogeneic:* Hematopoietic cells provided by human leukocyte antigen-matched donor (usually a sibling or other family member, but unrelated donors are used as well).
- *Syngeneic:* Hematopoietic cells provided by an identical twin.
- *Peripheral Blood Cells (PBC):* Blood cells, collected from the peripheral blood instead of the marrow, are given instead or in addition to marrow. Both autologous and allogeneic PBC transplants are being performed and are more

Table 3–17 Five Key Phases in Hematopoietic Cell Transplantation

Phases	Day in Relation to Transplant	Common Processes and Complications Seen in Key Phases
Preparation	2 months to day 10	Disease staging Donor selection Plan of care development Blood cell mobilization and collection or marrow harvest (autologous transplant recipients) Initial nutrition assessment and intervention as needed in nutritionally depleted patients
Cytoreductive	Day 10 to day 0 Hematopoietic cells are infused/transplanted on day 0	Administration of chemotherapy and radiation Fluid and electrolyte imbalances Tumor lysis syndrome Nausea and vomiting Anorexia and early satiety may begin
Neutropenic	Day 0 to day +20	Infections (bacterial, fungal) Organ dysfunction, including gastrointestinal toxicities (mucositis common during this phase) Hyperacute graft-versus-host disease (GVHD)
Engraftment/early recovery	Day +20 to Day +70	Acute GVHD Infections (viral, fungal)
Late recovery	Day +70 to > 1 year	Chronic GVHD Infertility Delayed growth and development in pediatric patients Relapse Secondary malignancies

common than use of hematopoietic cells collected from the marrow.

- *Nonmyeloablative HCT:* Uses lower doses of chemotherapy and/or TBI than employed in conventional HCT. This approach leads to a mixed chimerism (both patient and donor cells present) with the intent to induce a remission through the graft-versus-tumor effect. Because the toxicity of the chemotherapy and TBI are lessened, this type of transplant allows HCT in older patients and patients with less than optimal organ function. HCT patients undergoing nonmyeloablative transplant may not have extensive nutritional problems in the early posttransplant period. However, once they develop graft-versus-host disease, their nutritional problems and con-

cerns are very similar to conventional HCT patients.

Cause

HCT is used to treat a variety of diseases including hematological disorders and malignancies, genetically determined diseases, and solid tumors.

NUTRITIONAL ASSESSMENT

Objective Parameters

Available objective data is often invalid due to the effects of the treatment and medications on organ function, fluid status, and immune function. Table 3–18 outlines factors that must be taken into consideration when objective parameters are used to assess nutritional status.

Subjective Parameters

A complete nutrition/medical history is essential to an accurate nutritional assessment in HCT patients. Obtain the following information from the patient and medical record for the initial nutritional assessment:

- Current and recent appetite
- Usual weight/ideal body weight/recent weight changes—one study has shown patients who are at < 95% of ideal body weight have increased risk of nonrelapse morality following HCT
- Gastrointestinal (GI) complaints affecting oral intake (now and with previous oncological therapies)
- Vitamin/mineral, herbal, and other dietary supplement use
- Food allergies or intolerances
- Special diet
- Recent activity level (ability to perform normal activities)
- Oral nutritional supplement use (current and past)
- Diabetes history (personal and family)
- Recent or current medications
- Previous need for nutrition support
- Physical exam (muscle loss, caloric reserves)

Problems

Nutritional complications and their causes are shown in Table 3–19.

Medical Complications

- Hepatic veno-occlusive disease (VOD)
  1. The incidence is 20%.
  2. VOD results from damage to hepatocytes by high-dose chemotherapy.
  3. The small intrahepatic veins become obstructed by fibrous material.
  4. The symptoms usually begin 1–3 weeks posttransplant.

5. The symptoms may include increased bilirubin with low to moderate increases in LFT's, significant weight gain due to fluid retention, hepatomegaly, right-upper quadrant pain, jaundice, ascites, encephalopathy, and sodium and fluid retention.

- Infection
  1. Opportunistic infections are common in the early posttransplant phase due to profound neutropenia following intensive chemotherapy/TBI and use of immunosuppressive medications to prevent graft-versus-host disease (GVHD).
  2. Mulitple antimicrobial agents are prescribed to prevent and treat infections.

- Acute GVHD
  1. This major complication of allogeneic transplant usually occurs within 100 days posttransplant.
  2. The donor's T cells (from the graft) attack the recipient (host).
  3. The organs most affected are the skin, GI tract, and liver.
     –*Skin:* macropapular rash appearing on trunk, palms, soles, and ears; can progress to generalized erythroderma with desquamation and bullae (burn-like injury).
     –*GI tract:* secretory diarrhea, guaiac-positive stools, abdominal cramping, nausea and vomiting, GI protein losses, hypoalbuminemia, and ileus.
     –*Liver:* elevated LFTs and serum bilirubin, cholestasis, malabsorption, ascites, encephalopathy, and decreased synthesis clotting factors.

- Chronic GVHD
  1. This multisystem autoimmune disease develops after 100 days posttransplant.
  2. It may involve the skin, liver, eyes, mouth, esophagus, skeletal muscle, and respiratory tract.
  3. It is treated with immunosuppressive medications including corticosteroids.
  4. Nutritional problems may include weight loss, muscle wasting, failure-to-thrive, stomatitis, dysphagia, xerostomia, anorexia, diarrhea, steatorrhea, and dysgeusia.

Table 3–18 Objective Nutritional Assessment Parameters and Confounding Factors

Parameter	Confounding Factors
• Laboratory measures	
–Serum albumin	Hydration, capillary leak syndrome, skin and GI GVHD, hepatic function, albumin infusion, high-dose corticosteroid use, blood loss, blood component transfusions.
–Serum prealbumin	Infection, inflammation, hepatic function, renal function, hydration
–Serum transferrin	Hydration, hepatic function, renal function, iron overload, blood component transfusions, zinc deficiency
• All three of the above serum proteins follow a trend of dropping significantly after the intensive chemotherapy/ radiation and returning toward normal with engraftment (recovery of the hematopoietic cell function).	
–Serum retinol-binding protein	Hydration, renal function, hepatic function, hyperthyroidism, vitamin A supplementation or deficiency
–Total lymphocyte count	Immunosuppressed state due to intensive chemotherapy/radiation, infection, cancer, immunosuppressive medications
• Anthropometric measures—most useful if serial measurements are followed	
–Body weight	Hydration, capillary leak syndrome, veno-occlusive disease, splenomegaly; significant weight loss is common in the posttransplant period
–Height	Multiple myeloma can shorten height due to vertebral compression. Use of pre-illness height may be appropriate for calculation of ideal body weight
–Triceps skinfold	Hydration, age, evaluator's technique
–Midarm circumference	Hydration, evaluator's technique
• Other objective measures	
–Skin antigen testing	Immunosuppressed state due to intensive chemotherapy/ radiation, immunosuppressive medications
–Creatinine-height index	Renal function, liver function, aging, protein intake, presence of diarrhea mixed with urine
–Nitrogen balance	Renal function, protein intake, diuretic use, presence of diarrhea mixed with urine, significant nitrogen losses with stool as seen in GI GVHD
–3-Methylhistidine excretion	Age, sex, protein intake, renal function, infection
–Indirect calorimetry	Presence of mucositis indication for use of hood system; most useful in critically ill, long-term TPN or GVHD patients

Table 3–19 Nutritional Complications of Hematopoietic Cell Transplantation and Their Causes

GI Side Effects	*Possible Causes*
• Nausea and vomiting	Chemotherapy/TBI, medications, dehydration, electrolyte imbalances, mucositis, GI GVHD, GI infections, high serum glucose or amino acid levels
• Oral mucositis and esophagitis	Chemotherapy, TBI, infections, GVHD, methotrexate (used for GVHD prophylaxis)
• Xerostomia	TBI, antiemetics, chronic GVHD, narcotics
• Early satiety	Decreased gastric motility due to prolonged absence of enteral nutrition, narcotics, high-dose chemotherapy
• Thick, viscous saliva	TBI, intensive chemotherapy
• Dysgeusia	TBI, intensive chemotherapy, antimicrobials, narcotics
• Diarrhea and steatorrhea	TBI, intensive chemotherapy, antibiotics, GI and liver GVHD, intestinal infections, such as *Clostridium difficile* and cytomegalovirus
• Anorexia	Disease state, intensive chemotherapy, TBI, drug toxicities, infections, fluid and electrolyte imbalances, psychological and environmental factors
• Micronutrient abnormalities	Medications, vomiting, diarrhea, decreased oral intake, altered absorption

• Organ failure—refer to the sections on organ failure.

A variety of medications taken by HCT recipients have nutritional implications:

• Refer to the section Solid Organ Transplantation for side effects of immunosuppressive medications. In HCT recipients, the most commonly used immunosuppressive medications are cyclosporine, tacrolimus, corticosteroids, and mycophenolate mofetil. Zenapax is under investigation for its effectiveness in treating GVHD, and OKT-3 and ATG are sometimes used in steroid-resistant GVHD.
• Methotrexate (given in the first week posttransplant to prevent GVHD) can cause mucositis, nausea, vomiting, diarrhea, and hepatotoxicity.
• Antibiotics, antivirals, antifungals can lead to nausea, vomiting, diarrhea, anorexia, dysgeusia, electrolyte imbalances, and nephrotoxicity.

TREATMENT/MANAGEMENT

Nutritional Complications

• Nausea and vomiting
  1. Consider etiology.
  2. Encourage clear liquids, salty foods, and cold bland foods as tolerated.
  3. Avoid foods with high fat content and strong odors.
  4. Encourage slow drinking and eating.
  5. Monitor fluid and electrolyte status with excessive vomiting.
  6. Use antiemetics—either scheduled doses or prior to meals to control nausea with or without vomiting.
• Xerostomia
  1. Good mouth care is very important due to the absence of antimicrobial effects of saliva.
  2. Saliva substitutes or mouth moisturizers may help.

3. Increase fluid content of foods with addition of gravy, broth, and sauces.

4. Drink liquids with meals and throughout the day.

5. If salivary glands are minimally functional, citric acid (in lemonade or sugarless lemon drops) may stimulate saliva production.

- Mucositis or esophagitis
  1. Limit intake to cool or room temperature liquids and soft foods when inflammation is significant.
  2. Acidic foods and liquids are not recommended. Bland foods work best.
  3. Diluted liquids are sometimes more tolerable.
  4. Topical swish-and-spit combination liquid medications can help decrease oral discomfort, although intravenous narcotics are often necessary due to the severity of the inflammation.
  5. Resolution of mucositis/esophagitis usually occurs within a week of white blood cell recovery. Both chronic GVHD and oral infections can result in mucositis at other times posttransplant.

- Early satiety
  1. Encourage small frequent feedings.
  2. Limit liquids with meals.
  3. Encourage high carbohydrate liquids as snacks between meals.
  4. Choose nutrient-dense foods.
  5. Consider use of a prokinetic medication to increase gastric emptying.

- Thick, viscous saliva
  1. Temporary liquid diet may be helpful.
  2. Club soda, hot tea with lemon, or sour lemon drops may help break up the mucus.
  3. Encourage high fluid intake.
  4. Milk products may be difficult to swallow but have not been proven to increase the mucus thickness.
  5. Rinse frequently with physiological saline to clear secretions and freshen mouth.
  6. Usually resolves with engraftment and healing of oral mucosa. Recurrence after this may be caused by dehydration or medications.

- Dysgeusia
  1. Encourage cold or room temperature foods and beverages.
  2. Strongly flavored foods, whose taste can better be detected, are recommended in patients with minimal/no mucositis or nausea.
  3. Use of plastic utensils may help if foods taste metallic.
  4. Adding sauces and spices to foods may be helpful.
  5. Rinse mouth often with physiological saline.
  6. Recovery of taste usually occurs 45 to 60 days posttransplant.

- Diarrhea and steatorrhea
  1. Provide adequate fluid intake orally or parenterally. Monitor fluid and electrolyte status.
  2. Avoid high-fiber and high-fat foods.
  3. Lactose intolerance may be present. Use of lactase enzyme replacement may be beneficial.
  4. With documented steatorrhea, use of low-fat diet, with supplements of water-miscible fat-soluble vitamins and MCT oil may be indicated.
  5. Consider use of antidiarrheal medications after each loose stool or as a scheduled medication. Treatment will vary depending on etiology of diarrhea.

- Anorexia
  1. Attempt to determine etiology of anorexia; if psychological, intervention by social worker or psychologist is needed.
  2. Encourage small, frequent high-calorie meals (every 2 hours).
  3. Light exercise may help stimulate the appetite.
  4. Drink high-nutrient liquids—avoid liquids with no nutritional value.
  5. Consider use of an appetite stimulant.

- Micronutrient abnormalities—patients should take an iron-free multivitamin/mineral supplement at least until all transplant medications are discontinued to prevent deficiencies during periods of inadequate oral intake.

1. Vitamins
   - Supplement to recommended daily intake (DRI).
   - Provide vitamin K weekly to those patients on parenteral nutrition support
   - The following vitamins may be depleted: thiamin, vitamin B_{12}, folic acid, vitamin A, vitamin E, and vitamin D.
2. Minerals
   - Supplement to DRI.
   - The following minerals are likely to be affected by medications and GI side effects: calcium, phosphorus, zinc, magnesium, and potassium.

Nutrition Support

Nutrient Needs

- *Calories:* 25–35 calories per kilogram or 1.3–1.5 × BEE.
- *Protein:* 1.5–2.0 grams per kilogram depending on stress factors (infection, GVHD) and corticosteroid dose (doses ≥ 1 gram/kg increase protein requirements).

- Oral diet
  1. Oral diet indicated when GI dysfunction is minimal. During the first two phases of HCT, oral intake is usually poor due to GI toxicities.
  2. In-between-meal snacks, oral nutritional supplements, and encouragement necessary to obtain an acceptable oral intake.
  3. Although still used by some HCT centers, the low-microbial diet is not universally prescribed. Well-washed fresh fruits and vegetables are now allowed at many HCT centers. Certain foods, such as aged cheeses and herbal supplements, can be contaminated with fungal organisms and are not recommended in immunosuppressed patients.
  4. Education for patients and caregivers regarding safe food handling practices is essential.
  5. Refer to Table 3–20 for oral diet guidelines for the HCT recipient.
  6. Nutrition support often needed due to the presence of nutritional and medical problems.

Table 3–20 Oral Diet Guidelines for Hematopoietic Cell Transplant Recipients (Should be utilized as long as in an immunosuppressed state)

Suggested Food Restrictions in Immunosuppressed Patients Following HCT

- Aged cheeses (e.g., Brie, Camembert, Blue, Roquefort, Sharp Cheddar, Stilton)
- Farmers and feta cheese as well as cheese with chili peppers or other uncooked vegetables
- Unwashed fresh fruits and vegetables and those with visible mold
- Raw and unpasteurized dairy products
- Fresh salad dressings containing aged cheese (e.g., Blue cheese) or raw eggs
- Raw or unpasteurized honey
- Miso products, tempeh, maté tea
- Untested well water; should be tested yearly and found safe prior to use
- Unpasteurized fruit and vegetable juices
- Undercooked or raw meats, poultry, fish, shellfish, hot dogs, lunch deli meats, tofu, sausage, bacon, eggs
- Cold smoked fish (salmon) and lox; pickled fish
- Alfalfa sprouts
- Unpasteurized beer
- Unroasted raw nuts and roasted nuts still in shell
- All moldy and outdated foods
- Nontraditional herbal and dietary supplements, uncooked brewer's yeast

7. *Oral glutamine*—research results are inconsistent regarding the efficacy of oral glutamine in HCT recipients. More research, including data on relapse and survival, is needed to evaluate this practice before it can be recommended as a standard therapy.

- Enteral feedings (EFs) (early—during the first 1–3 weeks posttransplant)
  1. EFs are not used extensively due to GI dysfunction, thrombocytopenia, and infection risk associated with the feeding tube and enteral feeding system.
  2. While some HCT centers report the use of tube feedings in adults in the early posttransplant period, this is more the exception than the rule. Theoretically, EFs could provide a more cost-effective and physiological feeding route in HCT recipients, if GI toxicities and infectious complications could be managed adequately to allow tolerance of EF.
  3. If EF is used during the early posttransplant period, continuous feedings via a nasointestinal feeding tube may be best tolerated.
  4. Combined enteral and parenteral nutrition support may be needed if adequate nutrition cannot be tolerated enterally.
  5. To reduce microbial contamination of the enteral feeding system, use only commercial sterile products, avoid mixing formula, and limit hang time to 8 hours.
  6. If thrombocytopenia is present, provision of a platelet transfusion prior to placement of the feeding tube is recommended.
- EF (late; > 3 weeks posttransplant)
  1. EF should be used in patients who have marrow engraftment and minimal/controllable GI side effects.
  2. HCT recipients who may require EF during this period includes those with GVHD, sepsis, infection, VOD, ARDS, or who require lengthy hospitalization or readmission.
  3. Placement of a percutaneous endoscopic gastrostomy (PEG) tube may be beneficial in patients requiring long-term EF.

4. Recommended formula selection (for both early and late EF): polymeric formulas can be tried initially. If not tolerated, use of an elemental or small peptide formula may be indicated. Other formula characteristics that will increase tolerance include lactose free, isotonic, and high nitrogen content.
- Total parenteral nutrition (TPN)
  1. Commonly used in the early posttransplant period and with acute GVHD of the GI tract.
  2. Concentrated formulas often needed due to volume overload.
  3. Dextrose: 50%–60% of total calories; hyperglycemia common due to the combination of stress, immunosuppressive medications, and TPN.
  4. Amino acids: 20%–25% of total calories; may need to decrease percentage in severe renal or liver dysfunction but not always necessary.
  5. Lipids: 25%–30% of total calories; hypertriglyceridemia can arise due to immunosuppressive medications as well as liver and renal dysfunction. Research in HCT patients has shown that provision of lipids in these amounts will not increase infectious complications.
  6. Glutamine-supplemented TPN: evidence from research to date does not support the routine use of glutamine-supplemented TPN in HCT patients.

NUTRITIONAL CONSIDERATIONS WITH MEDICAL COMPLICATIONS

- VOD
  1. Concentrate volume of nutrition support.
  2. Diuresis without depletion of intravascular volume.
  3. Fluid and sodium restriction may be necessary.
  4. Protein restriction not always needed in encephalopathy. Patients need protein to decrease muscle breakdown and contribution of endogenous protein to the urea pool.
  5. Use of liver failure amino acids may be trialed with encephalopathy, if en-

cephalopathy is related to administration of protein.

6. Discontinuation or decrease in provision of copper and manganese from TPN may be indicated with persistent cholestasis. Monitor copper and manganese levels to prevent deficiencies or toxicities.
7. Monitor lipid utilization.
8. Use of vitamin E and oral glutamine has been reported in 1 VOD case. More research is needed to determine the role of these supplements in VOD.

• Infection
1. Nutrition support and route will depend on the clinical status of the patient
2. Consider metabolic and volume status.
3. Evaluate type and severity of organ dysfunction.
4. Consider side effects of antimicrobial agents.
5. Provide at least $1.3 - 1.5 \times$ BEE.
6. Provide protein at 1.5 gm/kg.
7. Sodium restriction and concentrated nutrition support may be indicated.

• Acute GVHD
1. Severe skin GVHD
   –Meet increased calorie and protein needs (possibly up to 50 kcals/kg and 2 g protein/kg).
   –Provide adequate vitamin C (500–1000 mg) and zinc (based on serum zinc level) for healing.
   –Meet increased fluid needs.
2. Gastrointestinal GVHD
   –NPO + TPN until diarrhea < 500 ml/day.
   –Meet increased fluid and zinc requirements (provide 1 mg zinc/100 ml of stool output).
   –Hypocupremia may occur with excessive diarrhea. Monitor level and give supplemental dose if deficiency present (1 mg/day)
   –Meet elevated nutrient needs (same as listed above for severe skin).
   –Maintain serum albumin > 2.0 g/dl.
   –Control of GI side effects with antiemetics and H_2 blockers.

–Antidiarrheals may be contraindicated, but octreotide is often effective in controlling volume of diarrhea.
–When an oral diet is appropriate, restriction of fat, fiber, lactose, acidic foods, gastric irritants is usually recommended. Also, gradual addition of normal, solid foods will aid in determining which foods are tolerated versus those that exacerbate symptoms or increase diarrhea output.

3. Liver GVHD
–Avoid overfeeding with TPN and use EF when possible.
–Monitor tolerance of IV lipids.
–Maintain adequate blood glucose control (keep dextrose load to < 5 mg/kg/min if on TPN).
–When significant hyperbilirubinemia is present for > 1 week, check copper and manganese status and remove from TPN if levels are above normal. Hypocupremia can occur with diarrhea and hypermagnanesia has been reported in HCT patients.
–Provide adequate vitamin K.
–Sodium and fluid restrictions may be necessary.
–Liver failure amino acids may be trailed if the patient's encephalopathy occurs with administration of protein.
–For patients on EF or oral diet, watch for indicators of fat malabsorption. If fat malabsorption present, intervene with a low-fat diet, water-miscible fat-soluble vitamins, and MCT oil.

• Chronic GVHD
1. Nutrition support regimen prescribed should be dependent on severity and type of organ involvement.
2. Provide calories for weight gain or maintenance, whichever is appropriate
3. Provide 1.5 g/kg protein.
4. Monitor potassium, magnesium, calcium with steatorrhea, corticosteroid treatment and cyclosporine/tacrolimus.
5. Oral supplements and/or EF should be used with poor oral intake and inappropriate weight and lean body mass loss.

6. Oral and esophageal involvement requires avoidance of acidic foods and use of bland liquids and soft foods.

7. Liver involvement
   –If steatorrhea is present, moderate fat restriction (50–70 g/day) may be needed.
   –Water-soluble forms of fat-soluble vitamins sometimes necessary with fat-malabsorption.

8. Pulmonary involvement
   –Patient often unable to meet increased nutrient requirements via oral intake.
   –Encourage use of oral supplements and small frequent meals including high-calorie foods.
   –EF may be indicated if weight loss is persistent.

9. Pancreatic insufficiency also possible cause of malabsorption and weight loss. Treat with pancreatic enzymes.

10. Consider nutritional side effects of corticosteroids, the most commonly used medication to treat chronic GVHD.

MEDICATION SIDE EFFECTS

- Treat GI side effects with antiemetics, antidiarrheals, and nutrition interventions.
- Replace electrolytes when depleted.
- Modify nutrition support, as needed, if organ dysfunction occurs due to medications.

REFERENCES

Akpek G, Valladares JL, Lee L, et al: Pancreatic insufficiency in patients with chronic graft-versus-host disease. *Bone Marrow Transplant.* 2001;27:163–166.

Anderson PM, Ramsay NKC, Shu XO, et al: Effect of low-dose oral glutamine on painful stomatitis during bone marrow transplantation. *Bone Marrow Transplant.* 1998;22:339–344.

Antin JH: Long-term care after hematopoietic-cell transplantation in adults. *New Engl J Med.* 2002;347:36–42.

Appelbaum FR: Hematopoietic cell transplantation as a form of immunotherapy. *Int J Hematol.* 2002;75:222–227.

Chan LN: Drug-nutrient interactions in transplant recipients. *JPEN.* 2001;25:132–141.

Cheney CL, Abson KG, Aker SN, et al: Body composition changes in marrow transplant recipients receiving total parenteral nutrition. *Cancer.* 1987;59:1515–1519.

Coughlin Dickson TM, Wong RM, Offrin RS, et al: Effect of oral glutamine supplementation during bone marrow transplantation. *JPEN.* 2000;24:61–66.

Deeg HJ, Seidel K, Bruemmer B, et al: Impact of patient weight on non-relapse mortality after marrow transplantation. *Bone Marrow Transplant.* 1995;15:461–468.

Fredstrom S, Rogosheske, Gupta P, et al: Extrapyramidal symptoms in a BMT recipient with hyperintense basal ganglia and elevated manganese. *Bone Marrow Transplant.* 1995;15:989–999.

Fuhrman MP, Herrmann V, Masidonski P, et al: Pancytopenia after removal of copper from total parenteral nutrition. *JPEN.* 2000;24:361–366.

Geibig CB, Ponting-Owens J, Mirtallo JM, et al: Parenteral nutrition for marrow transplant recipients: evaluation of an increased nitrogen dose. *JPEN.* 1991;16:184–188.

Guidelines for the use of parenteral and enteral nutrition in adults and pediatric patients. *JPEN.* 2002;26(suppl):83SA–85SA.

Hasse J, Roberts S: Transplantation. In: Rombeau JL, Rolandelli RH, eds. *Clinical Nutrition Parenteral Nutrition,* 3rd ed. Philadelphia, PA: WB Saunders Co; 2001:529–561.

High KP, Legault C, Sinclair JA, et al: Low plasma concentrations of retinal and α-tocopherol in hematopoietic stem cell transplant recipients: The effect of mucositis and the risk of infection. *Am J Clin Nutr.* 2002;76:1358–1366.

Iestra JA, Fibbe WE, Zwinderman AH, et al: Body weight recovery, eating difficulties and complicance with dietary advice in the first year after stem cell transplantation: A prospective study. *Bone Marrow Transplant.* 2002;29:417–424.

Jacobsohn DA, Margolis J, Doherty J, et al: Weight loss and malnutrition in patients with chronic graft-versus-host disease. *Bone Marrow Transplant.* 2002;29:231–236.

Jebb SA, Marcus R, Elia M: A pilot study of oral glutamine supplementation in patients receiving bone marrow transplants. *Clin Nutr.* 1995;14:162–165.

Lenssen P, Aker SN: Adult hematopoietic stem cell transplantation. In: Hasse JM, Blue LS, eds. *Comprehensive Guide to Transplant Nutrition.* Chicago, IL: American Dietetic Association; 2002:123–152.

Lenssen P, Bruemmer B, Bowden RA, Gooley T, Aker S, et al: Intravenous lipid dose and incidence of bacteremia and fungemia in patients undergoing bone marrow transplantation. *Am J Clin Nutr.* 1998;67(5):927–933,.

Lenssen P: Hematopoietic cell transplantation. In: Matarese LE, Gottschlich MM, eds. *Contemporary Nutrition Support Practice,* 2nd ed. St. Louis, MO: WB Saunders Co; 2003:574–594.

Lenssen P, Sherry ME, Cheney CL, et al: Prevalence of nutrition-related problems among long-term survivors of allogeneic marrow transplantation. *JADA.* 1990;90: 835–842.

McDiarmid S: Nutritional support of the patient receiving high-dose therapy with hematopoietic stem cell support. *Can Oncol Nurs J.* 2002;12:102–115.

Mulder POM, Bouman JG, Gietama JA, et al: Hyperalimentation in autologous bone marrow transplantation for solid tumors. *Cancer.* 1989;64:2045–2052.

Nattakom TV, Charlton A, Wilmore DW: Use of vitamin E and glutamine in the successful treatment of severe veno-occlusive disease following bone marrow transplantation. *Nutr Clin Pract.* 1995;10:16–18.

Oliver MR, Van Voorhis WC, Boeckh M, et al: Hepatic mucormycosis in a bone marrow transplant recipient who ingested naturopathic medicine. *Clin Infect Dis.* 1996;22: 521–524.

Peters E, Beck J, LeMaistre C: Changes in resting energy expenditure (REE) during allogeneic bone marrow transplantation. *Am J Clin Nutr.* 1990;51:521.

Piccirillo N, De Matteis S, Laurenti L, et al. Glutamine-enriched parenteral nutrition after autologous peripheral blood stem cell transplantation: Effects on immune reconstitution and mucositis. *Haematologica.* 2003; 88:192–200.

Pytlik R, Benes P, Patorkova M, et al. Standardized parenteral alanyl-glutamine dipeptide supplementation is not beneficial in autologous transplant patients: A randomized, double-blind, placebo-controlled study. *Bone Marrow Transplant.* 2002;30:953–961.

Roberts S, Miller J: Success using PEG tubes in marrow transplant recipients. *Nutr Clin Pract.* 1998;13:1–5.

Roberts S, Vanzee J: Nonmyeloablative stem cell transplantation (NMSCT) and its nutritional consequences. *Support Line.* 2003;25:3–9.

Schloerb PR, Skikne BS: Oral and parenteral glutamine in bone marrow transplantation: A randomized, double-blind study. *JPEN.* 1999;23:117–122.

Scolapio JS, Tarrosa VB, Stoner GL, et al: Audit of nutrition support for hematopoietic stem cell transplantation at a single institution. *Mayo Clin Proc.* 2002;77:654–659.

Sefcick A, Anderton A, Byrne JL, et al: Naso-jejunal feeding in allogeneic bone marrow transplant recipients: Results of a pilot study. *Bone Marrow Transplant.* 2001;28: 1135–1139.

Slavin S, Or R, Aker M, et al: Nonmyeloablative stem cell transplantation for the treatment of cancer and life-threatening nonmalignant disorders: Past accomplishments and future goals. *Cancer Chemother Pharmacol.* 2001;48(suppl):79–84.

Stern JM: Solution center: Nutritional assessment and management of malabsorption in the hematopoietic stem cell transplant patient (Response by Roberts SR). *JADA.* 2002;102:1812–1816.

Szeluga DJ, Stuart RK, Brookmeyer R, et al: Energy requirements of parenterally fed bone marrow transplant recipients. *JPEN.* 1985;9:139–143.

Szeluga DJ, Stuart RK, Brookmeyer R, et al: Nutritional support of bone marrow transplant recipients: Randomized clinical trial comparing total parenteral nutrition to an enteral feeding program. *Canc Res.* 1987;47: 3309–3316.

Tabbara IA, Zimmerman K, Morgan C, et al: Allogeneic hematopoietic stem cell transplantation: Complications and results. *Arch Intern Med.* 2002;162:1558–1566.

Weisdorf SA, Lysne J, Wind D, et al: Positive effect of prophylactic total parenteral nutrition on long-term outcome of bone marrow transplantation. *Transplantation.* 1987;43:833–838.

Ziegler TR, Young LS, Benfell K, et al: Clinical and metabolic efficacy of glutamine-supplemented parenteral nutrition after bone marrow transplantation. *Ann Int Med.* 1992;116:821–828.

Otolaryngology

Karen Masino, RD, RN

DESCRIPTION: DISEASES OF THE ORAL CAVITY

Diseases of the oral cavity and structures in the neck can significantly impact the nutritional status of the patient. The mouth is the main portal of entry to the body and provides a formidable defense in preventing invading pathogens from entering the body. If the tissues of the oral cavity become compromised due to illness or injury, the mouth can become the source of the pathological process and ultimately impact the nutritional status of the individual. Further, nutritional deficiencies and many systemic diseases can present with alterations in the oral cavity alerting the clinician to the need for further assessment. Also, alterations in smell and taste can indicate possible disease and negatively impact nutritional status. Poor oral health in geriatric populations can lead to life-threatening conditions, including malnutrition and dehydration, valvular heart disease, joint infections, and pneumonia. Many pharmaceuticals and other therapies commonly used in treating systemic conditions can also produce alterations in the integrity of the oral mucosa and impact nutritional status as well.

Lifestyle behaviors that affect general health can affect oral and craniofacial health and are associated with an increased risk for craniofacial birth defects, oral and pharyngeal cancers, periodontal disease, dental caries, and candidiasis, among other oral health problems.

Oral health is related to well-being and quality of life as measured along functional, psychosocial, and economic dimensions. Poor oral health and craniofacial disease can contribute to loss of productivity and impaired quality of life due to interference with social interaction, verbal communication, and pain, and contribute to anxiety and depression. Clinicians should be aware of physical problems that can occur as a result of disease and how this will affect the nutrition management of the patient.

GENERALIZED NUTRITION ASSESSMENT

- See Chapter 1, Screening and Assessment
- *History:* appetite, GI symptoms (diarrhea/nausea/vomiting/constipation), presence of soreness, burning, toothache pain, halitosis, painful opening/closing of mouth, chewing/swallowing difficulty, smell and taste alterations, salivation ability or xerostomia, tobacco and recreational drug use, weight history
- *Past medical history:* pneumonia, diabetes, cancer, chemotherapy, radiation therapy to head or neck region, tracheostomy, HIV/AIDS, Sjögren's syndrome, mandibular fracture/surgery, Crohn's disease.
- *Medications:* see table of medications with nutrition implications in oral health.
- *Nutrition history:* calorie/protein intake, alcohol use, fruit and vegetable intake, sucrose and simple sugar intake, vitamin/mineral intake, herbal and nutrition supplement use.
- *Physical exam:* cracked lips, ulcerations, dentition or how well dentures fit, facial weakness, drooling, oral lesions or ulcerations, dental prosthesis, coughing with eating or drinking, presence of masses or swelling, gingival dysplasia.

Evaluate for signs and symptoms of vitamin and mineral deficiency. See Table 3–21 for signs and symptoms of vitamin and mineral deficiency.

For patients with olfactory complaints, a smell identification test can be completed.

A taste test evaluating sweet (sucrose), salty (sodium chloride), bitter (quinine), and sour (citric acid) can be helpful to determine taste alterations.

- Laboratory measurements are necessary for metabolic monitoring in the unstable patient but can also contribute to baseline assessment and exclude specific pathological states or focus the diagnostic approach.
  - Visceral proteins are utilized to assess protein status. See Chapter 1, Screening and Assessment.
  - Baseline serum electrolytes, phosphorus, magnesium, and complete blood count may be useful in evaluating nutritional status. For suspected liver disease, a hepatic panel including bilirubin and transaminases is indicated. If thyroid disease is suspected, a thyroid panel should be completed. If anemia is detected, further workup should include an evaluation of TIBC, ferritin, iron, transferrin saturation, and reticulocyte count.
- A swallowing evaluation should be considered for patients with dysphagia or symptoms of dysphagia which may include a wide range

Table 3–21 Signs and Symptoms of Vitamin and Mineral Deficiencies

Vitamin	Deficiency Symptom	Vitamin	Deficiency Symptom
Thiamin	Beriberi	Iron	Microcytic anemia
	mental confusion		Fatigue
	weakness		Angular stomatitis
	peripheral neuropathy		Impaired wound healing
	Heart disease		Alopecia
	Wernicke's encephalopathy		Skin rash
Riboflavin	Angular stomatitis		Impaired taste
	Cheilosis	Vitamin B_{12}	Megaloblastic anemia
	Glossitis		Neuropathy
Niacin	Pellagra		Stomatitis
	diarrhea		Glossitis
	dementia		Anorexia
	dermatitis	Vitamin C	Diarrhea
	death		Hemorrhaging
	Scarlet tongue		Weakness
	Tongue fissuring		Irritability
Biotin	Skin rash	Vitamin A	Bleeding gums
	Alopecia		Poor night vision
	Lethargy		Bitot's spots
	Anorexia	Vitamin D	Xerosis
	Paresthesia		Osteomalacia
Folic Acid	Macrocytic anemia	Vitamin K	Rickets
	Stomatitis		Purpura
	Glossitis	Vitamin E	Bleeding
	Lethargy		Hemolysis
	Diarrhea		Anemia
Phosphorus	Cardiac failure	Calcium	Myopathy
	CNS dysfunction		Osteomalacia
	Respiratory failure		Rickets
Magnesium	Anorexia		Osteoporosis
	Hypokalemia		Tetany
	Hypocalcemia		
	Vomiting		

of problems from decreased saliva production to aspiration. See Table 3–22 for signs of dysphagia and aspiration.

- Functional status is often forgotten but is an essential part of a physical exam. All patients should be monitored for their strength and ability to obtain and prepare food. A decline in functional status often leads to decreased food intake and may necessitate a consult to social services to obtain assistance.

Assessment of Nutrition Requirements

- Calorie requirements can be estimated by 25–35 kcal/kg/day of ideal body weight (IBW). Estimates within this range are based on stress level, activity, and degree of malnutrition. Although these calculations are useful, they are only estimates and require adjustments according to weight changes. Indirect calorimetry is useful for patients for whom it is difficult to estimate calorie requirements,

Table 3–22 Signs of Dysphagia/Aspiration and Risk Factors for Aspiration

Signs of Dysphagia/Aspiration	Risk Factors for Aspiration
• Drooling excessive secretions • Pocketing of food • Poor control of tongue movements • Poor lip closure • Slowed oral transit time • Decreased oral sensation • Facial weakness/difficulty chewing • Slurred speech • Coughing before, during, or after swallowing food or fluids • Choking • Nasal regurgitation • Wet "gurgly" voice after swallowing foods or liquids • Hoarse or breathy voice • Absent swallow reflex • Delay or absence of laryngeal elevation • Complaints of food getting "stuck" • Poor control of head/body position • Inadequate food and fluid intake • Prolonged mealtime • Refusal to eat • Mucositis • Xerostomia	• Elderly age with degenerative cerebrovascular and neuromuscular disease • Dysphagia • Sedative medication • Absent cough reflex • Altered level of consciousness • Oropharyngeal tumors/radiation therapy to head and neck area • Esophageal motility disorders

Source: Adapted from Lofton J. (1999). Dysphagia: Etiologies, risk identification and assessment methods. *Support Line* 21:(6); 3–10.

such as those who are severely under or over IBW.

- Protein requirements range from 1.0–2.5 g/kg IBW. Postoperative patients require approximately 1.5 g of protein per kilogram per day. Adjustments can be initiated based on nitrogen balance studies. Stable patients who are several weeks postsurgery will require 1.0–1.5 g of protein per kilogram of body weight.
- Vitamin and mineral deficiency should be evaluated at initial evaluation if deficiency is suspected.
- Several methods are available to estimated fluid needs. A quick method is 30–35 ml/kg.
- Refeeding syndrome is a life-threatening event that occurs when a malnourished pa-

tient is aggressively fed. Patients with cancer of the head and neck region and dysphagia often delay treatment and present with significant nutritional depletion. For this reason, these patients can be at risk for refeeding syndrome. See Enteral Nutrition for further explanation, assessment, and refeeding recommendations discussed in the Nutrition Support in the Critically Ill Patient Section.

- Parenteral nutrition is not typically indicated for patients with head and neck disease. Refer to Parenteral Nutrition discussed in the Nutrition Support in the Critically Ill Patient Section for guidelines in patient selection and administration.

CAUSE

Disorders Associated with Altered Smell (Dysosmia) and Taste (Dysgeusia)

Our senses of taste and smell allow us to fully appreciate the aroma and taste of foods, aide in digestion, and protect us against potential environmental toxins such as polluted air, smoke, and spoiled food products. Alterations in taste and smell can impact nutrition status as well as quality of life. Certain populations are especially vulnerable to the effects of olfactory disturbances, such as the elderly and renal patients.

- Dysgeusia may be related to genetic disease, or neurological disorders such as Alzheimer's dementia, multiple sclerosis, Parkinson's disease, and damage to cranial nerves. Endocrine disorders such as thyroid dysfunction, diabetes, or renal disease may also impair olfactory sensation.
- Advancing age is associated with an increased incidence of impaired taste with a 60% incidence in people aged 65–80 years and an 80% incidence in people greater than age 80.

- Nutritional factors implicated as possible contributors to dysgeusia include vitamin deficiencies, anemia, and malnutrition.
- Some possible causes of dysosmia include injuries from head trauma, infections such as pneumonia, rhinitis and allergies, cocaine abuse, radiation to the head and neck area, brain malignancies, sinus or nasal polyps, systemic lupus erythematosus, and cranial nerve damage.
- Multiple medications can contribute to alterations in taste and smell. See Table 3–23.

Diseases of the Oral Cavity

- Oral and craniofacial diseases and conditions contribute to poor nutrition due to compromised chewing and swallowing ability, thereby limiting food selection. These conditions include tooth loss, diminished salivary function, oral–facial pain conditions such as temporomandibular disorders, alterations in taste, and functional limitations of prosthetic replacements.
- Because of the rapid turnover of the tissue in the oral mucosa, it is particularly susceptible

Table 3–23 Medications with Oral Nutrition Implications

Nutritional Sequelae	Drug Class	Medications
Xerostomia	Anxiolytics	Alprazolam, busipirone
	Anticholinergics	Atropine
	GI tract agents	Ranitidine
	Antidepressants	Amitriptyline, mirtazapines, ertraline
	Antihypertensives	
	Antipsychotics	Clozapine, risperadone
	Antihistamines	Loratadine, ceterizine
	Diuretics	Bumetanide, triamterene
	Opiates	Morphine, oxycontin
	Miscellaneous	Levodopa
Olfactory dysfunction	Antibiotics	Ampicillin, clarithromycin
	Antidepressants	Amitriptyline, doxepin
	Anti-inflammatory	Colchicine
	Bronchodilators	Albuterol, metaproterenol
	Cardiovascular	Captopril, HCTH hydrochlorothiazide triamterene
	Lipid-lowering	Cholestyramine, clofibrate
	Miscellaneous	Famotidine

to physiological systemic alterations in the body.

- Most nutrient deficiency disease states exhibit oral manifestations.
- Caries and inflammatory periodontal disease are the most prevalent oral diseases, both as a result of the activity of dental bacterial plaque. Periodontal disease is a general term describing bacterial infection of the gingiva (the oral mucosa covering the root and apical portion of the crown).
- Plaque is a complex of various microorganisms that adhere to teeth, particularly between them, along the gingival margin, and in fissures and pits. If plaque is not regularly removed the flora evolves, and plaque may calcify, forming tartar.
- Fermentation of sucrose and other nonmilk extrinsic sugars by plaque bacteria to lactic and other acids causes tooth decay (caries). The main causal organism is *Streptococcus mutans*.
- Untreated, caries can progress through the dentin to the pulp, causing pulpitis, which can eventually lead to necrosis forming an abscess, granuloma, or cyst.
- Accumulation of plaque and a change in the microflora may also cause gingival inflammation (gingivitis). If conditions are appropriate, this may progress to damage the periodontal membrane (chronic periodontitis) and lead to tooth loss.
- Tooth enamel can be damaged by grinding of teeth (bruxism) and continual exposure to abrasive surfaces such as using a hard toothbrush. Vigorous brushing can lead to exposure of the dentin, which can cause sensitivity to hot and cold temperatures.
- Tooth erosion is an increasing problem from consumption of carbonated and fruit drinks and occasionally from gastric regurgitation or repeated vomiting (as in bulimia, alcoholism, and gastroesophageal reflux). In most cases it results in little more than a loss of normal enamel contour, but in severe cases dentine or pulp may be damaged.
- Enamel hypoplasia may result from high levels of fluoride or from disturbances in calcium and phosphate metabolism, which can occur in hypoparathyroidism, gastroenteritis, celiac disease, and osteoporosis.
- Dentition can affect intake. Individuals with missing teeth, or partial or full dentures, are at risk for decreased nutrient quality of the diet with edentulous individuals eating less fiber, fewer vegetables, and more cholesterol and saturated fat.
- Salivary secretions provide protection to the oral mucosa against pathogens. Damage to the oral mucosa from mechanical trauma, infection, or salivary dysfunction can result in derangements in increased risk of infection and may be the result of chemotherapy, radiation, and medications causing hyposalivation. The salivary glands are also frequently involved in tuberculosis and histoplasmosis infections.
- Swollen parotid glands are a cardinal sign of infection with the mumps virus and can also be seen in individuals with Sjögren's syndrome and HIV.
- Salivary hypofunction can result in dysphagia and dysgeusia, leading to alterations in dietary selection that may compromise nutritional status.
- Animal- and population-based studies have demonstrated an association between periodontal diseases and diabetes, cardiovascular disease, stroke, peripheral artery disease, respiratory disease, and adverse outcomes in the immunosuppressed and hospitalized patients. Possible mechanisms to explain why individuals with diabetes may be more susceptible to periodontitis include vascular changes, alterations in gingival crevicular fluid, alterations in connective tissue metabolism, altered host immunological and inflammatory response, altered subgingival microflora, and hereditary patterns. Poor oral health has also been correlated as a potential risk indicator of all-cause mortality.
- A potential mechanism of respiratory infection relates to the hypothesis that some oral pathogens, in particular periodontal pathogens, could facilitate colonization of the airways by pulmonary pathogens. Colonization of dental plaque was highly predictive of concurrent or subsequent nosocomial infection.

- Dissemination of oral bacteria into the blood-stream (bacteremia) can occur after most invasive dental procedures, including tooth extractions, endodontic therapy, periodontal surgery, and scaling and root planing.

- See Table 3–24 for abnormal oral findings and associated local and systemic diseases.

Table 3–24 Abnormal Oral Findings and Associated Local and Systemic Diseases

Clinical Feature	Associated Findings	Associated Disorders	Nutritional Considerations
Xerostomia	Excessive dental caries Candidiasis Dysphagia Burning mouth/tongue	Drug-induced Sjögren's syndrome Connective tissue disorders Diabetes	Push fluids, evaluate caries potential of diet, modify consistency and avoid dry foods, limit spicy, hot acidic, and seasoned foods
Burning mouth/ tongue	With or without associated erythema, edema (stomatitis)	Anemia Diabetes Candidiasis Neuropathy Parkinson's disease	Determine etiology of deficiency Evaluate source of poor glycemic control, modify diet Push fluids Evaluate caries potential of diet Evaluate for dysgeusia/ dysphagia
	Glossitis	R/o iron deficiency, folate, B_6, B_{12}, niacin, and/or riboflavin	Determine etiology Add supplements, modify diet as needed
	Pale atrophic smooth tongue	R/o iron deficiency, B_{12}, folate	As above
Angular fissures of lips	Dry, cracked lips	R/o niacin, riboflavin, B_6, iron deficiency Dehydration	Determine etiology
Thrush	White patches on palate or buccal mucosa when wiped off leave red, bleeding, sore surface	Candidiasis	See above
Difficulty biting/ chewing food	Partial or total edentulism Lack of occlusion Ill-fitting dentures		Modify diet consistency Loss of anterior occlusion–modify for difficulty biting Loss of posterior occlusion–modify for difficulty chewing
Sore throat	Gingival bleeding Petechiae	Strep throat EBV Infectious mononucleosis	Modify texture of diet and temperature of food

continues

Table 3–24 continued

Clinical Feature	Associated Findings	Associated Disorders	Nutritional Considerations
Lichen planus	White striae in mouth Occasional mucosal ulcers and erosive gingivitis	Drug-induced NSAIDs hepatitis, leukoplakia, lupus erythematous, graft-versus-host disease Malignant transformations	Modify consistency, temperature of food, and avoid irritants
Aphthous ulcers	Single or clusters of painful round or oval ulcers, with a grayish yellow, crateriform base surrounded by an erythematous halo of inflamed mucosa For 24–48 hours preceding the appearance of an ulcer, most patients have a pricking or burning sensation in the affected area	Trauma, stress, hormonal alterations, infection, HIV nutritional deficiencies–iron, folic acid, zinc, and vitamins B_1, B_2, B_6, and B_{12}, food allergy, neutropenia, Crohn's, ulcerative colitis, celiac disease, malignant ulcers, medications	Modify consistency and temperature of foods; avoid acidic foods and irritants; adjust diet for associated conditions as appropriate; multi-vitamin mineral supplementation may be helpful
Pemphigoid (oral mucous membrane)	Gray-white collapsed vesicles or bullae surrounded with erythema; initially may present as desquamative gingivitis, bleeding, pain, peeling of oral mucosa, and dysphagia; may affect tongue, palate, buccal mucosa, and floor of mouth		Adjust consistency and temperature of foods, avoid irritants
Erythema multiforme	Raised edematous papules with mucous membrane erosion	Herpes simplex; adverse drug reaction	Adjust consistency and temperature of foods, avoid irritants

Source: Adapted from Touger-Decker R. & Sirois D. (1996). Physical assessment of the oral cavity. *Support Line.* 18: (5);1–6.

MEDICAL NUTRITION THERAPY

Oral Disease

- Good oral hygiene can prevent periodontal disease and halitosis.
- Primary prevention of many oral, dental, and craniofacial diseases and conditions is possible with appropriate diet, nutrition, oral hygiene, and health-promoting behaviors, including the appropriate use of professional services.
- Health care providers can successfully deliver tobacco cessation and other health promotion programs in their offices, contributing to both oral health and overall health.
- Saliva buffers may counter plaque acids, and thus chewing sugar-free gum or cheese after meals may be of value. Fresh fruit and vegetables can also confer some protection against oral cancer. However, smoking or chewing tobacco and some other habits may contribute to periodontal disease and oral malignancy, and some chewed products containing sugars may predispose to caries.
- Fluorides protect against caries by inhibiting mineral loss, promoting remineralisation of decalcified enamel, and reducing formation of plaque acids. Water fluoridation has consistently been shown to be the most effective, safe, and equitable means of preventing caries and can reduce the prevalence of caries by about half.
- See Table 3–25 for strategies to reduce caries.

DESCRIPTION

Mandibular Fracture

- Mandibular fracture occurs most commonly in adolescents and young adults aged 16–30 years. Treatment involves intermaxillary fixation (wiring of teeth/mandible). The mandible may remain wired for an average of six weeks. Blenderized and liquid foods in addition to supplements are recommended so that patients can maintain their nutritional status.

CAUSE

Mandibular Fracture

- Typically due to trauma such as during an altercation or a motor vehicle accident.

MEDICAL NUTRITION THERAPY

Mandibular Fracture

- Initially postsurgery, intake will be minimal due to increased edema of the oral cavity.
- Patients' diets can usually be progressed from liquids to blenderized foods over 48 to 72 hours.
- Weight loss can be a concern for patients if they rely only on liquids for the duration that the jaw is wired. The dietetics professional needs to provide education on the importance of maintaining nutrition by using a blenderized diet and supplements.

Table 3–25 Strategies to Reduce Caries

- Brush teeth thoroughly twice daily with a fluoride toothpaste and clean between teeth with dental floss.
- Effective plaque removal is essential to prevent periodontal disease.
- Toothbrushing alone cannot prevent dental caries, but fluoride toothpastes offer major benefits.
- Drink fluoridated water.
- Have an oral examination every year with dental cleaning every 6 months. More frequent examinations may be indicated for patients at risk for increased caries due to xerostomia or for whom oral disease presents an increased risk such as heart disease.

Table 3–26 Nutrition Guidelines for a Blenderized Diet

- Refer to instruction manual with the equipment for proper care and cleaning instructions.
- To prevent overblending and overworking equipment, blend food in 15–20 second cycles. Repeat cycles as necessary to obtain desired consistency.
- Food to be blenderized should be cut into small pieces so it blends more readily.
- Place liquid into container before adding solids.
- To puree foods, mix two parts solid to one part liquid. Foods with a high water content such as fruits and vegetables may need very little additional water.
- To liquefy foods, mix equal amounts of solids and liquids.
- Some foods may be difficult to blend such as meat with gristle, nuts, seeds, and very fibrous foods such as celery.
- A syringe or straw may be easier to use to push food through openings in the teeth, but a spoon can also be used.
- Weight loss can occur due to a decreased intake because of the filling effect of liquids. Smaller, more frequent meals may be necessary.
- Nutrition supplements may also be necessary to provide adequate nutrition.
- There is potential for increased gas ingestion with the use of a straw or a syringe. Patients should be encouraged to ask their physician or health care provider about the use of simethicone.

- See Table 3–26 for nutrition guidelines for a blenderized diet.
- Patients need to follow their oral surgeon's guidelines for the care of their teeth while the jaw is wired, but generally are advised to rinse their mouth with a baking soda and water rinse, or a therapeutic rinse, after eating or as directed.

DESCRIPTION—CANCERS OF THE HEAD AND NECK

- Cancers of the head and neck region include structures of the oral cavity, oropharynx, hypopharynx, nasopharynx, larynx, parotid gland, and cervical esophagus.
- Most cancers of the head and neck are squamous cell (epidermoid), but may include sarcomas, lymphomas, and melanoma.
- Head and neck cancers typically metastasize locally to lymph nodes or to adjacent or contralateral structures, however distant metastasis can occur late in the disease.

- Head and neck cancers overall tend to occur more commonly in men $>$ age 59 years, with the exception of salivary gland tumors.
- Many patients with head and neck cancer may present with malnutrition due to the location of the lesion and possible interference with either mastication or swallowing of food. Also, some patients may be malnourished because of alcoholism and poor intake associated with long-standing poor dental hygiene.
- *Oral cancers.* Early lesions may be asymptomatic, but more advanced tumors can severely inhibit oral intake. Tumors of the mandible or retromolar trigone can result in loose teeth, trismus (muscle spasm), and pain with mastication. Advanced lesions of the tongue can inhibit the ability to propel food boluses. Often oral lesions are irritated by dentures and foods, especially sour, salty, spicy, and hot foods. Such discomfort and difficulties can cause the patient to restrict intake.
- *Oropharyngeal cancers.* Advanced lesions of the soft palate can result in oronasal fistulas.

Tonsillar lesions can cause dysphagia, odynophagia, and sore throat. Tumors in the base of the tongue may cause dysphagia by restricting tongue mobility. Large base-of-tongue tumors can result in greatly diminished intake, weight loss, and malnutrition.

- *Laryngeal cancers.* Laryngeal cancer typically presents as hoarseness progressing to sore throat and odynophagia. More advanced lesions cause dysphagia, hemoptysis, and weight loss.
- Patients with head and neck cancer will likely have multimodal therapy involving both radiation and chemotherapy, and possibly surgery. Treatment has the potential to negatively impact the nutritional status of the head and neck cancer patient.
- Common side effects of radiation therapy to the head and neck area include mucositis, xerostomia or thickened saliva, taste dysgeusia or hypogeusia and dysphagia, with mucositis being the most commonly occurring toxicity. See Table 3–27 for nutrition sequelae of radiation therapy to the head and neck.
- Historically it was believed that mucositis developed as a result of injury to the epithelium of the oral mucosa; however newer research indicates that mucositis results from a series of dynamic and interactive molecular and cellular events that involve all the elements of the mucosa, and in fact occurs in several stages.
- It is important to culture oral lesions of patients undergoing immunosuppressive therapy since these lesions can be caused by fungal, bacterial, or viral lesions, and they will not heal without appropriate therapy.
- The use of combination radiation and chemotherapy is increasing to promote preservation of structures in the head and neck and to improve cure rates. Patients may experience additional and more intense side effects from chemotherapy given concurrently with radiation therapy.
- Radiation can cause irreversible damage to the salivary glands, resulting in dramatic increases in dental caries. Oral mucosal alterations may become portals for invasion by

pathogens, which may be life-threatening to immunosuppressed or bone-marrow-suppressed patients.

- Surgery can include: partial, supraglottic, or total laryngectomy; glossectomy; or neck dissection and resection of other involved structures. Patients with a supraglottic laryngectomy are at increased risk for aspiration. Some patients will also have creation of a flap for future reconstructive surgery. Recently, the use of "total" chemotherapy-radiation therapy treatment, the appropriate application of the newer chemotherapy active agents, and the inclusion of the biological and the specific targeted compounds as part of therapy in these patients has improved the prospect for organ preservation.
- Many patients will need to have a temporary or permanent tracheostomy placed to maintain patency of their airway.
- A significant number of patients with tracheostomies will be at risk for aspiration depending upon the type of tracheostomy, so swallowing should be evaluated prior to feeding to assure competence of the swallow mechanism.
- Patients that have had a total laryngectomy will lose the ability to speak until they either learn esophageal speech or master the ability to use an electrolarynx. Communication from the patient will have to be accomplished by using a writing table or, if the patient is illiterate or speaks a foreign language, the speech pathologist can assist communication through the use of a picture board. Patients can become frustrated at times and communication can take longer. Patients can be very frightened by their inability to summon help when they need it or express concerns. It is important to convey patience and an accepting attitude to allow the patient adequate time to communicate concerns. The patient may develop fatigue from writing, so questions that require a yes/no or minimal response may be indicated to obtain necessary information. The use of several framed instead of open-ended questions may assist in obtaining necessary history.

Table 3–27 Nutrition Sequelae of Therapy for Head and Neck Cancer

Therapy	Potential Complications	Nutrition Therapy
Radiation to mouth	Xerostomia	Adequate fluids Artificial saliva Sugar-free candy or gum to stimulate saliva
	Diminished taste	Increased flavor of foods
	Metallic, bitter, salty or altered taste	Add salt to decrease sweetness, add sugar for bitter taste, use plastic utensils
	Dental caries	Good oral hygiene, soft toothbrush, fluoride
	Mucositis/stomatitis	Soft to pureed nonacidic, nonirritating foods, baking soda/H_2O rinses, evaluate for infection, foods at room temperature
	Osteoradionecrosis	Mouth rinses
Radiation to neck	Esophagitis	Adjust texture/temperature of foods, nonacidic, nonirritating
	Dysphagia	Adjust texture, possible swallow study
	Stricture	Adjust texture, dilatation, possible enteral feeding
Anterior tongue/floor of mouth resection	Slight difficulty manipulating food	Eat from nonoperative side Check mouth for food after meals Soft food/thick liquids until swelling subsides
Resection of hard palate	Nasal regurgitation food/fluids	Intraoral prosthetic device
Mandibular resection	Difficulty chewing	Ground/pureed diet, thick liquids
	Drooling, difficulty with mastication	Mandibular reconstruction
Partial glossectomy	Dependent on resection—if lengthwise initially, soreness and tongue swelling eventually resolve	Soft foods, eat from nonsurgical side
Resection of base of tongue, tonsil, or structures in pharyngeal wall	Potential dysphagia pending structures removed with difficulty propelling bolus	Enteral feeding until incision heals Swallow study prior to initiating oral feeding with swallow therapy
Laryngectomy		
Hemi	Removal of arytenoid cartilage may cause aspiration in small number of patients	Possible need for swallow evaluation prior to feeding
Partial	Usually no risk of aspiration Possible stricture	No specific diet unless develops stricture
Supraglottic	High risk of aspiration especially if edema present postoperatively	Swallowing evaluation Possible extended time for enteral feeding
All neck surgeries	Postoperative swelling Tracheostomy may interfere with swallowing Stricture	Enteral feedings until safe to feed by mouth, dilatation

- Patients may be at risk for dysphagia depending upon the structures affected by the surgery and the area of the head and neck receiving radiation. Dysphagia is a general term that describes difficulty swallowing and is due to disease or dysfunction in one or more areas of the swallowing mechanism.
- Although dysphagia can be suspected if it's noted that the patient coughs or chokes when eating, silent aspiration can occur, in which a patient aspirates material into the bronchus without any overt signs of aspiration. See Table 3–22 for signs and symptoms of dysphagia and risk factors for aspiration.

CAUSE

Cancers of the Head and Neck

Head and neck cancer is correlated with:
- alcohol abuse and tobacco
- infrequent fruit and vegetable consumption
- chronic irritation of the oral cavity due to sharp teeth, ill-fitting dentures, or use of a pipe
- poor dental hygiene
- oral leukoplakia (mucosal lesion with white-plaque-type appearance)
- excessive sun exposure (lip cancer)

MEDICAL NUTRITION THERAPY

Head and Neck Cancer

- Assessment and management of dysphagia requires a team approach which includes the physician, nurse, speech-language pathologist, radiologist, and registered dietitian.
- If dysphagia is suspected, a bedside swallow evaluation should be done, and if necessary a video fluoroscopic swallow study (VFSS), since a bedside evaluation does not always detect silent aspiration. Many patients will have VFSS completed postsurgery, prior to initiating oral feedings.
- The VFSS can provide information including the degree of aspiration, bolus transit time, the integrity of the swallow, whether dysphagia is present, and any motility problems. From the results of the VFSS, the speech/language pathologist can determine with the dietetics professional the appropriate texture of solid and liquid foods and if any precautions for feeding are indicated.
- Common techniques to prevent aspiration include upright positioning for feeding, chin-down positioning when swallowing liquids, drinking small amounts, and dry swallow to clear the pharyngeal cavity.

Diets for dysphagia have been standardized by the National Dysphagia Diet Task Force (NDDTF), a group of Registered Dietitians, Speech-Language Pathologists and researchers. Four levels of liquid and solid consistency have been identified.

- Thickening agents may be necessary for patients requiring thickened liquids. Commercially available products as well as readily available foods from the grocery store can be used as thickeners. Table 3–28 lists commonly used thickeners with suggestions for their use.
- The speech-language pathologist can also determine if specific exercises can be used to improve the swallowing ability of the patient.
- The more restrictive the diet is, the more difficult it may be for patients to obtain adequate nutrition. Adequacy of fluid intake should be monitored as well as adequacy of calories, protein, vitamins, and minerals. Patients may not readily accept thickened liquids and be at risk for dehydration. Enteral feeding may be necessary to provide adequate supplementary nutrition until the patient is able to take adequate amounts. (See the section on Enteral Nutrition earlier in Chapter 3.)
- Adding thickeners to liquids will increase the carbohydrate content of the liquid, and this must be considered when planning carbohydrate-restricted diets.
- Many patients will require enteral feeding in the immediate postoperative period to provide nutrition until the suture lines are healed well enough to tolerate the stress of eating. A swallow evaluation may be necessary prior to

Table 3–28 Consistencies and Thickeners

Standard liquid consistencies
- Thin—regular liquids—no adjustments needed
- Nectar—falls slowly from spoon and can be sipped through a straw or from a cup. Examples—buttermilk, tomato juice.
- Honey—drops from a spoon, but too thick to be sipped from a straw. Examples: honey, tomato sauce
- Spoon—maintains shape, needs to be taken with a spoon—too thick to drink. Example—pudding

Thickeners
- Commercial thickeners—Use for hot or cold foods. Follow manufacturer instructions to achieve desired consistency. Adds carbohydrate calories.
- Pureed vegetables or fruits—Alters the flavor of the foods. Vegetables best used in soups, sauces, gravies. Fruits best added to juices.
- Starches—tapioca, baby rice cereal, potato flakes. Need to be cooked into the foods added to. Best used for soups, gravies, sauces.
- Powdered skim milk—can be added to cream soups, milkshakes.

initiating feedings in some patients. Many patients will need to continue enteral feedings to meet partial or all of their nutrition needs post-discharge to provide adequate nutrition during subsequent radiation and chemotherapy. (Refer to the enteral feeding and discharge planning sections in the Nutrition Support in the Critically Ill Patient Section.)

Nutrition and oral health are strongly linked to overall health and well-being. People can be motivated to change their health habits, including eating habits, through aggressive health promotion and disease prevention programs. The dietetics professional has an important and vital role in the management and prevention of diseases of the head and neck area and should be included in programs and services to improve the oral health of individuals.

REFERENCE

1. Shepherd, A. (2002). The impact of oral health on nutritional status. *Nursing Standard 16* (27), 37–38.
2. Jansson, L., Lavstedt, S., Frithiof, L., & Theobald, H. (2001). Relationship between oral health and mortality in cardiovascular diseases. *Journal of Clinical Periodontology 28* (8), 762–768.
3. Terpenning, M. & Shay, K. (2002). Oral health is cost-effective to maintain but costly to ignore. *Journal of the American Geriatrics Society 50* (30), 584–585.
4. Ritchie, C., Joshipura K., Hung H., & Douglass C. (2002). Nutrition as a mediator in the relation between oral and systemic disease: associations between specific measures of adult oral health and nutrition outcomes. *Critical Reviews in Oral Biology & Medicine 13* (3), 291–300.
5. Petzold, G., Einhaupl, K., & Valdueza J. (2003). Persistent bitter taste as an initial symptom of amyotrophic lateral sclerosis. *Journal of Neurology, Neurosurgery & Psychiatry, 74* (5), 687–688.
6. Odaka, M., Yuki, N., Nishimoto, Y., & Hirata K. (2002). Guillain-Barre syndrome presenting with loss of taste. *Neurology 58* (9), 1437–1438.
7. Shay, K., & Ship, J. (1995). The importance of oral health in the older patient. *Journal of the American Geriatric Society 43,* 1414–1422.
8. Coleman, P. (2002). Improving oral health care for the frail elderly: A review of widespread problems and best practices. *Geriatric Nursing 23* (4), 189–199.
9. Karuza, J., Miller, W., Lieberman, D., Ledenyi, L., Thines, T. (1995). Oral status and resident well-being in a skilled nursing facility population. *Gerontologist 35,* 104–112.

10. Mojon, P., & Bourbau, J. (2003). Respiratory infection: How important is oral health? *Current Opinion in Pulmonary Medicine 9* (3), 166–170.

11. Yoneyama, T., Yoshida, M., Matsui, T., Sasaki, H. (1999). Oral care and pneumonia. Oral care working group. *Lancet 354* (9177), 515.

12. Bartzokas, C., Johnson, R., Jane, M., Martin, M., Pearce, P., Saw, Y. (1994). Relation between mouth and haematogenous infection in total joint replacements. *British Medical Journal 309,* 506–508.

13. Joshipura, K., Rimm, E., Douglass, C., Trichopoulos, D., Ascheriio, A., & Willett, W. (1996). Poor oral health and coronary heart disease. *Journal of Dental Research 75,* 1631–1636.

14. Miller, C. (2000). Medications and sensory function. *Geriatric Nursing 21 (6),* 328–329.

15. Lissowska, J., Pilarska, A., Pilarski, P., Samolczyk-Wanyura, D., Piekarczyk, J., Bardin-Mikollajczak, A., Zatonski, W., Herrero, R., Munoz, N., & Franceschi, S. (2003). Smoking, alcohol, diet, dentition and sexual practices in the epidemiology of oral cancer in Poland. *European Journal of Cancer Prevention 12* (1), 25–33.

16. Holt, R., Roberts, G., & Scully, C. (2000). Dental damage, sequelae, and prevention. *British Medical Journal 320* (7251), 1717–1719.

17. Johnson, N., & Bain, C. (2000). Tobacco and oral disease. EU-Working Group on Tobacco and Oral Health. *British Dental Journal 189,* 200–206.

18. Scully, C., & Porter, S. (2000). Swellings and red, white, and pigmented lesions. *British Medical Journal 321* (7255), 225–228.

19. Karuza, J., Miller, W., Lieberman, D., Ledenyi, L., & Thines, T. (1992). Oral status and resident well-being in a skilled nursing facility population. *Gerontologist 35,* 104–112.

20. Coleman, P. (2002). Improving oral health care for the frail elderly: a review of widespread problems and best practices. *Geriatric Nursing 23 (4),* 189–199.

21. Gardiner, D. & Raigrodski, A. Psychosocial issues in women's oral health. (2001). *Dental Clinics of North America 45* (3), 479–490.

22. Locker, D., Clarke, M., & Payne B. (2000). Self-perceived oral health status, psychological well-being, and life satisfaction in an older adult population. *Journal of Dental Research 79 (4),* 970–975.

23. Miwa, T., Furukawa, M., Tsukatani, T., Costanzo, R., DiNardo, L., & Reiter E. (2001). Impact of olfactory impairment on quality of life and disability. *Archives of Otolaryngology—Head & Neck Surgery 127 (5),* 497–503.

24. Perros, P., MacFarlane, T., Counsell, C., & Frier B. (1996). Altered taste sensation in newly-diagnosed NIDDM. *Diabetes Care 19 (7),* 768–770.

25. Kho, H., Lee, S., Chung, S., & Kim, Y. (1999). Oral manifestations and salivary flow rate, pH, and buffer capacity in patients with end-stage renal disease undergoing hemodialysis. *Oral Surgery, Oral Medicine, Oral Pathology, Oral Radiology, & Endodontics 88 (3),* 316–319.

26. Bromley, S. (2000). Smell and taste disorders: A primary care approach. *American Family Physician 61 (2),* 427–436.

27. Hoffman, H., Ishii, E., & MacTurk, R. (1998). Age-related changes in the prevalence of smell/taste problems among the United States adult population. Results of the 1994 disability supplement to the National Health Interview Survey (NHIS). *Annals of the New York Academy of Sciences 855,* 716–722.

28. Depaola, D., Faine, M., & Palmer, C. (1995). Nutrition in relation to dental medicine. In Shils, M., Olson, J., Shike, M., & Ross, C.A. (Eds.) *Modern Nutrition in Health and Disease* (pp. 1099–1124). Philadelphia, Baltimore, New York, London, Buenos Aires, Hong Kong, Sydney, Tokyo: Lippincott Williams & Wilkins.

29. Feihn, N., Gutshik, E., Larsen, T., & Bangsborg, J. (1995). Identity of streptococcal blood isolates and oral isolates from two patients with infective endocarditis. *Journal of Clinical Microbiology 33,* 1399–1401.

30. Sebring, N., & McCarthy, G. (1995). As cited in Shils, M., Olson, J., Shike, M., & Ross, C. *Modern Nutrition in Health and Disease.* 1999, 1117. Philadelphia: Lea & Febiger.

31. Ship, J., Pillemer, S., & Baum, B. (2002). Xerostomia and the geriatric patient. *Journal of the American Geriatrics Society 50* (3), 535–543.

32. Lash, A. (2001). Sjögren's syndrome: Pathogenesis, diagnosis, and treatment. *Nurse Practitioner 26 (8),* 53–58.

33. Greenspan, D., & Greenspan, J. (1996). HIV-related oral disease. *Lancet 348* (9029), 729–733.

34. Grossi, S., & Genco, R. (1998). Periodontal disease and diabetes mellitus: A two-way relationship. *Journal of Periodontology 3* (1), 51–61.

35. Taylor, G., Loesche, W., & Terpenning, M. (2000). Impact of oral diseases on systemic health in the elderly: Diabetes mellitus and aspiration pneumonia. *Journal of Public Health Dentistry 60,* 313–320.

36. Fourrier, F., Duvivier, B., Boutigny, H., & Roussel-Delvallez, M. & Chopin, C. (1998). Colonization of dental plaque: A source of nosocomial infections in intensive care unit patients. *Critical Care Medicine 1998, 26,* 301–308.

37. Hung, H., Willett, W., Merchant, A., Rosner, B., Ascherio, A., Joshipura, K. (2003). Oral health and peripheral arterial disease. *Circulation: Journal of the American Heart Association 107* (8) 4, 1152–1157.

38. Abe, S., Ishihara, K., & Okuda, K. (2001). Prevalence of potential respiratory pathogens in the mouths of

elderly patients and effects of professional oral care. *Archives of Gerontology and Geriatrics 32,* 45–55.

39. Scannapieco, F., Papandonatos, G., & Dunford, R. (1998). Associations between oral conditions and respiratory disease in a national sample survey population. *Annals of Periodontology 3,* 251–256.

40. Hujoel, P., Drangsholt, M., Spiekerman, C., & De-Rouen, T. (2000). Relationship between oral health and mortality rate, periodontal disease and coronary heart disease risk. *Journal of the American Medical Association 284* (11), 1406–1410

41. Scannapieco, F., & Ho, A. (2001). Potential associations between chronic respiratory disease and periodontal disease: Analysis of National Health and Nutrition Examination Survey III. *Journal of Periodontology 72,* 50–56.

42. Scannapieco, F. Role of oral bacteria in respiratory infection. (1999). *Journal of Periodontology 70,* 793–802.

43. Lacassin, F., Hoen, B., Leport, C., Selton-Suty, C., De-lahaye, F., Goulet, V., Etienne, J., & Briancon S. (1995). Procedures associated with infective endocarditis in adults. A case control study. *European Heart Journal 16 (12),* 1968–1974.

44. Holt, R., Roberts, G., & Scully, C. (2000). Dental damage, sequelae, and prevention. *British Medical Journal 320* (7251), 1717–1719.

45. Azevedo, A., Trent, R., & Ellis, A. Population-based analysis of 10,766 hospitalizations for mandibular fractures in California, 1991 to 1993. (1998). *Journal of Trauma-Injury Infection & Critical Care 45* (6), 1084–1087.

46. Gaziano, J. (2002). Evaluation and management of oropharyngeal dysphagia in head and neck cancer. *Cancer Control 9* (5), 400–409.

47. Vissink, A., Jansma, J., Spijkervet, F., Burlage, F., & Coppes, R. (2003). Oral sequelae of head and neck radiotherapy. *Critical Reviews in Oral Biology & Medicine 14,* 199–212.

48. Sonis, T. (2004). The pathobiology of mucositis. *Nature Reviews Cancer 4* (4), 277–284.

49. Nicolatou-Galitis, O., Dardoufas, K., Markoulatos, P., Sotiropoulou-Lontou, A., Kyprianou, K., Kolitsi, G., Pissakas, G., Skarleas, C., Kouloulias, V., Papanicolaou, V., Legakis, N., & Velegraki, A. (2001). Oral pseudomembranous candidiasis, herpes simplex virus-1 infection, and oral mucositis in head and neck cancer patients receiving radiotherapy and granulocyte-macrophage colony-stimulating factor (GM-CSF) mouthwash. *Journal of Oral Pathology & Medicine 30* (8), 471–480.

50. Pannunzio, T. (1996). Aspiration of oral feedings in patients with tracheostomies. *Advanced Practice in Acute and Critical Care 7* (4), 560–569.

51. Happ, M., Roesch, M., & Kagan, S. (2004). Communication Needs, Methods, and Perceived Voice Quality Following Head and Neck Surgery: A Literature Review. *Cancer Nursing 27* (1), 1–9.

52. Smith, C., Logemann, J., Colangelo, L., Rademaker, A., & Pauloski, B. (1999). Incidence and patient characteristics associated with silent aspiration in the acute care setting. *Dysphagia 14,* 1–7.

53. National Dysphagia Task Force. (2002). *National dysphagia diet: Standardization for optimal care.* American Dietetic Association, Chicago, Illinois.

54. Touger-Decker, R., & Sirois, D. (1996). Physical assessment of the oral cavity. *Support Line 18* (5) 1–6.

55. Gorsky, M., Raviv, M., Moskona, D., Laufer, M., & Bodner L. (1996). Clinical characteristics and treatment of patients with oral lichen planus in Israel. *Oral Surgery, Oral Medicine, Oral Pathology, Oral Radiology, & Endodontics 82,* (6), 644–649.

56. Fishman, T. (1999). Wound assessment and evaluation . . . bullous pemphigoid. *Dermatology Nursing 11* (6), 436–437.

57. Barrons, R. (2001). Treatment strategies for recurrent oral aphthous ulcers. *American Journal of Health-System Pharmacy 58* (1), 41–53.

58. Dayan, S., Simons, R., & Ahmed, A. (1999). Contemporary issues in the diagnosis of oral pemphigoid: A selective review of the literature. *Oral Surgery, Oral Medicine, Oral Pathology, Oral Radiology, & Endodontics 88* (4), 424–430.

59. Salvi, G., Collins, J., Yalda, B., Arnold, R., Lang, N., & Offenbacher, S. (1997). Monocytic TNF alpha secretion patterns in IDDM patients with periodontal diseases. *Journal of Clinical Periodontology 24* (1), 8–16.

60. Langmore, S., Terpenning, M., Schork, A., Chen, Y., Murray, J., Lopatin, D., Loesche, W., & Kaslick, R. (1998). Predictors of aspiration pneumonia: How important is dysphagia? *Dysphagia 13,* 69–81.

61. Taylor, G. (1999). Periodontal treatment and its effect on glycemic control. *Oral Surgery, Oral Medicine, Oral Pathology, Oral Radiology, & Endodontics 87,* 311–316.

HIV/AIDS

Jül L. Gerrior RD, LDN, Kimberly Dong RD, LDN, Kristy Hendricks RD, DSC, and Christine A. Wanke, MD

DESCRIPTION

According to the Centers for Disease Control and Prevention (CDC), 40 million people worldwide are estimated to be living with the human immunodeficiency virus infection (HIV), the virus that causes acquired immune deficiency syndrome (AIDS). Of these, 37 million are adults and 2.5 million are children under age 15 years. Nearly 1 million people are infected with HIV in the United States and approximately 40,000 new HIV infections occur each year. Seventy percent of those newly infected are men. Minority groups in the United States have been disproportionately affected by the epidemic. Approximately 23 million cases—the majority of HIV/AIDS cases worldwide—are in sub-Saharan Africa. However, populations on every continent except for Antarctica have been affected by the epidemic, and the cumulative total estimated number of deaths of persons with AIDS is 501,669, including 496,354 adults and adolescents and 5315 children under age 15 years.

Although the number of people living with HIV/AIDS continues to rise, dramatic advancements have been made on the management of the virus in countries where access to treatment is available. Most notably is the advent of highly active antiretroviral therapy (HAART), a combination of three or more anti-HIV agents acting on the virus's ability to replicate, and in many cases leading to nearly complete suppression of virus in the blood. The impact of these drugs on mortality rates associated with HIV disease has been spectacular, with a $\sim 50\%$ reduction of deaths since 1997. Although the optimal treatment of HIV is to achieve viral suppression in the blood, research has shown that HIV remains present in the lymph nodes, brain, testes, and retina, even in patients who have been treated successfully. This is noteworthy because many

individuals consider suppression of HIV to be synonymous with a cure and this is not true, as reservoirs of HIV remain present in other body tissues. In addition, HIV may be replicating at a low level when the virus is undetectable in blood by currently available technology.

With access to HAART, HIV infection may be considered a chronic manageable disease. Chronic treatment of HIV raises new issues such as adherence and tolerability of antiretroviral medications, emergence of viral resistance, and to sequencing of drug selection and treatment regimens. Many patients are living longer with HIV disease and may be susceptible to other diseases that are increasingly common with aging, such as cardiovascular disease, diabetes, and obesity. Traditional metabolic complications associated with HIV infection, such as hypertriglyceridemia, low high-density lipoprotein cholesterol, and weight loss, continue to occur in HIV-infected patients; however new abnormalities, such as regional alterations in body shape (the so-called lipodystrophy syndrome), increasing body weight, and other metabolic derangements such as high low-density lipoprotein cholesterol and insulin resistance, may also be present.

The CDC defines the stages of HIV infection according to three CD4+ T-cell lymphocyte categories:

- Category 1: ≥ 500 cells/mm^3
- Category 2: 200–499 cells/mm^3
- Category 3: < 200 cells/mm^3

The three clinical categories of HIV infection are as follows:

- *Category A:* One or more of the following conditions:
  1. Asymptomatic HIV infection
  2. Persistent generalized lymphadenopathy
  3. Acute (primary) HIV infection with

accompanying illness or history of acute HIV infection

- *Category B:* Symptomatic conditions that meet at least one of the following criteria:
  1. The conditions are attributed to HIV infection or are indicative of a defect in cell-mediated immunity.
  2. The conditions are considered by physicians to have a clinical course or to require management that is complicated by HIV infection.
- *Category C:* Clinical conditions listed in the AIDS surveillance case definition (e.g., *Pneumocystis carinii* pneumonia, candidiasis, cryptococcosis, Kaposi's sarcoma, cryptosporidiosis, cytomegalovirus, histoplasmosis, lymphoma, toxoplasmosis of the brain, progressive multifocal leukoencephalopathy, and wasting syndrome due to HIV)

CAUSES

Exposure to HIV occurs through contact with blood or other bodily fluids from an infected person. This may occur by sexual contact with an infected partner; intravenously through blood products or contaminated needles; or through maternal transmission in utero, at the time of delivery, or from breast milk. The mechanism of how HIV causes the immune system to break down is not completely understood. Most scientists believe that HIV causes AIDS by inducing cell death of the CD4+ T cells by interfering with their normal function. Consequently, this impaired immunity inhibits a person's immune function to fight infections normally. Much attention has been directed to the prevention of HIV transmission through education and awareness. Primary prevention factors include condom use, avoidance of shared needles with infected blood, early HIV testing, and abstinence.

ASSESSMENT

A nutrition assessment should be made early in the course of the disease in order to establish baseline parameters for the individual patient. The recognition of nutritional compromise or the lipodystrophy syndrome associated with HIV disease should be evaluated and monitored. Attention to body weight, body composition, total dietary intake, appetite status, regional body shape changes, gastrointestinal function and symptoms, metabolic markers, and hormone levels are all key areas to be assessed. The severity of the disease and condition will dictate how often follow-up assessments should be made. The American Dietetic Association developed a priority timeline for referral by categorized HIV nutritional risk. These categories include the following:

1. *High risk*—to be seen by a registered dietitian (RD) within one week
2. *Moderate risk*—to be seen by an RD within one month
3. *Low risk*—to be seen by an RD as needed

In general, high-risk patients include those with severe weight loss ($> 10\%$ within 4–6 months or $> 5\%$ within 4 weeks), pregnancy, poorly controlled diabetes, failure to thrive, patients on nutrition support, and those with chronic diarrhea, nausea, and vomiting. In addition, high-risk patients may be on dialysis or have severe dysphagia, chronic oral thrush, central nervous system (CNS) disease, food–drug–nutrient interactions, and patients suffering from acute opportunistic infections, and/or patients experiencing serious psychosocial problems that contribute to poor nutritional status. A patient who is described as having moderate risk may have evidence of fat redistribution syndrome, obesity, hyperlipidemia, osteoporosis, hypertension, controlled diabetes, excessive vitamin use, oral thrush, dental issues, possible food–drug–nutrient interactions, eating disorders, evidence for sedentary lifestyle or excessive exercise regimen, and unstable psychosocial situations. A low-risk patient is one who has weight stability, adequate and balanced diet, regular exercise regimen, normal lipid and glucose metabolism, normal renal and hepatic function, and psychosocial stability.

Common Assessment Parameters

Global Assessment

- Physical appearance and subjective global assessment
- HIV-associated wasting with evidence of periorbital and total body thinness
- Evidence of dorsocervical fat pad and increased abdominal girth; increased venous markings may indicate subcutaneous fat atrophy and regional body shape changes

Body and Body Composition Measurements

- Weight
  1. Current weight
  2. Weight history, including usual body weight and highest and lowest weights
  3. Percent weight change
  4. Estimated ideal weight and weight goals
  5. Estimated weight goals if overweight
- Height
- Calculated body mass index (BMI)
- Body composition as lean body mass, body cell mass, and fat mass
  1. Bioelectrical impedance analysis (BIA)

Anthropometric Measures

- Skinfold thickness measurements
  1. Triceps
  2. Subscapular
  3. Suprailiac
  4. Thigh
- Regional measurement of body fat and composition
  1. Chest circumference
  2. Waist circumference
  3. Hip circumference
  4. Thigh circumference
  5. Midarm Circumference
  6. Dual-energy x-ray absorptiometry (DXA), a measure of soft tissue and regional body composition specific to fat atrophy (typically done in research)
  7. CT scans and MRI imaging to quantify visceral and subcutaneous fat (typically done in research)

Biochemical Parameters

- Serum albumin concentrations
- Serum lipid concentrations
  1. Total cholesterol, high density lipoproteins, low density lipoproteins
  2. Serum triglycerides
- Serum electrolyte concentrations
- Complete blood count with differential
- Liver function studies
- Glucose and insulin levels (if visceral fat deposition/subcutaneous fat loss or other suspicion of glucose intolerance)
- Vitamin B_{12} (if symptoms of neuropathy and fatigue evident)
- Total/free testosterone levels (if weight loss, symptoms of fatigue, low sex drive, or loss of lean body mass evident)
- Other serum micronutrients, such as selenium or RBC folate (if available)
- Thyroid function (if weight loss and symptoms of fatigue present)

Immune/HIV-Related Parameters

- HIV viral load
- T-cell subsets
- Detection of HIV viral load to < 25 copies/ml of blood
- Viral resistance testing (if drug resistance evident)

Gastrointestinal Symptoms

To be checked routinely:

- Stool number and consistency
- Symptom log of abdominal cramping, bloating, or pain

To be performed when symptoms (weight loss, chronic diarrhea, anorexia, pain, or dysphagia) occur:

- Stool culture and/or stool examination for routine or opportunistic pathogens within the GI tract
- Stool nitrogen measurement
- Fecal fat measurement: qualitative or 72-hour fecal fat measurement following a 100-g fat diet

- D-xylose test
- Upper and lower endoscopy and biopsy (if necessary)

Appetite

- Presence of anorexia, nausea, vomiting, or diarrhea
- Difficulty swallowing or chewing
- Mouth sores
- Poor dentition
- Gum inflammation
- Taste changes

Diet History

- 3-day food record
- 24-hour recall
- Food frequency questionnaire
- Supplement use including macro- and micronutrients

Medications

- Antiretroviral therapies and history of drug regimens
- All other medications, including route of administration
- Nonprescription drugs, including complementary therapies (herbs)

Activities of Daily Living

- Workplace and schedule
- Exercise routine, including both aerobic and progressive resistance exercise as well as how often, duration of workouts, and intensity

Financial Status/Meal Planning

- Access to food, including shopping, delivered meals, soup kitchens, or food pantries
- Preparation and storage of food
- Support system

Alternative Therapies

- Mind/body classes
- Yoga
- Acupuncture
- Chiropractor
- Nontraditional medicine

Other Medical Diagnosis

- Pulmonary
  1. *Pneumocystis carinii* pneumonia (PCP)
  2. Tuberculosis (TB)
  3. Cytomegalovirus (CMV)
- Neurological
  1. CNS involvement
  2. Peripheral neuropathy (relating to HIV itself, or drug-induced)
  3. Visual impairments
- Hematological
  1. Anemia
  2. Neutropenia
  3. Thrombocytopenia
- Tumors
  1. Kaposi's sarcoma
  2. Lymphoma
- Cardiac
  1. Cardiomyopathy
  2. Atherosclerosis
  3. Angina
  4. Myocardial infarction
  5. Hypertension
     –Lifestyle: smoking, diet, exercise, obesity, age, family history
- Renal
  1. Nephropathy
  2. Dialysis
- Endocrine
  1. Testosterone insufficiency
  2. Adrenal insufficiency
  3. Lactic acidosis
  4. Glucose intolerance / diabetes
- Skeletal
  1. Osteopenia
  2. Osteoporosis
  3. Osteonecrosis
- Musculoskeletal
  1. Dorsocervical fat pad
  2. Increased visceral adipose tissue; umbilical hernia
  3. Lipomas
  4. Peripheral fat atrophy
- Other non–AIDS-related diagnosis

PROBLEMS

Unintentional Weight Loss

- Weight loss is still common despite effective treatment of HIV (30% of patients experience it)
- 10% weight loss is an independent predictor of death in HIV
- Loss of 5%–10% of weight is predictive of disease progression in HIV
- Disproportionate depletion of body cell mass compared to fat mass
- Timing of death has been related to loss of body cell mass (BCM), with death occurring when BCM is 54% of normal
- Fat mass depletion can also occur with end-stage disease and is different from fat atrophy associated with lipodystrophy
- Associated with elevated levels of cytokines (specifically tumor necrosis factor and interferon gamma) in some instances
- Possible causes:
  1. Impaired oral intake
  2. Malabsorption/diarrheal illness
  3. Metabolic alterations
  4. Hormonal disturbances
  5. Cytokine production

Diarrhea

- Chronic diarrhea defined as a change in bowel habits that persists for > 28 days
- Possible causes
  1. Although less common with the advent of HAART, potential gastrointestinal pathogens may be bacterial, parasitic, and viral; probably only seen with advanced, uncontrolled disease
     - *Common bacteria: Salmonella, Shigella, Mycobacterium avium,* and *campylobacter*
     - *Protozoa: Giardia, Cryptosporidium, isospora belli,* and *microsporidium*
     - *Common viral: cytomegalovirus, adenovirus,* and *herpes simplex virus*
  2. Gastrointestinal Kaposi's sarcoma
  3. Medication side effects

- *Common antiretroviral medications:* zidovudine, lamivudine, indinavir, nelfinavir, ritonavir, tenofovir, saquinavir, amprenavir, and lopinavir
- *Other medications:* sulfamethoxazole, acyclovir, nystatin, clotrimazole, ketoconazole, and fluconazole
4. Dysfunction of intestinal tract due to primary HIV infection.
5. 50%–80% of HIV infected patients have diarrhea; the majority of cases are chronic.
6. 30%–40% of HIV patients with chronic diarrhea have no recognizable etiology despite undergoing intensive intestinal workup, including biopsies.
   - Small intestinal diarrhea is usually frequent and high volume, often accompanied by umbilical pain, dehydration, and weight loss.
   - Large intestinal diarrhea is often marked by an urgent need to empty the bowel, accompanied by pain, cramping, and involuntary straining efforts.
   - May result in electrolyte imbalances and/or dehydration

Malabsorption

- Exacerbated by high-fat diet (particularly long-chain triglycerides (LCT).
- May interfere with absorption of other fat-soluble vitamins
- Can often inhibit absorption of other minerals and vitamins (e.g., zinc and vitamins B_1, B_6, and B_{12})
- Can be related to pathogen- or nonpathogen-related diarrhea illness
- Malabsorption may also be associated with GI mucosal edema from hypoalbuminemia, which may result from protein–calorie malnutrition
- Typical symptoms include multiple episodes of diarrhea daily with stools that are usually greasy, smelly, and floating

Anorexia

- Causes
  1. Fatigue

2. Depression
3. Medications
4. Cytokines (particularly tumor necrosis factor)
5. Malignancies
6. Opportunistic infections
7. Other HIV-related illnesses
• Results in progressive weight loss

Esophageal/Oral Lesions

• Causes
  1. Oral hairy leukoplakia
  2. Oral candidiasis
  3. Oral Kaposi's sarcoma or lymphoma
  4. Herpetic or apthous ulcers
  5. HIV-associated periodontitis or gingivitis
  6. HSV, CMV, or candidal esophagitis

Taste Changes

• Causes
  1. Medications (indinavir, ritonavir, acyclovir, amphotericin B, chemotherapy)
  2. Leads to decreased intake

Dysphagia

• Causes
  1. Oral and esophageal infections
  2. Leads to decreased oral intake

Nausea/Vomiting

• Causes
  1. Medications
  2. Gastritis/esophagitis
  3. Upper-small-bowel disease or infection
• May result in electrolyte imbalances and/or dehydration

Metabolic Derangements Relating to Weight Loss

• Causes
  1. Diarrhea
  2. Vomiting
• Cytokine activity leading to:
  1. Hypertriglyceridemia
  2. Decreased protein synthesis

3. Increased muscle breakdown
4. Increased energy expenditure in relation to body cell mass

Micronutrient/Trace Element Deficiencies

• Causes
  1. Poor intake
  2. Diarrhea
  3. Intestinal infections with impaired absorption
• May result in poor immune function and impaired protein synthesis

Anemia

• Types and causes
  1. *Macrocytosis:* vitamin B_{12} or folate deficiency due to enteropathy
  2. *Normocytic:* anemia or chronic disease secondary to HIV infection, bone marrow suppression by opportunistic infections, or medications (zidovudine, indinavir)
  3. *Microcytosis:* chronic blood loss from gastrointestinal tract secondary to neoplasms or infectious enteropathies

Pancreatitis

• Causes
  1. Medications (pentamidine, didanosine, stavudine, ritonavir)
  2. Hypertriglyceridemia
  3. Excessive alcohol consumption

Serum Lipid Abnormalities

• Types: hypertriglyceridemia, hypocholesterolemia (historical and current), and hypercholesterolemia.
• Causes
  1. Abnormal lipid metabolism in HIV-infected patients was described early in the epidemic with marked increases in triglycerides, decreases in HDL cholesterol.
  2. Elevated circulating levels of tumor necrosis factor (TNF) and interferon gamma increased adipose tissue lipolysis and hepatic lipogenesis.

3. Increased synthesis of very low density lipoproteins (VLDLs) in the liver and decreased lipoprotein lipase activity impair triglyceride clearance.
4. Hypertriglyceridemia is associated with malnutrition in the presence of wasting.
5. In the current era, hypertriglyceridemia is associated with antiretroviral therapy (primarily protease inhibitors).
6. Low high-density lipoproteins were associated with malnutrition in HIV infection and continue to persist in the current era.

Insulin Resistance/Glucose Intolerance

- Causes
  1. Increased visceral adiposity and lipoatrophy is often associated with significant insulin resistance; such observations have been observed among HIV-infected patients.
  2. It is unclear whether these findings are due to the regional shifts in body fat, antiretroviral therapy (specifically protease inhibitors), factors related to HIV, hormones, body composition, family history, or other factors that may predispose patients to developing insulin resistance.

Overweight and/or Obesity

- Causes
  1. Recent data suggests that some patients with HIV infection are gradually increasing their weight. Although weight gain and prevalence of overweight among such patients appears evident, the average BMI compared to the general population still remains lower.
  2. Such weight gain among these patients differs from the general population because they started out with a lower baseline body weight.
  3. Increased weight trends may also be associated with an abnormal energy balance with increased energy intake while macronutrient demands are less.

TREATMENT/MANAGEMENT

Unintentional Weight Loss

- Nutrition counseling for patients experiencing unintentional weight loss due to HIV infection and its associated complications
- High-calorie, high-protein diet
  1. *Caloric requirements:* 30–40 kcal/kg body weight
  2. *Protein requirements:* 1.2–2.0 g/kg body weight
  3. Focus on small, more frequent nutrient-dense meals throughout the day
  4. Appetite stimulation if necessary
     –Megestrol acetate
     –Dronabinol
  5. Appetite-enhancing strategies for patients with HIV-associated anorexia
     –Relaxing while eating
     –Eating favorite foods
     –Ordering take-out food, having somebody else cook, or eating out at a restaurant
- If significant weight loss occurs, enteral or parenteral support may be indicated.
- Oral nutrition supplements
  1. Standard, polymeric formulas may be used if no diarrhea or malabsorption are present.
  2. Elemental or partially hydrolyzed formulas with low amounts of LCT but abundant amounts of medium-chain triglyerides (MCT) are acceptable in the presence of diarrhea/malabsorption.
  3. Specialized diet for HIV infection and for AIDS patients: A diet with hydrolyzed proteins and fish oil may improve weight maintenance by reducing the effect on cytokine production, but more research is needed.
  4. Glutamine and β-hydroxy β-methylbutyrate (β-HMB) supplementation has been shown to increase lean body mass in HIV patients with wasting.
- Tube feeding
  1. Enteral nutrition should be reserved for patients who have a mechanical obstruction and whose gut is intact and functional.

2. Nasogastric or nasoenteric tube for short-term feeding or if patient is motivated to insert tube for long-term use.
3. Endoscopically or surgically placed gastrostomy or jejunostomy tube for long-term feeding.

- Total parenteral nutrition (TPN) is rarely used today for HIV-associated weight loss; however, patients with evidence of malabsorption, such as intractable vomiting or diarrhea, may benefit from TPN. The weight gain associated with TPN is predominantly fat mass.
- Anabolic therapies
1. Progressive resistance exercise (PRE) has been shown to improve body composition by increasing lean body mass in HIV-infected patients.
  –A 6- or 8-week program consisting of progressive resistance training 3 times a week increased muscle function and strength in arms and legs, as well as increased weight and lean body mass.
2. Human growth hormone is an anticatabolic therapy that has been shown to increase lean body mass while decreasing total fat mass in patients with AIDS wasting.
  –Side effects most commonly reported include arthralgia, myalgia, peripheral edema, and hyperglycemia
3. Recent prevalence estimates of testosterone insufficiency in men with HIV infection is approximately 20%, compared to 50% described in the pre-HAART era.
  –Testosterone replacement therapy in hypogonadal men and women with HIV-associated weight loss improves lean body mass and weight. However, given the potential risk with androgen use in women, general recommendations cannot be made until further studies are done.
4. Androgenic-testosterone analogues such as oxandrolone, oxymetholone, and nandrolone have been studied in patients with HIV-associated weight loss and have been shown to increase both weight and lean body mass.
  –Side effects mostly reported include liver dysfunction and alterations in lipids

- Anticytokine therapies
1. Cytokine modulators, such as thalidomide and pentoxifylline, have been studied as treatments for HIV-associated wasting.
  –Two studies of thalidomide in patients with and without wasting have shown increases in body cell mass and extracellular fluid, as well as decreases in urinary nitrogen excretion. Cytokine modulators are not approved therapies for HIV-associated wasting and remain experimental.

Diarrhea

- Low-fat diet (20% of total calories), or add limited amounts of MCT oil (up to 30 cc TID or QID) to foods.
- Low-lactose diet if lactose tolerance is present.
- Low-fat or MCT-rich oral liquid supplement (e.g., Lipisorb).
- Increase fiber (e.g., psyllium, pectin, or guar) intake.
- Increase electrolyte-repleting fluids such as broths, diluted fruit juices, and oral rehydration drinks.
- Small, frequent meals with vitamin supplementation.
- Avoid caffeinated beverages.
- Antidiarrheal medications.
- Parenteral nutrition may be indicated if severe persistent diarrhea with no identifiable etiology.
- Glutamine supplementation and use of probiotics may be useful but further investigation is required.

Malabsorption

- Low-fat diet.
- Use of MCT oil and/or MCT-containing oral supplements.
- Pancreatic enzymes.

Esophageal/Oral Lesions

- Soft foods, fluids with meals, and oral liquid supplements can allow nutrient intake without exacerbation of lesions.
- Highly acidic and extremely spicy or hot foods should be avoided.

- Cold foods may be soothing (e.g., Popsicles).
- Good oral and dental hygiene should be practiced.
- A topical anesthetic oral rinse may be helpful.

Taste Changes

- Medications that are taste-altering should be taken between meals if possible.
- Addition of spices and flavorings can be added to food.
- Avoid supplements in metal cans if supplements taste metallic.

Dysphagia

- Sauces can moisten foods.
- Soft foods should be provided.
- Foods that are difficult to swallow should be avoided (e.g., peanut butter or other sticky foods).
- Adequate fluids should be taken with solids.
- Use of artificial saliva may be useful.

Nausea/Vomiting

- Meals should be small and frequent.
- Treat dehydration and electrolyte imbalances before taking calorie-rich foods and beverages.
- Patients should be seated upright for at least 30 minutes after eating.
- Food should be served at room temperature to diminish food odor.
- Foods with strong odors (e.g., fish, coffee) should be avoided.
- Clear, cool liquids and gelatin may be tried between meals.
- The patient should eat slowly.
- Low-fat foods should be chosen over greasy, fried foods.
- Dry, salted, high-carbohydrate foods should be eaten between meals (e.g., crackers, salted pretzels).
- Take medications with food to avoid nausea on an empty stomach.
- The patient should take antiemetic medications prior to meals.

Metabolic Derangements

- If diarrhea is severe, supplementation with electrolytes is required.
- Cytokine suppressors described earlier may be useful.

Micronutrient/Trace Element Deficiencies

- All patients should take a daily multivitamin/mineral supplement that supplies 100% of the DRIs for each nutrient.
- Decreased plasma concentrations of zinc, selenium, and vitamins B_6, B_{12}, A, and E have been observed in HIV-infected patients and appear to be functionally relevant in maintaining the integrity of the immune system. Specific low-serum micronutrients are associated with disease progression in HIV. Based upon these observations of micronutrient status and possible physiological role in HIV/AIDS, supplementation with antioxidant vitamins (C, E, beta carotene, and selenium) may be warranted.
- In the presence of severe diarrhea, zinc and/or calcium supplementation may be needed.
- Adequate intakes of calcium and vitamin D should be promoted due to new and emerging data on bone health and HIV status.

Anemia

- Evaluate medications and other factors that may be contributing to anemia.
- Treat with erythropoietin, blood transfusions, or granulocyte-macrophage colony-stimulating factor (GM-CSF) if warranted.
- Provide iron supplementation if iron-deficiency anemia is evident.
- Assess and provide B_{12} and/or folate supplementation if macrocytosis is evident.

Pancreatitis

- Evaluate medications.
- Avoid alcohol intake.
- Prescribe a low-fat diet if the patient's symptoms persist on a regular diet.
- On TPN, withhold intravenous lipids if serum triglycerides exceed 1000 mg/dL.

Hyperlipidemia

- Diet and exercise
  1. The National Cholesterol Education Program (NCEP) guidelines should be used for HIV-infected patients with lipid abnormalities.
  2. Structured exercise plus diet reduced triglyceride levels by 21% in HIV-infected patients.
  3. For patients with low HDL cholesterol, monounsaturated fats (e.g., canola and olive oils) should be substituted for saturated fats.
  4. For patients with high triglycerides, a very-low-fat diet, avoidance of simple sugars, and alcohol is suggested.
  5. Increasing intake of high-fiber foods may assist with high cholesterol.
  6. Fish oils (omega-3 fatty acid supplements) may decrease triglyceride synthesis.
  7. Weight reduction, particularly central obesity, is important in managing abnormal lipid levels.

Insulin Resistance

- Diet and exercise
  1. Increase intake of high-fiber foods such as fruits, vegetables, whole grains, and legumes.
  2. Focus on high-quality, low glycemic index carbohydrates.
  3. Structured exercise plus diet may lead to weight reduction, which is important in managing glycemic levels.
- Drug therapy for elevated LDL-C or non-HDL-C
  1. Hydroxymethylglutaryl coenzyme A (HMG-CoA) reductase inhibitors or statins can lower LDL-C. Pravastatin (20 mg daily) or atorvastatin (10 mg daily) may be used because they do not compete with the metabolism of other antiretroviral agents.
  2. Fibrates (gemfibrozil and fenofibrate) are alternative agents for the treatment of hypercholesterolemia accompanied by elevated triglycerides.
  3. Niacin lowers LDL-C and triglycerides but may produce cutaneous flushing.

Overweight

- Traditional approaches to weight reduction should be emphasized for persons with HIV infection. Such programs should include dietary counseling and appropriately recommended caloric goals, combined with continuous aerobic and anaerobic exercise. In addition, a multidisciplinary team approach to weight management is most beneficial with a committed health care team: psychosocial involvement, use of an exercise specialist and/or personal trainer (if available), and family support are strongly encouraged.

Regional Body Shape Changes (Lipodystrophy)

- Progressive resistance exercise and diet can reduce visceral adiposity in HIV-infected patients with lipodystrophy.
- The nucleoside agent (Zerit or D4T) may be associated with fat atrophy. If severe fat atrophy is present, a switch in nucleosides may be warranted if the option is available while maintaining optimal control of virus.
- Under investigation:
  1. Human growth hormone may reduce visceral fat and improve hyperlipidemia.
  2. Metformin and rosiglitazone (oral hypoglycemic agents) may improve insulin resistance and lower total body weight.
  3. Plastic surgery to remove buffalo hump or implant surgery to augment facial fat atrophy.
  4. Other switch studies of antiretroviral agents.

REFERENCES

Batterham M, Garsia R, Greenip P. Dietary intake, serum lipids, insulin resistance and body composition in the era of highly active antiretroviral therapy 'Diet FRS Study.' *AIDS*. 2000;14:1839–1843.

Baum MK, Shor-Posner G. Micronutrient status in relationship to mortality in HIV-1 disease. *Nutri Reviews.* 1998; 56:S135–S139.

Bell SJ, Chavali S, Forse RA. Cytokine influence on the human immunodeficiency virus (HIV): Action, prevalence, and treatment. In: Forse RA, Bell SJ, Blackburn GL, Kabbash LG, eds. *Diet, Nutrition, and Immunity.* Boca Raton, FL: CRC Press; 1994:115–126.

Bell SJ, Mascioli EA, Forse RA, et al. Nutrition support and the human immunodeficiency virus (HIV). *Parasitol.* 1993;107:553–567.

Carr A, Samaras K, Burton S, et al. A syndrome of peripheral lipodystrophy, hyperlipidemia, and insulin resistance in patients receiving HIV protease inhibitors. *AIDS.* 1998; 12:F51–F58.

Carr A, Samaras K, Thorisdottir A, et al. Diagnosis, prediction, and natural course of HIV-1 protease-inhibitor-associated lipodystrophy, hyperlipidemia, and diabetes mellitus: A cohort study. *Lancet.* 1999;353:2093–2099.

Chlebowski RT, Beall G, Grosvenor M, et al. Long-term effects of early nutritional support with new enterotropic peptide-based formula vs. standard enteral formula in HIV-infected patients: Randomized prospective trial. *Nutr.* 1993;9:507–512.

Chlebowski RT, Grosvenor MB, Bernhard NH, et al. Nutritional status, gastrointestinal dysfunction, and survival in patients with AIDS. *Am J Gastrol.* 1989;84:1288–1293.

Currier J, Carpenter C, Daar E, et al. Identifying and managing morphologic complications of HIV and HAART. *AIDS Reader.* 2002;12:114–125.

Dube MP, Sprecher D, Henry WK, et al. Preliminary guidelines for the evaluation and management of dyslipidemia in HIV-infected adults receiving antiretroviral therapy. Recommendations of the Adult ACTG Cardiovascular Disease Focus Group. *Clin Infect Dis.* 2000;31: 1216–1224.

Dwyer JT, Bye RL, Holt PL, et al. Unproven nutrition therapies for AIDS: What is the evidence? *Nutr Today.* March/April 1988;25–33.

Ellis W, Basinger G, Paul J, et al. The use of home total parenteral nutrition in a patient with AIDS. *AIDS Patient Care.* 1994;8:6–10.

Expert Panel on Detection Evaluation and Treatment of High Blood Cholesterol in Adults. Executive summary of the third report of the National Cholesterol Education Program (NCEP) Expert Panel on Detection, Evaluation and Treatment of High Blood Cholesterol in Adults (Adult Treatment Panel III). *JAMA.* 2001; 285:2486–2497.

Feingold KR, Serio MK, Adi S, et al. Tumor necrosis factor stimulated hepatic lipid synthesis and secretion. *Endocrinol.* 1989;124:2236–2342.

Gerrior J, Kantaros J, Coakley E, et al. The fat redistribution syndrome in patients infected with HIV: Measurements of body shape abnormalities. *J Am Diet Assoc.* 2001; 101:1175–1180.

Gerrior J, Wanke C. *Nutrition and Acquired Immunodeficiency Syndrome (AIDS),* Nutrition in the Prevention and Treatment of Disease. Authors include J Gerrior, C. Wanke. Edited by Ann Coulston, Cheryl Rock, and Elaine Monsen. San Diego, CA: Academic Press; 2001.

Grinspoon S, Corcoran C, Lee K, et al. Loss of lean body and muscle mass correlates with androgen levels in hypogonadal men with acquired immunodeficiency syndrome and wasting. *J Clin Endocrin Metab.* 1996; 81(1)4051–4058.

Grinspoon S, Mulligan K, for the Department of Health and Human Services Working Group on the Prevention and Treatment of Wasting and Weight Loss. Weight loss and wasting in patients infected with Human Immunodeficiency Virus. *Clin Infect Dis.* 2003;36(Suppl 2):S69–S78.

Grunfeld C, Kotler DP, Shigenaga JK, et al. Circulating interferon-alpha levels and hypertriglyceridemia in the acquired immunodeficiency syndrome. *Am J Med.* 1991; 90:154–162.

Hadigan C, Jeste S, Anderson E, et al. Modifiable dietary habits and their relation to metabolic abnormalities in men and women with human immunodeficiency virus infection and fat redistribution. *Clin Infect Dis.* 2001; 33:710–717.

Hadigan C, Miller K, Corcoran C, et al. Fasting hyperinsulinemia and changes in regional body composition in human immunodeficiency virus-infected women. *J Clin Endocrinol Metab.* 1999;84:1932–1937.

Hendricks KM, Dong KR, Tang A, et al. High-fiber diet in HIV-positive men is associated with lower risk of developing fat deposition. *Am J Clin Nutr.* 2003;78:790–795.

Knox T, Zafonte-Sanders M, Fields-Gardner C, et al. Assessment of nutritional status, body composition, and human immunodeficiency virus-associated morphologic changes. *Clin Infect Dis.* 2003;36(Suppl 2):S63–S68.

Kosmiski L, Kuritzkes D, Lichtenstein K, et al. Fat distribution and metabolic changes are strongly correlated and energy expenditure is increased in the HIV lipodystrophy syndrome. *AIDS.* 2001;15:1993–2000.

Kotler DP. Nutritional effects and support in the patient with acquired immunodeficiency syndrome. *J Nutr.* 1992; 122:(Suppl 3):723–727.

Kotler DP, Tierney AR, Wang J, Pierson, RN. Magnitude of body-cell mass depletion and the timing of death from wasting in AIDS. *Am J Clin Nutr.* 1989;50:444–447.

Kotler DP, Wang J, Pierson RN. Body composition studies in patients with acquired immunodeficiency syndrome. *Am J Clin Nutr.* 1985;42:1255–1265.

Krauss R, Eckel R, Howard B. AHA scientific statement: AHA Dietary Guidelines Revision 2000: Statement for healthcare professionals from the Nutrition Committee of the American Heart Association. *J Nutr.* 2001;131: 132–146.

Lichtenstein K, Delaney K, Armon C, et al. Incidence of and risk factors for lipoatrophy (abnormal fat loss) in ambulatory HIV-1-infected patients. *JAIDS.* 2003; 32:48–56.

Moyle G, Baldwin C, Phillipot M. Managing metabolic disturbances and lipodystrophy: Diet, exercise, and smoking advice. *AIDS Reader.* 2001;11:589–592.

Mulligan K, Grunfeld C, Tai VW, et al. Hyperlipidemia and insulin resistance are induced by protease inhibitors independent of changes in body composition in patients with HIV infection. *J Acquir Immune Defic Syndr.* 2000; 23:35–43.

Position of the American Dietetic Association and Dietitians of Canada: Nutrition intervention in the care of persons with human immunodeficiency virus infection. *J Am Diet Assoc.* 2000;100:708–717.

Sattler F. Body habitus changes related to lipodystrophy. *Clin Infect Dis.* 2003;36(Suppl):S84–S90.

Schambelan M, Benson C, Carr A, et al. Management of metabolic complications associated with antiretroviral therapy for HIV-1 infection: Recommendations of an International AIDS Society–USA Panel. *JAIDS.* 2002; 31:257–275.

Shevitz A, Wanke C, Falutz J, and Kotler D. Clinical perspectives on HIV-associated lipodystrophy syndrome: an update. *AIDS.* 2001;15:1917–1930.

Shor-Posner G, Baum MK. Nutritional alterations in HIV-1 seropositive and seronegative drug users. *Nutr.* 1996; 12:555–556.

Stack JA, Bell SJ, Burke PA, Forse RA. Use of supplements in patients with human immunodeficiency virus infection. *J Amer Diet Assoc.* 1996;96:337–341.

Tang AM, Graham N, Semba RD, Saah AJ. Association between serum vitamin A and E levels and HIV-1 disease progression. *AIDS.* 1997;11:613–620.

Von Roenn J, Armstrong D, Kotler DP, et al. Megestrol acetate in patients with AIDS-related cachexia. *Ann Inter Med.* 1994;121:393–399.

Wanke C. Epidemiological and clinical aspects of the metabolic complications of HIV infection: The fat redistribution syndrome. *AIDS.* 1999;13:1287–1293.

Wanke C, Falutz J, Shevitz A, et al. Clinical evaluation and management of metabolic and morphologic abnormalities associated with human immunodeficiency virus. *Clin Infect Dis.* 2002;34:248–259.

Wanke CA, Pleskow D, Degirolami PC, et al. A medium-chain triglyceride-based diet in patients with HIV and chronic diarrhea reduces diarrhea and malabsorption: A prospective, controlled trial. *Nutri.* 1996;12:766–771.

Wirfalt E, Hedblad B, Gullberg B, et al. Food patterns and components of the metabolic syndrome in men and women: A cross-sectional study within the Malmo Diet and Cancer cohort. *Am J Epidemiol.* 2001;154: 1150–1159.

Yarasheski KE, Tebas P, Stanerson B, et al. Resistance exercise training reduces hypertriglyceridemia in HIV-infected men treated with antiviral therapy. *J Appl Physiol.* 2001;90:133–138.

Obesity

Linda Veglia, MA, RD, LDN, RN, Anne McNamara, RN, and Edward Hatchigian, MD

DESCRIPTION

More that 129 million adults (64.5%) are overweight or obese. Obesity is the second leading cause of preventable deaths in the United States, and is associated with comorbid conditions such as heart disease, type 2 diabetes, stroke, sleep apnea, asthma, depression, and breast and colon cancers.

Prevalence

The prevalence of obesity is highest in minority populations, women, and those with low socioeconomic status.

Childhood obesity has reached epidemic proportions: 16% of adolescents 12–19 years old were overweight (defined as a BMI $\geq$ 95th percentile of the sex-specific BMI for age growth charts) in 1999–2002, an increase of nearly 50% over the last decade.

Childhood obesity can be a predictor of adolescent and adult obesity. Factors associated with childhood obesity include the environment, socioeconomic status, family size, and activity patterns.

In cases of childhood obesity:

• Medical causes (metabolic/genetic) should be ruled out.

- Use of anti-obesity medication is not recommended outside the context of clinical trials.
- Gastric restrictive surgery, though effective, should be considered as a last resort in those with life-threatening complications of obesity.

Family Influence

Treatment requires positive family support and lifestyle changes that involve the whole family. Family involvement and support are key to success. Food preferences are influenced by parental eating habits early on and remain constant into adulthood. Activity (or inactivity) levels of children are learned from parents, and an inactive lifestyle can persist into adulthood.

CAUSES

Genetic

Studies indicate a large genetic component to obesity. Heredity may account for 25% to 40% of individual differences in body fat mass. Age-related changes in body fat and distribution of body fat demonstrate a strong genetic influence as seen in studies of adopted children, twins, and ethnic/racial groups.

Environmental

Environmental factors include:

- Widespread availability of low-cost, energy-dense foods that taste good and can be consumed with little or no preparation.
- Increased number of eating events in restaurants and fast-food establishments, especially for those in the 19- to 39-year-old age group.
- Increased frequency of snacking, especially among children and adolescents.
- Super-sized portions of commercially-prepared foods.
- Sedentary lifestyles. Nearly 50% of children ages 8 to 16 watch three–five hours of television daily; these children have the highest rates of obesity.
- Labor-saving devices (e.g., computers, video games).

- Increased consumption of sweetened beverages, with a corresponding decrease in milk consumption among children and adolescents.
- Televised marketing of food via advertising targeted to children.

Medications

Certain medications are known to increase body weight, including selective serotonin reuptake inhibitors (e.g., Paxil, Prozac), atypical antipsychotic agents (in particular, olanzipine and clozapine), tricyclic antidepressants, and monoamine oxidase inhibitors. Other medications that may influence weight gain include some that are used to treat seizure disorders, migraine, neuropathic pain, bipolar disorder, and diabetes.

PROBLEMS

Health

Overweight and obesity are associated with

- hypertension
- coronary heart disease
- stroke
- type 2 diabetes
- insulin resistance
- hyperinsulinemea
- dyslipidemia
- metabolic syndrome
- venous stasis ulcers
- osteoarthritis/degenerative joint disease
- gallbladder disease
- respiratory disorders (sleep apnea, asthma)
- menstrual irregularities
- stress incontinence
- complications of pregnancy
- hirsutism
- increased risk for surgical procedures
- certain cancers (prostate, colon, breast, endometrial)

Risks of morbidity and mortality start to increase at BMI > 25; at BMI > 30, risk of mortality from all causes (especially heart disease) increases 50%–100% over that of individuals with BMI of 20–25.

Economics

Based on figures from 2000, the economic cost of obesity to the United States is $117 billion ($61 billion direct; $56 billion indirect). The cost in lost productivity among Americans aged 17–64 years is an estimated $3.9 billion. The direct cost of physical inactivity is estimated to be as high as $24.3 billion.

DIAGNOSIS

Measurement

The most common ways to measure obesity are Body Mass Index (BMI) and waist circumference (WC). BMI is obtained by dividing weight in kilograms by height in meters squared (kg/m^2).

- *Ideal weight:* BMI of 18.5 to 24.9
- *Overweight:* BMI of 25.0 to 29.9
- *Class I obesity:* BMI of 30.0 to 34.9
- *Class II obesity (severe):* BMI of 35.0 to 39.9
- *Class III obesity (extreme):* BMI $\geq$ 40

WC is a marker for visceral adiposity and metabolic syndrome, a cluster of risk factors for diabetes and cardiovascular disease. Cutoff points for risk (prediabetic) are:

- Women: WC > 35 in (> 88 cm)
- Men: WC > 40 in (> 102 cm)

ASSESSMENT

Thorough assessment of nutritional requirements includes review of factors that include physiological, psychological, socioeconomic, environmental, cultural, and educational.

History

Weight

- age of onset
- range of adult weight
- pattern of gain and loss
- weight > last five years
- previous diets
- nutrition knowledge

Medical

- past history
- comorbidities (patient and family)
- current medications (including herbal and OTC)
- food or drug allergies

Mobility

- frequency, duration, intensity
- Activities of Daily Living (ADLs)

Psychological

- eating disorders—binging, purging, or anorexia
- other mental health problems—depression, substance abuse, bipolar
- goals, motivations, readiness to change
- environmental triggers
- stressors—e.g., economic status, employment, family issues
- support system (work, home, religious, social)

Diet

- Food Record Analysis
  1. Meal frequency—e.g., snacks, grazing, night grazer
  2. Meal composition—protein, fat, carbohydrates, fiber, fluid
  3. Alcohol intake—what, how much, how often

NONSURGICAL TREATMENT OPTIONS

Overview of Calorie-Restricted Diets

- Starvation diet (0–200 kcal/day)
- Very-low-calorie diet (VLCD; 200–800 kcal/day)
- Low-calorie diet ($\geq$ 800 kcal/day)

Starvation diets and/or fasting diets have been associated with loss of lean muscle mass, fluid, and electrolyte abnormalities. Very-low-calorie diets (VLCDs) are contraindicated during pregnancy, after recent myocardial infarction, severe congestive heart failure, unstable angina, severe psychiatric disturbances (including eating disorders and substance abuse), and in children and the elderly. Low-carbohydrate diets (< 60 g/day) produce rapid weight loss largely by diuresis and low-carbohydrate diets (< 50 g/day) promote ketosis, which when prolonged, may cause bone demineralization. Further research is needed to determine the long-term effects on health and weight from low carbohydrate diets.

Other Diets

- Meal replacement (shakes, bars, or meals); calories range from 300–800
- Portion control (self-measured, meal replacements)

Nutrition—Macronutrients

Dietary Reference Intake (DRI) is the new term for Recommended Daily Allowance (RDA). It includes the RDA, the Estimated Average Requirement (EAR), the Adequate Intake (AI), and the Tolerable Upper Intake Level (UL).

Carbohydrates

RDA for adults and children is 130 g/day.

Fiber

AI for total fiber intake for adults is:

- 38 g for men, 25 g for women (aged 19–50)
- 30 g for men, 21 g for women (aged 51 and older)

AI for total fiber intake for children aged 9 and older is:

- 31 g for boys, 26 g for girls (aged 9–13)
- 38 g for boys, 36 g for girls (aged 14–18)

Fats

Approximately 20%–25% of total kcals; fat intake of less than 15% of total kcals provides no health benefits or performance advantage. A minimum fat intake of 10% of total kcals is required for absorption of fat-soluble vitamins.

- cholesterol < 200 mg/d
- polyunsaturated fat around 10%
- saturated fat $< 7\%$

(Cholesterol, saturated fat, and monounsaturated fats are synthesized by the body; therefore, no AI, EAR, or RDA have been set.)

Essential Fatty Acids (EFA)

Because they are not synthesized by the body, linoleic acid (LA n-6) and alpha linoleic acid (ALA n-3) are required in the diet. LA is metabolized to arachidonic acid (AA-n6). ALA is metabolized to eicosapentaenoic acid (EPA) and docosahexaenoic acid (DHA). Recommendations vary regarding optimal ratio of LA (n-6) to ALA (n-3). The NIH recommendations are based on proposed AIs of 2:1–3:1.

- LA deficiency is associated with dry, scaly skin; dermatitis; and abnormal hair loss
- ALA deficiency is associated with neurological impairments such as tingling sensations in arms and legs and decreased visual acuity

Minimum requirements of essential fats for adults:

- EFA: 0.33 kg/IBW/day or 0.66 g/lb/ IBW/day
- AI for LA:17 g/day for men, 12 g/day for women (aged 19–50)
- AI for ALA: 1.6 g/day for men, 1.1 g/day for women (aged 19–70)

Trans Fatty Acids

Trans fatty acids are found in partially hydrogenated, unsaturated vegetable oils. They have been reported to inhibit metabolism of essential fatty acids.

Protein

RDA for adults

- Minimum of 0.8 g/kg/d of IBW
- Up to 1.5 g/kg/d of IBW (for obese individuals, to preserve lean body mass, especially when consuming VLCD < 800 kcal/d)

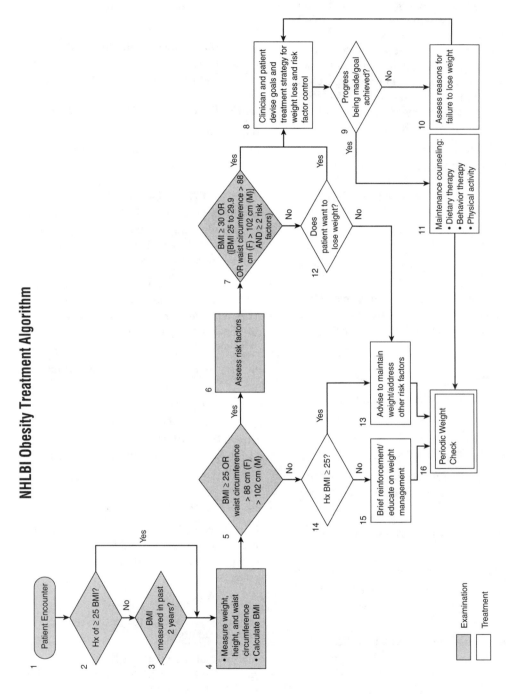

Figure 3–3 An evidence-based conceptual scheme showing the process of evaluating patients for obesity and selecting treatment.

*This algorithm applies only to the assessment for overweight and obesity and subsequent decisions based on that assessment. It does not include any initial overall assessment for cardiovascular risk factors or diseases that are indicated.

Fluid

Fluid requirements vary with age, activity, and body size. Adjusted body weight has been used to assess fluid requirements in individuals with obesity. The average-sized adult requires 30–40 ml/kg.

Exercise

Physical activity is related to successful weight loss and maintenance more than diet alone. To achieve optimal impact on body weight regulation, recommendations vary from 30–60 minutes per day on most days to 300 minutes per week of moderately intense exercise.

Pharmaceutical

Currently, two anti-obesity medications are approved for long-term use in the United States and Europe: Sibutramine (a selective serotonin reuptake inhibitor) and Orlistat (a pancreatic lipase inhibitor). A sustained weight loss of 10% has been shown to reduce or delay incidence of obesity-related comorbidities, such as type 2 diabetes and coronary artery disease.

Treatment guidelines recommend that weight loss medication be limited to patients with BMI > 30 kg/m^2 without obesity-related comorbid conditions or BMI 27 kg/m^2 with significant risk factors (Figure 3–3).

Behavioral Therapy

Behavioral therapy helps patients increase awareness of environmental cues and their consequences on eating and activity patterns. It typically incorporates some or all of the following factors:

- Dietary and exercise counseling
- Self-monitoring through food and activity recording
- Frequent person-to-person contact with the interventionist
- Long-term contact with the interventionist

GASTRIC RESTRICTIVE SURGERY

Gastric Bypass

The most common and successful (many patients can lose 40%–70% of their body weight) procedure is the Roux-en-Y gastric bypass (RYGB). It can be performed by either open or laparoscopic incisions (Figure 3–4). The procedure creates a small stomach pouch. A section of small intestine attached to the pouch allows food to bypass the power stomach, duodenum, and the first part of the jejunum. Gastric bypass is a major surgical procedure with risk of perioperative and long-term complications. Candidates for surgery:

- BMI > 40 (morbid obesity) with a history of failed attempts with diets and other nonsurgical weight-loss methods
- BMI 35–40 with significant comorbid conditions (e.g., Type 2 diabetes, obstructive sleep apnea)

Laparoscopic Adjustable Gastric Banding (LAGB)

In the LAGB procedure (Figure 3–5), a band is placed around the upper end of the stomach, creating a small pouch that empties via a narrow passage into the remainder of the stomach. The band can be tightened or loosened over time by increasing or decreasing saline solution via a portal device in the abdomen under the surface of the skin. Weight loss is much slower with the lapband procedure than with gastric bypass surgery.

POSTSURGICAL NUTRITION

Micronutrients

RYGB alters digestion and absorption as it bypasses the main gastric acid-producing areas of the stomach and the primary absorptive areas of the small bowel (duodenum and approximately two-thirds of the jejunum). Seventy-five to 150 cm of small bowel may be bypassed. As

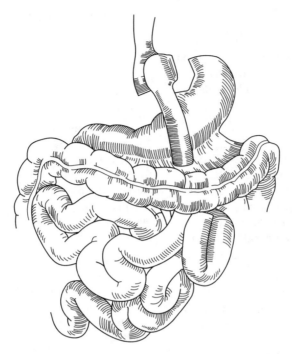

Figure 3–4 Roux-en-Y Gastric Bypass Surgery. The most common and successful (many patients can lose 40%–70% of their body weight) procedure is the Roux-en-Y gastric bypass (RYGB). The procedure creates a small stomach pouch. A section of small intestine attached to the pouch allows food to bypass the power stomach, duodenum, and the first part of the jejunum. Gastric bypass is a major surgical procedure with risk of peri-operative and long-term complications. Candidates for surgery include those with intractable obesity and a BMI over 40 kg/m^2, and individuals with BMI 35–40 with significant comorbid conditions (e.g., type 2 diabetes, obstructive sleep apnea).

a result, several nutrients are at risk for deficiency, such as iron, B$_{12}$, folate, and calcium. The distribution of these deficiencies in RYGB patients is as follows:

- *B$_{12}$:* deficiency seen in approximately 26%–70%
- *Folate:* deficiency seen in approximately 20%
- Iron deficiency occurs in approximately 33%–50%

Recommendations for Vitamin B$_{12}$, Folate, Calcium, Vitamin D, Iron, and Thiamin following RYGB

- *B$_{12}$*—Monitor Serum B$_{12}$
  1. Supplementation varies with form of B$_{12}$

  –*Sublingual:* 350 mcg per day
  –*Nasal:* 500 mcg weekly
  –*IM:* 100 mcg per month (maintenance); 1000 mcg for repletion
- *Folate*—Monitor Serum Folate
  1. Folate deficiency resulting from RYGB can be easily prevented by providing 800–1000 mcg per day. Folate is found in most regular MVI @ 400 mcg per dose and is present in higher doses in most standard prenatal multivitamins (1 mg)
- *Calcium*—Monitor serum calcium, phosphorus, ionized calcium, parathyroid hormone (PTH), and alkaline phosphatase
  1. Calcium recommendations are > 1200 mg (calcium plus vitamin D) per day in di-

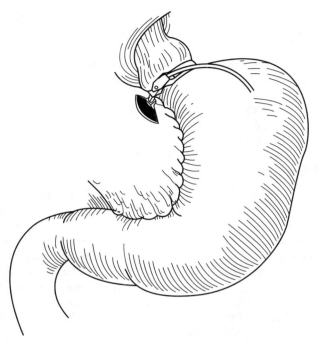

Figure 3–5 Laparoscopic Adjustable Gastric Banding (LAGB). The adjustable gastric band is placed around the upper end of the stomach, creating a small pouch that empties via a narrow passage into the remainder of the stomach. The band can be tightened or loosened over time by increasing or decreasing saline solution via a portal device in the abdomen under the surface of the skin.

vided doses at mealtimes; chewable form preferred. Upper limits (UL) set at 2500 mg per day. Calcium citrate is more soluble in a nonacid environment. Calcium carbonate is better absorbed following surgeries that maintain gastrointestinal circuit and physiology such as in the LAGB procedure.

2. Take steps to maximize utilization and absorption of calcium. Iron interferes with calcium absorption.

3. Obese individuals are at risk for osteoporosis as weight loss increases; therefore, bone density screening (DEXA scan) should be performed routinely.

• *Vitamin D*—Monitor 25 (OH) vitamin D

1. Vitamin D regulates calcium absorption from the gut

2. Vitamin D recommendations are 400–800 IU (10–20 μg) per day

• *Iron*—Monitor iron, ferritin, % iron saturation, and TIBC. In pregnancy ($\sim$ 28–32 weeks) the transferrin receptor concentration may be a useful tool; it is elevated with iron deficiency

1. Iron recommendations are 45–100 mg per day of elemental iron for premenopausal, menstruating women and 180–220 mg of elemental iron daily for repletion

2. Ferrous fumarate is best tolerated and most effective when the duodenum is bypassed

3. Men and postmenopausal women are at less risk for iron deficiency in the presence of consistent multivitamin intake with iron; however, monitoring is required to avoid deficiency or excess iron

- *Thiamin*—Thiamin is a conditional nutrient risk and should be monitored
    1. Patients who present with uncontrollable vomiting should be given supplemental thiamin to avoid deficiency
    2. Patients who present with neurological symptoms such as mental confusion, double vision, bilateral facial weakness, and/or polyneuropathy should be given 100 mg IV or IM for 7–14 days followed by 10 mg per day orally until full recovery

Macronutrients

The post-GBP (Table 3–29) advances through several stages, starting with thin liquids and advancing to pureed/soft food to regular healthy food. These diet stages are designed to provide general guidelines, and, although they may vary slightly among health care institutions, desired outcomes are similar. The patient's tolerance to the diet determines the progression. (See Table 3–30.)

Food should be nutrient-dense, containing high-quality protein, carbohydrate, and essential fat:

- *Protein* (fish, egg whites, low-fat dairy, soybean products, and lean meat): Meat should be moist and tender; consistency-modified per stage of diet (pureed, ground, soft).
- *Carbohydrate:* Incorporate low-fat dairy, non-starchy vegetables, legumes, whole grains, and fruits; limit white, starchy foods (potato, rice, and pasta); avoid simple sugars and processed snacks and foods.
- *Fiber:* Gradual increase of total fiber; ≤ 5 g of fiber at one time

- *Fat:* Incorporate combinations of good sources of omega-3 and -6 (e.g., oils made with soybean [n-6, n-3], safflower, and sunflower [n-6], and flaxseed [n-3]). Store essential fats in a cool, dark place. Fats are sensitive to light, heat, and oxygen; do not fry or use them in cooking. Incorporate at the end of cooking, or put in salad dressing mix.

Fluid

Individuals with acute illness or chronic digestive diseases that promote fluid losses (watery diarrhea or excessive vomiting; perspiration), coupled with inadequate fluid intake, are at risk for dehydration. An isotonic, rice-based, polysaccharide and electrolyte salt solution (ORS) may be a better choice for fluid and electrolyte replacement in those situations.

Post-GBP patients are at risk for dehydration due to gastric limitations and intolerances; therefore, it is essential that minimal fluid requirements be met. Fluid requirements vary according to age, body weight, environmental factors, illness, and activity. Fluid assessments are variable depending on which parameter is used—adjusted body weight (ABW) or ideal body weight (IBW).

Adequate fluid intake is better tolerated if consumed slowly throughout the day, as it is very difficult to catch up all at once!

Individuals should be taught to monitor signs and symptoms of dehydration such as

- dry mouth
- low urine output or dark concentrated urine
- chronic headache
- lightheadedness

Table 3–29 Long-Term Macronutrient Recommendations Post-Gastric Bypass (GBP)

Phase	Energy—Kcal/kg/IBW	% PRO	% CHO	% FAT
Weight loss	20–25	30–35	40–45	20–25
Weight maintenance	25–35	25–30	45–50	25–30

Source: Adapted from Krause's *Food, Nutrition, & Diet Therapy,* 10th Ed. and National Academies DRI's, 2002.

Table 3–30 Post-GBP Diet at BIDMC

Stage and Location	Diet	Items
Stage I—Hospital	Water	1 oz per hour, throughout the day IV Fluid
Stage II—Hospital	Modified clear liquids, low-sugar, noncarbonated and noncaffeinated	Broth, flat diet ginger ale, water, sugar-free beverages ≤3 oz at one time, sip slowly, stop when full
Stage III—Hospital to Home	Modified low-fat, lactose, sugar, and high-quality protein	Protein supplement; low-fat, strained soup; light yogurt; sugar-free, low-fat custard and pudding; and blended cottage cheese
	Calorie goals: 600–800 kcal *Protein goals: 60–80 g*	
Stage IV—Home	Pureed/Ground No bread, rice, or pasta No protein bars until stage V	Moist, pureed meat, poultry, egg, soybean meat alternatives, and finely mixed tuna, chicken or egg salad. Soft, whipped vegetables (carrots, potato, winter squash). Pureed fruit (applesauce, pears, and peaches) and mashed banana. Fat from good sources of essential fatty acids (soybean) and to provide calories. Fiber from oatmeal, fruit, and vegetables listed above, and low-fat, refried beans. Spices
	Calorie goals: 800–1000 kcal *Protein goals: Individuals at* *1.0–1.5 g per kg IBW*	to taste (minced onion, celery, garlic), mustard, relish, ketchup, and lemon and lime juices
Stage V—Home	Regular healthy foods within reasonable portion size	Meat, poultry, pork, seafood, and soybean products (moist and tender). Limited white starchy foods (rice, pasta, and bread). Fruit and vegetables
	Calorie goals: 1000–1500 kcal *(higher with increased exercise)* Diet composition: *CHO: 40%–50%* *PRO and FAT: 25%–30%*	(avoid tough skin and large seeds)

Sample of Dietary Stages for Post-Bariatric Surgery Patients (Beth Israel Deaconess Medical Center, Boston, MA). The Patient's Tolerance to the Diet Determines the Progression. As the Patient Recovers from Surgery and Intestinal Adaptation Continues, Tolerance to a Variety of Food Is Enhanced. Stages May Vary in Time Frame Among Individual Patients.

- postural dizziness
- chronic fatigue

Beverages should be low-sugar, nonalcoholic, and noncarbonated. Alcohol may cause gastric irritation (GI). Caffeinated beverages are restricted for their diuretic effect and gastric distress in prone individuals.

If a patient demonstrates good hydration evidenced by urine output of approximately ≥ 1000 cc per day, is asymptomatic, and is without history of peptic ulcer disease, caffeine may be allowed in limited amounts (≤ 8 ounce/d).

Postsurgery Diet

The focus of nutrition support following bariatric surgery is to maintain adequate hydration and nutrition to effectively support homeostasis of bodily functions, promote wound healing, and preserve lean muscle mass without compromising anatomical structures or physiological milieu.

The patients experience a learning curve as they become more familiar and comfortable with their new anatomical restrictions. The following recommendations have proved to be beneficial:

- Hold liquids to 30 minutes before and after intake of solids to avoid vomiting, diarrhea, and premature satiety
- Eat slowly, allowing 10 minutes per ounce
- Eat four small meals per day with protein and calorie supplements as needed
- Chew foods very well
- Stop when full; protein is a priority
- Use child-sized dinner plate and tableware
- Keep foods moist; avoid drying out or frequent reheating in microwave; a baby food warmer keeps food warm while eating
- Avoid distraction and stress while eating; stay focused on body cues
- If food gets stuck, walk around to enhance stomach emptying and avoid washing it down
- If having difficulty advancing the diet, go back to the previously tolerated diet stage
- Initially avoid gum and hard candy (may cause swallowing of air or may get stuck)

Success Factors

Success is more likely for RYGB patients who have access to a bariatric surgical program that offers a multidisciplinary approach. It should include surgeons, physicians, nurses, dietitians, psychologists, and group support sessions.

Bariatric surgery is a tool that patients can use to manage their weight. Successful use of the tool requires motivation and a lifetime commitment to healthy eating habits and exercise.

EDUCATION AND POLICY

Reversing the epidemic of obesity will require commitment, financial resources, and a strong focus on prevention at all levels of society, including:

Families

- Increase at-home meals
- Limit TV viewing
- Engage in moderate-intensity leisure activities

School Systems

- Mandatory physical education
- Improved quality of school lunches
- Replace unhealthy vending machine fare with nutritious choices

Local and State Governments

- Safe, open recreational space
- Activity programs for all age groups
- Small tax on junk food items
- Use of tax money to fund enrichment and health programs

Academia

- Increase education in health sciences
- Encourage pertinent research
- Bridge the gap from research to clinical care
- Use stature to influence media, government, and industry

Health Care Industry

- Increase emphasis on prevention
- Improve reimbursement for obesity treatment

Media, Food, and Agricultural Industries

- Promote development and submission of news releases/stories focusing on nutrition and health
- Limit snack food advertising aimed at children
- Improve food labeling (e.g., fast-food packaging)
- Downsize portions
- Decrease hidden fats and concentrated sweeteners in products

Government

- Adjust farm subsidies for nutrient-dense foods and fresh produce
- Regulate special interest contributions to legislators
- Restrict scope of food marketing to children
- Pursue multiagency national public health campaigns

REFERENCES

Blackburn, G.L. Benefits of weight loss in the treatment of obesity. *Am J Clin Nutr,* 1999. 69: p. 347–349.

Blackburn, G.L. Weight gain and antipsychotic medication. *J Clin Psychiatry,* 2000. 61: p. 36–41.

Bravata, D.M., Sanders, L., Huang, J. et al. Efficacy and safety of low-carbohydrate diets: a systematic review. *JAMA,* 2003. 289(14): p. 1837–1846.

Bray, G.A. Low-carbohydrate diets and realities of weight loss. *JAMA,* 2003. 289: p. 1853–1855.

Bray, G.A. Medical consequences of obesity. *J Clin Endocrinol Metab,* 2004. 89: p. 2583–2589.

Bray, G.A., Champagne, C.M. Obesity and the metabolic syndrome: implications for dietetics practitioners. *J Am Diet Assoc,* 2004. 104: p. 86–89.

Bouret S.G., Simerly R.B. Minireview: leptin and development of hypothalamic feeding circuits. *Endocrinology,* 2004. 145: p. 2621–2626.

Charles, P. Calcium absorption and calcium bioavailablility. *J Internal Med,* 1992. 231:161–168.

Coates, P.S. Gastric bypass surgery for morbid obesity leads to an increase in bone turnover and a decrease in bone mass. *J Clin Endocrinol Metab,* 2004. 89: p. 1061–1065.

Collene, A.L., Hetzler, S. Metabolic outcomes of gastric bypass. *Nutrition in Clinical Practice,* 2003, April. 18: p. 136–140.

Cotton, P.A. et al., Dietary sources of nutrients among US adults, 1994 to 1996. *J Am Diet Assoc,* 2004. 104: p. 921–930.

Cummings, S., Parham, E.S. and Strain, G.W. Position of the American Dietetic Association: weight management. *J Am Diet Assoc,* 2002. 102: p. 1145–1155.

Dietz, W.H. Overweight in childhood and adolescence. *N Engl J Med,* 2004. 350: p. 855–857.

Diliberti, N. et al. Increased portion size leads to increased energy intake in a restaurant meal. *Obes Res,* 2004. 12: p. 562–568.

Ebbeling, C.B., Pawlak, D.B. and Ludwig, D.S. Childhood obesity: public-health crisis, common sense cure. *Lancet,* 2002. 360: p. 473–482.

Elliot, K. Nutritional considerations after bariatric surgery. *Crit Care Nurs Q,* 2003. 26: p. 133–138.

Goode, L.R., Brolin, R.E., Chowdhury, H.A., and Shapses, S.A. Bone and gastric bypass surgery: effects of dietary calcium and vitamin D. *Obes Res,* 2004, Jan. 12(7): p. 40–47.

Halford, J.C. et al., Effect of television advertisements for foods on food consumption in children. *Appetite,* 2004, 42: p. 221–225.

Institute of Medicine. Dietary Reference Intakes for Energy, Carbohydrate, Fiber, Fat, Fatty Acids, Cholesterol, Protein, and Amino Acids. 2002, Washington, DC: National Academy of Sciences.

Inzucchi, S.E. Diseases of calcium metabolism and metabolic bone disease. *WebMD Scientific American® Medicine.* Retrieved April 24, 2003.

Jakicic, J.M. Exercise in the treatment of obesity. *Endocrinol Metab Clin North Am,* 2003. 32: p. 967–980.

Kushner, R. Managing obese patient after bariatric surgery: a case report of severe malnutrition and review of the literature. *JPEN,* 2000, Mar.–Apr. 24(2): p. 126–132.

Ladiopo, O.A. Nutrition in Pregnancy: mineral and vitamin supplements. *Am J Clin Nutr,* 2000. 72(Suppl): p. 280S–290S

Manson, J.E., Skerrett, P.J., Greenland, P., VanItallie, T.B. The escalating pandemics of obesity and sedentary lifestyle. A call to action for clinicians. *Arch Intern Med,* 2004. 164: p. 249–258.

Marcason, W. What are the dietary guidelines following bariatric surgery? *J Am Diet Assoc,* 2004. 104: p. 487–488.

McTigue, K.M. et al. Screening and interventions for obesity in adults: summary of the evidence for the U.S.

Preventive Services Task Force. *Ann Intern Med,* 2003. 139: p. 933–949.

Millen, A.E., Dodd, K.W. and Subar, A.F. Use of vitamin, mineral, nonvitamin, and nonmineral supplements in the United States: the 1987, 1992, and 2000 National Health Interview Survey results. *J Am Diet Assoc,* 2004. 104: p. 942–950.

Mun, E.C., Blackburn, G.L. and Matthews, J.B. Current status of medical and surgical therapy for obesity. *Gastroenterology,* 2001. 120: p. 669–681.

National Institutes of Health. *The Practical Guide: Identification, Evaluation, and Treatment of Overweight and Obesity in Adults.* Washington, DC, 2000.

Nestle, M. and Jacobson, M.F. Halting the obesity epidemic: a public health policy approach. *Public Health Rep,* 2000. 115: p. 12–24.

Snyder, E.E. et al. The human obesity gene map: the 2003 update. *Obes Res,* 2004. 12: p. 369–439.

St-Onge, M.P., Keller, K.L. and Heymsfield, S.B. Changes in childhood food consumption patterns: a cause for concern in light of increasing body weights. *Am J Clin Nutr,* 2003. 78: p. 1068–1073.

Weigle, D.S. Pharmacological therapy of obesity: past, present, and future. *J Clin Endocrinol Metab,* 2003. 88: p. 2462–2469.

Pediatric Conditions

Lucille Beseler, MS, RD, LD

DESCRIPTION

Feeding the pediatric patient poses a unique challenge to the health professional. Feeding and nutrition support become more multifaceted in the child who is still developing. Growth is a critical determinant of how a child is progressing. Because of this pediatric nutrition interventions are often highly complex and require individual evaluation. The following information is presented as a general overview. (For more specific guidelines, please refer to the list of references at the end of this section.) Criteria for feeding the pediatric patient should be based on medical history and the stage of development. The goal of medical nutrition therapy for all pediatric patients includes:

• Normal growth and development
• Adequate macro-/micronutrient intake
• Nutrition rehabilitation with catch-up growth
• Improved clinical outcomes

Pediatric Patients Are Classified Based on the Following Ages

Each age group may have unique characteristics.

• *Infants:* birth to 1 year
• *Preschoolers:* 1–5 years
• *School-age children:* 6–10 years
• *Adolescents:* 11–18 years

Unless otherwise noted, references to pediatric patients will encompass all age categories.

Infancy (birth to 1 year)

• Most rapid time of growth and development

Toddlers (2 years and older)

• Appetite patterns change
• Weight gain slows → average/year 2–3 kg.
• Linear growth slows → average linear growth/year 6–8 cm.

Adolescence (11–18 years)

• Onset of puberty
• Rapid growth
• Sexual maturation
• Changes in body composition
  –*Females:* ↑ Body fat mass
  –*Males:* ↑ muscle bone mass

CAUSES

Nutritional Problems in the Pediatric Patient

A wide range of pediatric disorders require nutrition intervention. Advances in medical technology have made it possible for infants and children with comprehensive congenital anomalies and chronic catastrophic disease to survive. The existence of any chronic disease can interfere with a pediatric patient's nutritional status, including the following:

- Allergies
- Burns
- Cancer
- Cardiac disease or anomalies
- Craniofacial anomalies
- Developmental disabilities
- Diabetes
- Eating disorders
- Failure to thrive
- Gastrointestinal diseases
- HIV/AIDS
- Inborn errors of metabolism
- Malabsorption syndromes
- Prematurity
- Pulmonary disease
- Renal disease

Screening criteria should be established to identify the pediatric patient at nutritional risk. Patients identified at nutritional risk should undergo a comprehensive nutrition assessment.

ASSESSMENT

Review of Medical History to Identify if a Comprehensive Assessment Is Necessary

Include the following:

- Gestational age
- Gastrointestinal symptoms, stool patterns, emesis
- Growth/weight history
- Social history
- Existence of developmental delay
- Stage of development
- Activity level
- Medications; any drug/nutrient interactions (e.g., of anticonvulsant drugs)
- Vitamins, mineral supplements

Anthropometry and Assessment of Growth

The measurement and evaluation of growth is a key component in assessment and essential in evaluating a child's nutritional status.

Growth patterns are influenced by:

- Genetics
- Nutrition
- Environment

Anthropometrics should be measured and plotted on a standard gender-specific National Center for Health Statistics (NCHS) growth chart.

Growth charts:

- Collection of growth data is essential for pediatric assessment
- Accuracy is essential to determine weight/height percentile
- Gender-specific charts should be used
- Accuracy is necessary when plotting age
- Correct for gestational age
- Disease-specific growth charts

The procedure for weighing and measuring should be consistent, using appropriate instrumentation. The patient should be gowned; infants should be measured without clothes. A stadiometer should be used for children over 3 years of age and a recumbent stadiometer should be used for children under 3 years of age.

The following measures should be taken:

- Weight for age (correct for gestational age; 40 weeks is baseline age for full-term gestation). Compares weight to standard reference.
- Height/length for age (recumbent length for children up to 3 years old). Compares length to standard reference.
- Weight for height/length evaluates child's individual weight compared to his/her own height. Determine if child's weight is proportionate for height.
- Head circumference (up to 36 months of age; adjust for prematurity up to 18 months old).

Affected by nutritional status, but weight/height deficits would be evident earlier.

Additional measures that can be used if child is at nutritional risk:

- Midarm circumference
- Midarm muscle circumference
- Triceps skinfold

Body Mass Index

The Body Mass Index is the most accurate measure for assessing obesity in patients and for monitoring changes in body weight. In the pediatric population it must be plotted on a BMI chart for percentile.

$$BMI = \frac{weight\ (kg)}{height\ (m^2)}$$

Interpretation of Growth Problems

- Wasting (acute malnutrition) = Low weight:height
- Stunting (chronic malnutrition) = Low height:age

Undernutrition and Overnutrition Can Effect Growth

Measure growth accurately to identify abnormalities in order to provide immediate intervention if necessary.

Normal Growth Patterns

- Weight gain: Infants double their birth weight by 6 months and triple their birth weight in one year
- Linear growth: Infancy (birth to 1 year): Length should increase 50% or approximately 10 inches
- Head circumference: The brain doubles its size from birth by 12 months and increases 5 cm from 12–24 months of age

Average Daily Weight Gain

- 0–3 months: 20–30 g/day
- 3–6 months: 15–21 g/day

- 6–12 months: 10–13 g/day
- 1–6 years: 5–8 g/day
- 7–10 years: 5–11 g/day

Weight Change

Weight changes in children may be cause for concern. Significant weight loss in children:

- 2% in one week
- 5% in one month
- 7.5% in 3 months
- 10% in 6 months

Assessment of Nutritional Intake

Dietary intake analysis can be derived from the following methods, using standardized questionnaires:

- 24-hour recall
- 3-day intake
- 7-day intake
- food frequency

Include a feeding history, with attention to the following:

- Food aversions
- History of oral-motor problems
- Allergies/intolerances
- Hunger opportunities
- Fluid intake
- Timing of snacks and meals
- Determine frequency and duration of meals and snacks
- Evaluate presentation of meals and portion sizes

Identify caretaker or/and feeder and determine:

- Parental/caretaker food beliefs
- Socioeconomic/religious or ethnic factors that may influence intake
- Method of feeding by caretaker
- Assess feeding environment, where meals are consumed, and food preparation practices
- Determine consequences for inappropriate feeding behavior

For infants, feeding history questions should cover:

- Type of feeding—formula or breast milk
- Volume and frequency of feeding
- Formula preparation
- Whether type and quantity of food are appropriate for age
- Whether method of feeding is appropriate and whether there are inadequate feeding practices or formula dilution errors
- Description of the location and equipment used during feeding

Problem feeding regimes for infants:

- Cow's milk unmodified: excess protein
- Skim milk: inadequate fat
- Goat's milk: inadequate folic acid
- Evaporated milk: excess protein

Drug–Nutrient Interaction

- Evaluate alteration in nutrient requirements due to drug therapy
- Evaluate side effects of drug therapy that may affect intake or gastrointestinal function

Laboratory Data

Lab measures may include:

- Hemoglobin/hematocrit
- Albumin or prealbumin
- Other nutritionally significant laboratory findings based on specific disease

PROBLEMS UNIQUE TO PEDIATRIC POPULATION

- Failure to thrive (FTT): Defined by a drop of 2 percentiles in 6 months for weight or height; the evaluation and treatment of FTT may require a multidisciplinary evaluation that includes a pediatric gastroenterologist
- Intolerance of feeding protocol
- Nutritional risk secondary to chronic disease preventing normal growth
- Family or patient's inability to achieve goals of medical nutrition therapy
- Financial inability to purchase special formulas or supplements

TREATMENT MANAGEMENT

Establishing Dietary Requirements

- Evaluate nutrient requirements—calories, protein, fat, carbohydrate, fluid, vitamins, and minerals—using Recommended Dietary Allowances (RDAs) for age (Table 3–31).
- In establishing nutrient requirements, an evaluation of activity level, disease state, and the need for catch-up growth must be considered. The RDAs must be adjusted on the basis of this information. In the case of children with developmental disabilities, caloric requirements may differ from RDAs. To estimate caloric requirements for catch-up growth, use the following equation:

$$\frac{\text{Ideal weight:}}{\text{Actual weight}} \times \text{RDA kcal/kg for weight age}$$

Weight age refers to the age at which present weight would equal the 50th percentile on the NCHS growth chart.

Table 3–31 Recommended Dietary Allowances of Protein and Calories for Infants, Children, and Adolescents

	Age	Protein g/kg	Cal/kg
Infants	0–6 mo	2.2	108
	6–12 mo	1.6	98
Children	1–3 yr	1.2	102
	4–6 yr	1.1	90
	7–10 yr	1.0	70
Females	11–14 yr	1.0	47
	15–18 yr	0.8	40
Males	11–14 yr	1.0	55
	15–18 yr	0.9	45

Source: Reprinted with permission from *Dietary Reference Intakes for Energy, Carbohydrates, Fiber, Fat, Fatty Acids, Cholesterol, Protein, and Amino Acids Macronutrients* © 2002 by the National Academy of Sciences, courtesy of the National Academies Press, Washington, D.C.

Classification of Malnutrition

Waterlow Criteria

- Most useful indicator for acute and chronic malnutrition
- Assess type of malnutrition present (acute vs. chronic)

Acute nutritional status

$$= \frac{\text{Actual weight} \times 100}{\text{50th percentile weight/height}}$$

Chronic nutritional status

$$= \frac{\text{Actual height} \times 100}{\text{50th percentile height/age}}$$

Results can be used to determine degree of malnutrition:

Nutritional Status	Acute	Chronic
Stage 0 (normal)	> 90%	> 95%
Stage 1 (mild)	81%–90%	90%–95%
Stage 2 (moderate)	70%–80%	85%–89%
Stage 3 (severe)	< 70%	< 85%

Fluid Requirements

- Assessment must also include evaluation of fluid needs. Review existence of conditions requiring fluid restriction or fluid replacement.
  1. Children 1–10 kg = 100 ml/kg/d
  2. Children 11–20 kg = 1000 ml plus 50 ml/kg for each kg above 10
  3. Children > 20 kg = 1500 ml plus 20 ml/kg for each kg above 20

General Guidelines for Medical Nutrition Therapy

- Establish goals of medical nutrition therapy, including the need for nutrient modification.
- Carefully consider if nutrient modification will cause inadequate intake or compromise the integrity of the child's diet.
- Develop a nutrition care plan based on assessment data and the disease process, with rec-

ommendations for how the plan can be implemented (oral or tube feeding).
- Set realistic goals for the caregiver.
- Evaluate the adequacy of the child's weight gain, on the basis of average weight gain for age, while the child is in the hospital and as an outpatient at regular intervals (monthly) until growth pattern improves to catch-up levels.
- Refer to a community-based health agency if you are unable to provide ongoing follow-up care.
- Revise the nutrition care plan to parallel changes in stage of development.
- Evaluate the parents' and the patient's understanding of nutrition care plan, including infant formula preparation.
- Provide anticipatory guidance on effective feeding techniques and diet for age based on recommendations from the Academy of Pediatrics. Discourage early feeding of solid foods to infants and toddlers. Food selection should be based on the infant's or toddler's chewing and swallowing ability. Early introduction of solid food has many disadvantages, including a potential for increased risk of allergies. A method for identification of food allergies should be outlined.

Treatment/Management for Infants with Growth Failure (Failure to Thrive)

- Evaluate appropriateness of formula with regard to type and caloric density.
  1. Standard infant formulas are available in ready-to-feed, concentrated, or powdered preparations. Standard caloric density of infant formulas is 20 kcal/oz. Breast milk is 20 cal/oz. Pumped breast milk can be altered to increase the caloric density. The caloric density of infant formulas often needs to be altered to meet the unique requirements of the medically complex pediatric patient. This may include patients with increased caloric needs or fluid restriction. Addition of modular fat, carbohydrate, and/or protein may be necessary.

Infant formulas may be concentrated to 24 kcal/oz or more in special circumstances.

2. Guidelines for altering caloric density of infant formula:
   –Concentrate formula base to 24 kcal/oz (concentrate or powdered formula).
   –Add modular fat as medium-chain triglyceride (MCT) oil/corn oil/emulsified safflower oil.
   –Add carbohydrate as glucose polymers/maltodextrin.

3. Evaluate
   –Renal solute load
   –Macronutrient distribution (should remain within normal range: CHO 35%–65%, protein 7%–16%, and fat 30%–55%; > 3% as essential fatty acids)
   –Osmolality (not to exceed 400 mOsm/kg H_2O)

• Determine if formula appropriate for special nutritional needs:
  1. Protein hydrolysate formulas:
     –*Alimentum* (Ross Labs): indicated for protein intolerance/allergy and fat malabsorption
     –*Nutramigen* (Mead Johnson): indicated for protein intolerance/allergy and sucrose intolerance
     –*Pregestimil* (Mead Johnson): indicated for protein intolerance/allergy, sucrose intolerance, and fat malabsorption

• Evaluate the possibility of improving nutrient composition of oral intake. To alter the caloric density of infant food:
  1. Encourage use of energy-dense infant foods, and discourage use of infant foods with low caloric density such as fruit, desserts, and juice.
  2. Add fat such as corn oil or safflower oil to boost calories of infant food if tolerated.

Noninvasive Nutrition Intervention for Poor Intake

• Feeding modifications:
  1. Structure meals, snacks, and beverages
  2. Adjust feeding environment
  3. Limit fluid intake
  4. Limit duration of feeding
  5. Provide examples of positive reinforcement
  6. Encourage consistent feeding techniques
  7. Evaluate need for age-appropriate nutritional supplements or modulars
  8. Don't punish or coax or threaten with invasive therapies or intervention
  9. Withhold other meals or snacks

• Altering oral intake for children and adolescents:
  1. Increase oral feedings and include calorically dense snacks.
  2. Increase caloric density of food with calorie boosters.
  3. Evaluate need for oral supplements, including homemade and commercial varieties.

• Evaluate the need for vitamin/mineral supplementation, including iron, calcium, and fluoride.

Monitoring Efficacy of Medical Nutrition Therapy

• Growth and weight gain compare to normal weight gain and growth patterns
• Improvement in nutrient intake
• Nutritional Labs WNL

NUTRITIONAL SUPPORT

In cases of growth failure unresponsive to oral nutrition therapy, consider the need for tube feedings for the pediatric patient with a functioning gastrointestinal tract.

Tube Feedings

• Enteral feedings are indicated for the pediatric patient when oral intake is contraindicated or nutritional rehabilitation cannot occur without nutritional support, due to inadequate oral intake or hypermetabolic needs. Hospitalized, normally nourished children with suboptimal nutrient intake for 5–7 days should receive nutritional support. Consultation with a pediatric gastroenterologist is necessary.

1. Determine need for feedings/conditions that may require tube feedings:
   –Growth failure secondary to a chronic disease such as cystic fibrosis
   –Short bowel syndrome
   –Neurological impairment
   –Coma
   –Ventilator-dependent
   –Surgery
2. Select formula (many pediatric formulas are available; this is an abbreviated list):
   –*Pediasure/Pediasure with fiber,* 30 kcal/oz (Ross Laboratories): for children aged 1–6 years; tube feeding or oral supplement
   –*Kindercal,* 30 kcal/oz (Mead Johnson): for children aged 1–10 years; tube feeding or oral supplement
   –*Nutren Junior/Nutren Junior with fiber,* 30 kcal /oz (Clintec): for children aged 1–10 years, tube feeding or oral supplement.
   Elemental formulas (for children aged 1–10)
   –*Peptamen Junior,* 30 kcal/oz (Clintec)
   –*Vivonex Pediatric,* 24 kcal/oz (Sandoz)
   –*Neocate One+,* 30 kcal/oz (Scientific Hospital Products)
3. Select mode of delivery

Nasogastric Tube Feedings

- Indicated for patients requiring:
  1. Short-term feeding
  2. Continuous infusion feedings or nocturnal feedings to supplement oral intake
- Contraindicated for patients at risk for aspiration, including those with gastroesophogeal reflux, neurological disorders, recurrent vomiting, impaired gastric emptying, and esophageal injury
- Guidelines
  1. Use small-bore, soft pediatric nasogastric tube (#5–#8 French).
  2. Monitor gastric residuals.
  3. Secure tube to prevent patient removal.
  4. Position patient to minimize risk of aspiration.

Gastrostomy Tube Feedings

- Indicated in cases of prolonged use in children unable to attain adequate oral intake, on the basis of increased nutrient needs:
  1. Neurological inability to suck or swallow
- Can be used for bolus or continuous feeds. Determine which method should be used on the basis of nutrient needs, GI function, and existence of fundoplication.

Jejunostomy Tube Feedings

- There is impaired gastric function with normal distal bowel.
- Pediatric elemental or semi-elemental formula is required.

Other Considerations for Pediatric Enteral Feedings

- If tube feeding will require home management, consider the parents' and/or caregiver's and child's lifestyle/schedule. Evaluate the parents' and the child's ability to handle complexity of nutritional support. Recommend social service evaluation if psychosocial problems prevail.
- Consider supplies, including formula, home care company, and cost–benefit factors. Is the home care company determined by insurance company? Communicate with the home care company. Refer to the federally funded program WIC to determine eligibility.
- Select the formula most appropriate and cost-effective if long-term use is necessary.
- Evaluate the need for pediatric multivitamins, including calcium and phosphorus (information on specific types can be found in the *Physician's Desk Reference Handbook on Nonprescriptive Drugs*).
- To preserve oral function and development, a speech/feeding therapy consult is recommended.
- Communicate with pediatric subspecialists and the primary care physician. Determine who will provide ongoing nutrition care for patient after discharge (e.g., outpatient services, community-based pediatric nutritionist).

To Initiate Continuous Tube Feedings

1. Start at 1–2 ml/kg/h.
2. Advance by 0.5–1.0 ml/kg every 8–12 hours as tolerated until final volume is achieved.
3. Do not advance formula volume and concentration simultaneously.

To initiate bolus feedings:

1. Start at 25%–50% of fluid volume per day.
2. Determine number of feedings (usually every 3–4 hours).
3. Divide volume equally between feedings.
4. Gradually advance.
5. Check residuals before each feeding.

Monitoring Efficacy of Enteral Feedings

- Growth/weight gain
- Stool output
- Fluid status
- Assessment of tolerance

The impact of tube feedings on oral feeding:

- Behavioral feeding disorders
- Oral aversions
- Delayed development of feeding skills

Intervention:

- Oral motor evaluation and therapy

If nutritional support will be continued after hospitalization, home care must be coordinated before hospital discharge. Once discharged from the hospital, the patient must be referred to an appropriate health professional for monitoring.

Pediatric Parenteral Nutrition

Total parenteral nutrition (TPN) represents a complex intervention for the pediatric patient and requires professionals skilled and experienced in this area. Refer to Queen and Lang's *Handbook of Pediatric Nutrition* for a comprehensive guide to this subject. Peripheral parenteral nutrition (PPN) is indicated when the pediatric patient is unable to obtain adequate nutrition via oral or enteral means.

- Use will be short term (2 weeks).

TPN is indicated when:

- the pediatric patient is unable to tolerate enteral feedings.
- there is limited peripheral access.
- nutrient needs are greater than PPN can supply.
- parenteral support will last longer than 2 weeks.
- there is a condition requiring fluid restriction.

NUTRITION INTERVENTION FOR SELECT PEDIATRIC CONDITIONS CYSTIC FIBROSIS (CF)

- genetic disorder
- dysfunction of the exocrine glands

Nutritional Implications

Pulmonary System (Figure 3–6)

GI Manifestations as a Result of Pancreatic Insufficiency:

Malabsorption of:

- fat
- protein
- fat soluble vitamins
- essential fatty acids

↑ Infections → ↓ Pulmonary Function → ↑ Metabolic Rate

Figure 3–6 Pulmonary System

Endocrine System

- CF-related diabetes

Malnutrition

Adversely affects:

- Pulmonary status
- Immune status
- Pulmonary defense mechanism
- Respiratory muscle strength and fatigability
- Body image
- Quality of life

Factors Affecting Oral Intake in an Individual with Cystic Fibrosis

- Recurrent vomiting from coughing
- Pulmonary function
- GER
- Chronic pulmonary infections
- Psychosocial issues
- Behavioral issues

Nutritional Implications of CF

- Calories: 150% RDA
- Protein: 150% RDA
- Vitamins: 2× RDA
- Minerals: increased needs
- Sodium: increased needs in hot climates

Medical Nutrition Therapy for Children with CF

- Hypercaloric diet
- Oral supplements
- Enzyme replacement therapy
- Vitamin/mineral supplementation
- Pancreatic enzyme replacement therapy
- Treatment for malabsorption
- Replaces pancreatic enzymes: lipase, protease, and amylase

Nutrition Assessment and Management of Developmental Disorders

Etiology of developmental disorders can be as a result of a genetic disease, trauma, congenital defects, or an insult in the prenatal period.

Common Problems in Children with Developmental Disabilities

- Drug–nutrient interaction
- Constipation
- Dentition
- UTI
- Emesis/reflux

The nutritional needs of the child with developmental disabilities are as variable as they are for children without special needs.

Nutritional Considerations in Children with Developmental Disorders

- Assessment of growth
- Energy balance
- Obesity/failure to thrive

Feeding Problems for Children with Developmental Disabilities

- Suck and swallow problems
- Oral cavity obstruction
- Unusual feeding behaviors
- Existence of primitive oral reflexes
- Oral hypersensitivity

ASSESSMENT

Additional Nutritional Considerations

- Feeding—duration of feeding event?
- Oral motor skills—Ability to feed orally?
- Feeding skills—Existence of feeding delay? Ability to self-feed?
- Behavioral problems
- Tube-feeding management

Energy Requirements

Condition	Calories
Ambulatory (5–12 yr)	13.9 calories/ cm height
Nonambulatory (5–12 yr)	11.1 calories/ cm height
Cerebral palsy (poor activity)	10 calories/ cm height

Condition	Calories
Cerebral palsy (normal or moderate activity)	15 calories/ cm height
Spastic cerebral palsy	Can be up to 6000 calories/ day

Medical Nutrition Therapy

After careful assessment therapy should be specific to child's condition.

REFERENCES

American Academy of Pediatrics, Committee on Nutrition. *Pediatric nutrition handbook.* 3rd ed. Elk Grove Village, IL: American Academy of Pediatrics; 1993.

American Society for Parenteral and Enteral Nutrition, Board of Directors. Guidelines for the use of parenteral and enteral nutrition in adult and pediatric patients. *JPEN.* 1993;17(no 4, suppl):15A–525A.

Bazarte M, Beseler L. *Nurturing with Nutrition: A Guide to Feeding Toddlers and Infants.* Gulfstream, FL. 2003.

Evkall S. *Pediatric Nutrition in Chronic Diseases and Developmental Disorders: Prevention, Assessment, and Treatment.* New York, NY: Oxford University Press; 1993.

Food and Nutrition Board, National Research Council. *Recommended Dietary Allowances.* 10th ed. Washington, DC: National Academy of Sciences; 1989.

Friscancho A. *Anthropometric Standards for the Assessment of Growth and Nutritional Status.* Ann Arbor, MI: University of Michigan Press; 1990.

Mahan L, Rees J. *Nutrition in Adolescence.* St. Louis, MO: Mosby-Year Book, Inc.; 1984.

Pipes P, Trahms C. *Nutrition in Infancy and Childhood.* 5th ed. St. Louis, MO: Mosby-Year Book, Inc; 1993.

Queen P, Lang C. *Handbook of Pediatric Nutrition.* Gaithersburg, MD: Aspen Publishers, Inc; 1993.

Walker A, Hendrick K. *Manuel of Pediatrics.* Philadelphia, PA: WB Saunders Co; 1985.

Waterlow JC. *Classification and delinition of protein energy malnutrition.* In: Boston GH, Bengoa JM, eds. *Nutrition in Preventative Medicine: The Major Deficiency Syndromes: Epidemiology and Approaches to Control.* Geneva, Switzerland: World Health Organization; 1976.

Williams CP. *Pediatric Manual of Clinical Dietetics.* Chicago, IL: American Dietetic Association; 1998.

Woolridge N, Spinozzi N. *Quality Assurance Criteria for Pediatric Nutrition Conditions: A Model.* Chicago, IL: American Dietetic Association; 1993.

Pulmonary Conditions

Denise Baird Schwartz, MS, RD, FADA, CNSD

DESCRIPTION

Patients with pulmonary disease are individuals who are at risk of pulmonary failure. This organ failure is the end result of many types of chronic lung disease. The condition can occur as a complication of severe trauma, septicemia, and other acute conditions. Pulmonary failure occurs when the lungs fail to oxygenate the arterial blood adequately and/or fail to prevent CO_2 retention ($P_{O_2} < 60$ torr (mm Hg) or $P_{CO_2} > 50$ torr).

CAUSES

Acute Lung Disease

- Fulminating viral or bacterial pneumonias
- Vascular disease, including pulmonary embolism
- Exposure to inhaled toxic substances

Neuromuscular Disorders/Conditions

- Drug therapy (e.g., barbiturate use)
- Encephalitis

- Poliomyelitis
- Guillain-Barré syndrome
- Myasthenia gravis
- Anticholinesterase poisoning
- Chest wall trauma

Acute or Chronic Lung Disease

- Chronic bronchitis
- Chronic emphysema
- Asthma
- Cystic fibrosis

Acute Respiratory Distress Syndrome (ARDS)

- Trauma with direct or indirect injury to the lung
- Septicemia—most significant risk factor for ARDS
- Associated with multisystem organ failure

Malnutrition

- Weight loss
- Changes in body composition
- Decreased respiratory muscle mass and contractility
- Altered respiratory drive and pulmonary mechanics
- Loss of pulmonary connective tissue
- Severe hypoalbuminemia decreasing colloid osmotic pressure and leading to pulmonary edema
- Impaired immunocompetence resulting in increased infections
- Surfactant deficit due to decreased secretion and synthesis
- Altered antioxidant defense system
- Electrolyte derangements and vitamin deficiencies

ASSESSMENT

Areas

- Drive mechanism
- Respiratory muscle function
- Gas-exchange process

- Hemoglobin-oxygen affinity
- Arterial blood gases
- Mechanical ventilation
- Ventilatory capacity and mechanics
- Pharmacological intervention
- Nutritional support therapy

Instruments

- Spirometer
- Ventilator
- Enteral feeding tube/formulas
- Enteral feeding bag/syringe
- Enteral pump
- Parenteral nutrition bag/solutions
- Parenteral pump

PROBLEMS

Motor

- Limitations on food procurement and meal preparation with dyspnea on exertion
- Involuntary weight loss may result in physical weakness and decreased respiratory muscle strength
- Easily fatigued and reduced endurance of respiratory muscles

Sensory

- Altered food taste with medication
- Pain with breathing
- Impaired gastric function, limiting appetite and tolerance to tube-feeding administration
- Early satiety, caused by flattened diaphragm or air swallowing
- Feeling of bloating and fullness
- Abdominal discomfort, caused by bronchodilator drugs or corticosteroids
- Meal-related oxyhemoglobin desaturation contributing to dyspnea when eating

Cognition

- Limited understanding of the disease process and the role of adequate nutrition to optimize remaining lung function

Intrapersonal

- Depression
- Anxiety due to shortness of breath

Interpersonal

- Focus on breathing and on limiting external responsiveness
- Increased dependency on significant other or caregiver as functional capacity is reduced
- Exhaustion, depression, and dyspnea, preventing alertness and receptive potential for interaction

Self-Care

- Activities of daily living curtailed, as the ability to breathe requires concentration
- Ability to shop for food or going out to eat limited, with shortness of breath restricting going outside the home
- Meal preparation restricted; use of more ready-prepared food items (which increases sodium content of diet)

Productivity

- More time required in order to perform most activities
- Frequent rest periods required with shortness of breath

Leisure

- Individual unable to participate in leisure activities due to shortness of breath
- Depression with curtailment of normal activities, limiting social interaction

TREATMENT/MANAGEMENT

Motor

- Increase tolerance to activities with breathing exercises
- Practice controlled-breathing techniques to slow down expiration and help break the vicious cycle of breathless panic and air trapping
- Obtain adequate rest to fight off infection

Cognition

- Have the individual pace his/her strength with rest periods
- Teach energy conservation and work simplification
- Use a calm, confident, reassuring approach
- Relation techniques, positioning, and assisting the individual if it is necessary to reduce energy expenditure

Intrapersonal

- Provide discussion groups to enhance verbalization of problems, lifestyle changes, ways to improve eating, balanced diet, and simply prepared, nutritious meals
- Use guidelines for appropriate meal pattern and selection of foods:
  1. 5–6 small meals per day
  2. Rest before and after meal to avoid fatigue
  3. Use oxygen during meals, if ordered by physician
  4. Separate liquid and dry foods at mealtime to avoid distention
  5. Use soft, easy-to-chew foods to avoid overexertion
  6. Sodium restriction, if ordered by physician
  7. Use canned nutrition supplements as necessary if meal preparation is exhausting
  8. Patients that complain of early satiety should avoid a high-fat diet, which prolongs gastric emptying

Self-Care

- Focus on the relationship between nutrition and pulmonary function and exercise; the importance of a balanced diet; ways to increase caloric intake; and management of dyspnea, fatigue, and early satiety.
- Work with the individual/family to determine the need for small frequent meals and canned nutrition supplements if oral intake is inadequate.
- Consider nightly tube feeding to supplement oral diet, if intake remains inadequate.
- Design a nutritional regimen for the individual with lung disease to provide a diet that

will minimize metabolic demands while maximizing functional improvements.

- Avoid cooking fumes if these are found to be a bronchial irritant.
- Take bronchodilators and steroids with food to avoid gastric irritation.
- Limit shopping for food or meal preparation if shortness of breath occurs with exertion.

Precautions

- Symptoms of increasing dyspnea, increasing coughing spells, fatigue, chills, tremors, tachycardia, and nervousness
- Signs of discolored sputum and sudden loss of appetite (could be related to bronchodilator toxicity)
- Excessive work of breathing, causing visible use of neck muscles
- Abdominal tensing on expiration and generally distressed appearance, including pursed-lip breathing and gasping inspiratory efforts
- Limitation of increase in carbon dioxide (especially excessive calories when providing a balanced diet of protein, fat, and carbohydrate) related to fuel provided either orally, by enteral feeding tube, or parenteral feeding—especially important during weaning from mechanical ventilation or for an individual with declining pulmonary function who may soon require ventilatory support

PROGNOSIS AND OUTCOME

- The person demonstrates knowledge of the disease process and its relationship to maintaining good nutrition.
- The person is able to maintain his/her weight (gradual muscle mass weight gain if individual is cachectic and weight loss only as it relates to overall health, if significantly above ideal body weight).
- The person is able to perform activities of daily living at a maximum level of independence within medical limitations.

- The person understands that the stable ambulatory individual with chronic obstructive pulmonary disease (COPD) has a hypermetabolic state of rest and needs to increase their nutrient intake.

REFERENCES

Chailleux E, Laaban JP, Deale D. Prognostic value of nutritional depletion in patients with COPD treated by long-term oxygen therapy. *Chest.* 2003;123:1460–1466.

Engelen MPKJ, Deutz NEP, Mostert R, et al. Response of whole-body protein and urea turnover to exercise differs between patients with chronic obstructive pulmonary disease with and without emphysema. *Am J Clin Nutr.* 2003; 77:868–874.

Hogg J, Klapholz A, Reid-Hector J. Pulmonary disease. In: Gottschlich MM, ed. *The Science and Practice of Nutrition Support. A case-based core curriculum.* Dubuque, IA: Kendall/Hunt Publishing Co; 2001:491–516.

Ionescu AA, Nixon LS, Luzio S, et. al. Pulmonary function, body composition, and protein catabolism in adults with cystic fibrosis. *Am J Respir Crit Care Med.* 2002;165: 494–500.

Marquis K, Debigare R, Lacasse Y, et al. Midthigh muscle cross-sectioned area is a better predictor of mortality than body mass index in patients with chronic obstructive pulmonary disease. *Am J Respir Crit Care Med.* 2002;166: 808–813.

Mizock BA. Nutritional support in acute lung injury and acute respiratory distress syndrome. *Nutr Clin Prac.* 2001;16:319–328.

Piitulainen E, Areberg J, Linden M, et al. Nutritional status and muscle strength in patients with emphysema and severe alpha$_1$-antitrysin deficiency. *Chest.* 2002;122: 1240–1246.

Schwartz DB. Pulmonary and cardiac failure. In: Matarese LE, Gottschlich MM, eds. *Contemporary Nutrition Support Practice.* 2nd ed. Philadelphia, PA: WB Saunders Co; 2003:396–411.

Thorsdottir I, Gunnarsdottir I. Energy intake must be increased among recently hospitalized patients with chronic obstructive pulmonary disease to improve nutrition status. *J Am Diet Assoc.* 2002;102:247–248.

Wagener JS, Headley AA. Cystic fibrosis: Current trends in respiratory care. *Respir Care.* 2003;48:234–247.

Renal Conditions

Michelle Romano, RD, LD, CNSD

INTRODUCTION

The kidney's main function is to serve as a filter which removes substances the body does not require, and eliminates them in the urine. In this way it maintains fluid, electrolyte, and acid-base balance and rids the body of metabolic waste products. The kidneys also help to maintain blood pressure, produce erythropoetin, and activate vitamin D.

The work of the kidney is done by the nephron. There are over one million nephrons in the kidney. Renal failure is due to loss of nephron function. This can occur over time (chronic) or suddenly (acute).

CHRONIC KIDNEY DISEASE

Description

Chronic kidney disease is the slow, irreversible loss of kidney function. The glomerular filtration rate (GFR) decreases, as well as the urine-concentrating ability and urea clearance. Kidney damage should be present for $\geq$ 3 months by either pathological or laboratory abnormalities, and GFR $<$ 60 ml/min/1.73 m^2

Cause

- Diabetes mellitus
- Obstruction of the urinary tract
- Hypertension
- Vascular disease
- Infection
- Nephrotoxic substances
- Rejection of transplanted kidney
- Autoimmune disease

Assessment

Diet History

- Dietary recall: assess for adequacy and compliance with potassium, phosphorus, protein, sodium, fluids, calories

- Weight changes
- Chewing/swallowing ability
- Nausea/vomiting/diarrhea/constipation
- Taste changes
- Food allergies/intolerances
- Adequacy of diet and compliance with sodium, potassium, phosphorus, calories, protein, fluids
- Compliance with medications (phosphate binders, vitamins, minerals)
- Intake of vitamin, mineral, or herbal dietary supplements

Subjective Global Assessment (SGA)

Social History

- Religious or ethnic beliefs
- Potential risk factors for malnutrition
  1. Lives alone
  2. Inadequate income
  3. Unable to buy own food
  4. Inadequate refrigeration or cooking facilities
  5. Alcohol/drug addiction

Anthropometrics

- Height/weight (without shoes or prosthesis)
- Body mass index (BMI)
- Dry weight refers to body weight when the patient is free from edema and fluid retention
- Weight gain of more than 0.5 to 1 kg/day usually represents fluid retention
- Triceps skinfold thickness (TSF): Lange skinfold calipers are used to estimate body fat; best when used long term, as acute changes in fluid status may skew results
- Midarm muscle circumference (MAC): measurement of calorie and protein stores, positive fluid balance may skew results

Physical Exam

- Muscle wasting
- Physical signs of nutritional deficiency

- Edema
- Ascites
- Decubitus ulcers

Laboratory Values

- Glomerular filtration rate (GFR):
Stage of chronic kidney disease can be determined by the GFR:
  1. Stage 1: Kidney damage with normal or ↑ GFR: ≥ 90 ml/min/1.73 m^2
  2. Stage 2: Kidney damage with mild ↓ GFR: 60–89 ml/min/1.73 m^2
  3. Stage 3: Moderate ↓ GFR: 30–59 ml/min/1.73 m^2
  4. Stage 4: Severe ↓ GFR: 15–29 ml/min/1.73 m^2
  5. Stage 5: Kidney failure: < 15 ml/min/1.73 m^2 (or dialysis)
- Creatinine clearance is readily calculated and has been used to approximate GFR.
  1. Cockcroft-Gault equation:
  2. Cl$_{creat}$ (ml/min)
  $$= \frac{(140 - \text{age}) \times \text{body weight}}{72 \times \text{serum creatinine}}$$
  3. The value for women is adjusted by multiplying the result by 0.85
- Abbreviated MDRD Study Equations
  1. $= 186 \times (S_{Cr})^{-1.154} \times (\text{age})^{-0.203} \times$ (0.742 if female) × (1.210 if African-American)
  2. $= \exp (5.228 - 1.154 \times \ln (S_{Cr}) - 0.20 \times \ln (\text{age}) - (0.299 \text{ if female}) + (0.192 \text{ if African-American}))$
- Serum albumin
  1. May be falsely elevated in dehydration and depressed in overhydration
  2. May be depressed because of chronic losses (nephrotic syndrome), poor intake, and acute stress
  3. May be elevated after patient receives whole blood, albumin, or plasma
  4. For GFR < 20 ml/min, trends in serum albumin levels should be routinely monitored
- Serum prealbumin (transthyretin)
  1. Levels are increased in renal failure, due to impaired degradation by the kidney

  2. Affected by nonnutritional factors as an acute-phase protein
- Blood urea nitrogen (BUN)
  1. Elevated with renal failure, excessive protein intake, and anything that increases body catabolism
  2. BUN is decreased with malnutrition
- Serum creatinine
  1. Elevated in renal failure
  2. Directly proportional to muscle mass
- Serum sodium
  1. Increased with dehydration
  2. Decreased with overhydration
- Serum potassium
  1. Cardiac arrhythmias can occur with potassium > 7.0
  2. Catabolism (trauma, injury, surgery, infection, fever, acidosis) can result in the release of potassium from the cell into the blood
- Serum chloride
  1. Normal or increased with metabolic acidosis, increased with dehydration, fever, renal insufficiency
- Serum calcium
  1. Decreased in renal failure due to elevated phosphorus levels, impaired vitamin D metabolism
  2. Increased with hyperparathyroidism
  3. 60% of calcium is bound to albumin; to determine the ionized calcium concentration: −(4.0 g/dl − patient's albumin level × 0.8) + serum calcium
- Serum phosphorus
  1. Elevated with renal failure, as the kidney is unable to excrete
  2. Calcium phosphorus product = s. phosphorus × s. calcium
  3. If > 60–70, increased risk of metastatic calcification
- Serum glucose
  1. Insulin is degraded by the kidney, therefore requirements may be decreased in diabetics
- Hemoglobin/hematocrit
  1. Chronically depressed in renal disease
- Ferritin
- Lipid profile

- Urinalysis (protein, creatinine clearance)
- Normalized protein nitrogen appearance (nPNA), if available
  1. Requires 24-hr urine collection for urea and protein
  2. Normalization should be done with "desirable" body weight

For patients with GFR < 20 ml/min, nutritional status should be evaluated by serial measurements of:

- Serum albumin
- Edema-free actual body weight; percent standard (NHANES II) body weight
- Subjective global assessment
- Normalized protein nitrogen appearance (nPNA) or dietary interviews

Problems

Uremia/Uremic Syndrome

- Uremia: toxic waste products in the blood, associated with renal insufficiency
- Uremic syndrome: a complex of symptoms caused by uremia; abnormal energy and protein metabolism; net protein catabolism; symptoms include:
  1. fatigue
  2. weakness
  3. decreased mental alertness
  4. muscular twitches
  5. muscle cramps
  6. anorexia
  7. nausea/vomiting
  8. stomatitis
  9. dysgeusia
  10. skin itch
  11. GI ulcers and bleeding are common in later stages
  12. reduced GI absorption of many nutrients
  13. reduced inactivation of many hormones, including insulin, parathyroid hormone, and glucagon
  14. reduced synthesis of active vitamin D and erythropoietin
  15. metabolic acidosis; increases catabolism

Protein-Calorie Malnutrition

- Higher prevalence with GFR < 60 ml/min/1.73 m^2
- Inadequate dietary intake due to anorexia associated with uremic toxicity
- Debilitating effects of chronic illness
- Depression
- Diet prescription is restrictive and/or unpalatable
- High incidence of superimposed catabolic illness
- Protein-rich blood loss due to frequent blood drawing for laboratory testing or gastrointestinal bleeding

Renal Osteodystrophy

- As phosphorus levels increase with renal disease, calcium levels decline, signaling parathyroid hormone to maintain blood levels. Eventually PTH becomes ineffective at reducing phosphorus levels. There is also decreased absorption of calcium from the gut and decreased calcium intake due to protein restrictive diets.

Diabetic Nephropathy/Glucose Intolerance

- Peripheral insulin resistance
- Hyperkalemia also occurs with hyperglycemia as potassium shifts from intracellular to extracellular space
- Other complications of neuropathy, retinopathy, gastroparesis, and amputation all increase malnutrition risk
- Proteinuria
- Hyperinsulinemia

Electrolyte Imbalance

- Hypokalemia can occur with diuretic use
- Hyperkalemia can occur when urine output decreases to below normal. This should be avoided, as the risk increases for cardiac arrythmia and arrest.
- Hypertension, edema, and heart failure may result from sodium retention
- Hypermagnesemia occurs secondary to decreased excretion by the kidney; avoid magnesium-containing antacids

Anemia

- Intestinal absorption of iron is impaired with uremia
- GI bleeding
- Limited production of erythropoietin
- Shortened red cell survival

Cardiovascular Disease

- High-risk group for cardiovascular disease
- Increased very low density lipoprotein (VLDL), normal to low low density lipoprotein (LDL), decreased high density lipoprotein (HDL), elevated triglycerides

Vitamin Deficiency

- Uremia can affect metabolism of nutrients

Treatment/Management

Nutrition therapy with the chronic kidney disease patient (see Table 3–32).

- Current recommendations are based on IBW or desirable body weight.
- According to the National Kidney Foundation's Dialysis Outcome Quality Initiative (NKF-DOQI) guidelines, adjusted edema-free body weight should be used for patients who have an edema-free body weight less than 95% or greater than 115% of the median standard weight, as determined from the NHANES II data:
  1. adjusted BW = actual BW + [(standard BW − actual BW) × 0.25]
  2. other predictive equations have been studied in the inpatient and outpatient setting, including the use of an average/mean weight with the Harris-Benedict equation
  3. there are no validated methods for estimating protein needs in the obese patient with renal failure
  4. clinical judgment should be used on an individual basis
- Goal of therapy
  1. control of nitrogen intake to minimize the accumulation of nitrogenous waste product
  2. provide adequate calories and nitrogen to prevent wasting of lean body mass

Table 3–32 Stages of Chronic Kidney Disease

Stage	Description	GFR (mL/min/1.73 m^2)
1	Kidney damage with normal or ↑ GFR	≥ 90
2	Kidney damge with mild ↓ GFR	60–89
3	Moderate ↓ GFR	30–59
4	Severe ↓ GFR	15–29
5	Kidney failure	> 15 (or dialysis)

Chronic kidney disease is defined as either kidney damage or GFR < 60 mL/min/1.73 m^2 for ≥ 3 months. Kidney damage is defined as pathologic abnormalities or markers of damage, including abnormalities in blood or urine tests or imaging studies.

Source: National Kidney Foundation. K/DOQI Clinical Practice Guidelines for Chronic Kidney Disease: Evaluation, Classification & Stratification. *Am J Kidney Dis.* 39:31–3000, 2002 (Suppl 1).

---

  3. slow the decline of GFR
  4. should be individualized to the patient's condition
- Protein
  1. low protein diets will slow progression of renal failure
  2. for GFR <25 mL/min/1.73 m^2, 0.60–0.75 g pro/kg/d
  3. for GFR 25–50 mL/min/1.73 m^2, 0.8 g pro/kg/d
  4. at least 50% should be of high biological value
  5. see Nephrotic Syndrome for protein needs with proteinuria
- Energy
  1. For GFR < 25 mL/min/1.73 m^2, 35 kcal/kg/d for those less than 60 years of age
  2. 30–35 kcal/kg/d for those who are greater than 60 years of age
  3. Liquid nutritional supplements may be indicated that are low in protein, such as *Suplena* (Ross), or modular supplements, such as *Polycose* (Ross) and *Moducal* (Mead-Johnson).

- Diabetic nephropathy
  1. attainment of reasonable body weight, as determined by the health care provider
  2. slow weight loss is recommended and has been shown to improve glucose tolerance and lipid levels (approximately 0.5 − 1 pound per week)
  3. blood glucose control; education in self-management
  4. protein intake of 0.8 g/kg
- Phosphorus
  1. Phosphate binders are often needed in addition to low phosphorus diet (e.g., calcium acetate and calcium carbonate)
  2. aluminum-containing binders should be limited as aluminum may deposit in bone and brain
- Calcium
  1. supplementation of 1-25 dihydroxyvitamin D_3, or its analogs will improve absorption of calcium
  2. monitor for hypercalcemia
- Hyperlipidemia
  1. low cholesterol/low saturated fat diet (follow National Cholesterol Education Program (NCEP) guidelines
  2. avoid excessive alcohol intake, smoking, obesity, hypertension
- Vitamins/minerals/trace elements
  1. water-soluble vitamin supplementation is needed with diets providing less than 50 g protein/day
  2. multivitamins for renal patients, such as *Nephro-Vite Rx* (R & D Laboratories) and *NephroCap* (Fleming) contain water-soluble vitamins and folate
  3. some evidence to support zinc supplementation, but only after adequacy of diet is ensured
  4. vitamin A should not be supplemented due to risk of toxicity
  5. oral iron should be supplemented as needed, and taken separately from phosphate binders

Outcome

- Reduced nitrogenous waste products in the blood

- Reduced catabolism of lean body mass
- Blood pressure control
- Provision of adequate calories to maintain weight or achieve reasonable weight
- Limitation of phosphorus to control hyperphosphatemia and renal osteodystrophy
- Decreased risk for cardiovascular disease
- Laboratory values stable/maintained

END-STAGE RENAL FAILURE— HEMODIALYSIS

Description

Hemodialysis removes wastes from the blood by passing it outside the body (via an artery) through tubing made of a semipermeable membrane, and then back into the body via a vein. Blood is cleared of toxins by diffusion and osmosis through the membrane.

Assessment

Anthropometric

- Height
- Dry weight (post-hemodialysis)
- Percent of usual post-dialysis weight
- Percent of standard (NHANES II) body weight
- BMI
- Interdialytic fluid gains
- TSF/MAMC as needed (less precise)
- DEXA as indicated

Laboratory

- BUN, serum creatinine pre- and postdialysis
- Serum creatinine/creatinine index
  1. Directly proportional to muscle mass.
  2. The predialysis serum creatinine level will be proportional to dietary protein intake and the somatic mass, thus a low level (less than 10 mg/dL) suggests decreased skeletal muscle mass and/or decreased protein intake.
  3. A low or declining creatinine index correlates with mortality independent of the cause of death.

- Predialysis serum albumin
  1. Low serum albumin ($<$ 4.0 g/dl) has been associated with increased mortality.
- Serum prealbumin
  1. Indicator of future mortality risk; if level less than 30 mg/dl, should be evaluated for malnutrition.
- Serum cholesterol, lipid profile
  1. In the dialysis population, low (150–180 mg/dl) or declining serum cholesterol concentrations are predictive of increased mortality risk, and should be investigated for nutritional deficits.
  2. Levels above 200–300 are associated with increased mortality risk.
- Serum calcium
- Serum phosphorus
  1. Calcium phosphorus product = s. phosphorus $\times$ s. calcium.
  2. If $>$ 60–70, increased risk of metastatic calcification
- Serum magnesium
- Parathyroid hormone (PTH)
- Protein equivalent of nitrogen appearance (PNA)
  1. Determined by fat-free, edema-free body mass, and therefore is "normalized" (nPNA) to some function of body weight.
  2. Provides valid estimate of protein intake in the steady state (i.e., with anabolism, PNA will underestimate protein intake).
  3. Can be performed from urea kinetic modeling during hemodialysis session.

Physical Exam

- Ascites, edema
- Nutritional deficiencies
- Decubitus ulcer(s)
- Muscle/fat stores

Social History

- Religious or ethnic beliefs
- Potential risk factors for malnutrition
  1. Lives alone.
  2. Inadequate income.
  3. Unable to shop for food.

4. Inadequate refrigeration or cooking facilities.
5. Alcohol/drug addiction.

Diet History

- Dietary recall: assess for adequacy and compliance with potassium, phosphorus, protein, sodium, fluid, calories
- Tolerance to oral diet
- Vitamin/mineral, herbal, or other supplements
- Nutrient/drug interactions
- Assess knowledge of disease state and diet guidelines

Subjective Global Assessment (SGA)

Problems

- Protein-calorie malnutrition
  1. Average estimated prevalence is approximately 40%.
  2. Associated with increased morbidity and mortality.
  3. Anorexia; multifactorial.
  4. Delayed gastric emptying in diabetic and non-diabetic patients.
  5. Increased serum leptin levels.
  6. Protein loss during treatment.
  7. Side effects of dialysis treatments include hypotensive episodes, vomiting, headache; intake may be decreased on these days.
  8. Activation of acute phase response, which in turn may suppress appetite and lead to catabolism of lean body mass.
- Anemia; blood loss associated with dialysis procedure and laboratory testing
- Hyperlipidemia
  1. Type IV hyperlipidemia, increased triglycerides, VLDL, decreased HDL; total cholesterol elevated or unaffected; LDL decreased or unaffected.
- Renal osteodystrophy
- Diabetes
  1. Protein-calorie malnutrition may occur with diabetic gastroparesis.
  2. High blood levels of glucose may lead to increased thirst.

Treatment

See Table 3–33.

- Protein intake for stable patients is 1.2 g/kg/d
  1. At least 50% should be of high biological value.
- Energy
  1. 35 kcal/kg/d for those under 60 years of age.

2. 30–35 kcal/kg/d for those over 60 years of age, due to more sedentary lifestyle.
3. Adjusted edema-free body weight should be used for dialysis patients who have an edema-free body weight less than 95% or greater than 115% of the median standard weight, as determined from the NHANES II data.

Table 3–33 Daily Nutrient Recommendations for Patients with Chronic Renal Failure, Hemodialysis, and Peritoneal Dialysis

Nutrient	ESRD Pre-Dialysis	Hemodialysis	Peritoneal Dialysis
Protein	0.6–0.75 g/kg 50% high biological value 0.8–1.0 (nephrotic syndrome)	1.2 g pro/kg 50% high biological value	1.2–1.3 g pro/kg 50% high biological value
Energy	35 kcal/kg for > 60 years 30 kcal/kg for < 60 years	HBE × 1.2–1.3 30–35 kcal/kg for > 60 years 35 kcal/kg for > 60 years	35 kcal/kg for > 60 years 30–35 kcal/kg for > 60 years Adjust for dialysate calories
Fat	NCEP guidelines	NCEP guidelines	NCEP guidelines
Fluids	Maintain hydration	500–750 ml + urine output	to maintain fluid balance
Sodium	1–3 g/day	2–3 g/d	2–4 g/d
Potassium	Individualized	40 mg/kg	Individualized per labs
Calcium	Individualized	Individualized 1000–1500 mg/d	Individualized 1000–1500 mg/d
Phosphorus	Individualized; 8–12 mg/kg IBW may require phosphate binder	Individualized; < 17 mg/kg	
Niacin	14 mg female; 16 mg male	14 mg female; 16 mg male	14 mg female; 16 mg male
Thiamin	1.1 mg female; 1.2 mg male	1.1 mg female; 1.2 mg male	1.1 mg female; 1.2 mg male
Riboflavin	1.1 mg female; 1.3 mg male	1.1 mg female; 1.3 mg male	1.1 mg female; 1.3 mg male
Pantothenic acid	5 mg	5 mg	5 mg
Pyridoxine	10 mg	10 mg	10 mg
Biotin	30 μg	30 μg	30 μg
Folic acid	800–1000 mg	800–1000 mg	800–1000 mg
Vitamin B_{12}	6 μg	6 μg	6 μg
Vitamin C	75–100 mg	75–100 mg	75–100 mg
Vitamin D	Individualized	Individualized	Individualized
Vitamin A	0	0	0
Vitamin E	Information insufficient	Information insufficient	Information insufficient
Vitamin K	0	0	0

Adjusted BW = actual BW
$$+ [(\text{SBW} - \text{actual BW}) \times 0.25]$$

4. For patients whose weight is between 95% and 115%, use the actual edema-free weight.
5. Other predictive equations have been studied in the inpatient and outpatient setting, including the use of an average/mean weight with the Harris-Benedict equation.
6. There are no validated methods for estimating protein needs in the obese patient with renal failure.
7. Clinical judgement should be used on an individual basis.
- Nutrition counseling should encourage adherence to protein, potassium, sodium, phosphorus, and fluid allowance as well as meeting caloric needs
- Support from significant others may improve motivation to comply with diet
- Vitamins/minerals
  1. Water-soluble vitamin supplements are needed, as some are lost through dialysis and limited on restrictive diets.
  2. Multivitamins for renal patients, such as *Nephro-Vite Rx* (R & D Laboratories) and *NephroCap* (Fleming), contain water-soluble vitamins and folate.
  3. Vitamin C is limited due to oxalate formation.
  4. Supplementation of vitamin A can lead to toxicity in renal failure.
  5. Zinc may be deficient in dialysis patients who complain of anorexia and dysgeusia; however, therapeutic doses are not clearly defined. Doses > 50 mg/d (elemental) can decrease copper absorption.
  6. Optimizing B_{12}, B_6, and folic acid may have cardioprotective effects.
  7. Oral iron supplementation as needed, taken separately from phosphate binders.
- Phosphate is poorly dialyzed by the artificial kidney
- Calcium
  1. Follow serum level, supplement as needed.
- Hyperlipidemia

1. Low cholesterol/low saturated fat diet (NCEP guidelines).
2. Carbohydrates should be complex.
- Inadequate calorie-protein intake
  1. Nutritional supplementation may be needed to meet nutritional needs, and/or diet should be liberalized.
  2. Tube feedings for patients that are malnourished and unable to meet > 50% nutritional needs orally.
     –Standard formulas may be used with monitoring, or may use formulas that take into account fluid and mineral restrictions, such as *Magnacal Renal* (Mead Johnson), *Novasource Renal* (Novartis), or *Nepro* (Ross).
  3. Intradialytic parenteral nutrition (IDPN) if tube feedings are not used
     –Should be considered short-term therapy
     –May be of benefit if the following criteria are met:
     a. Evidence of protein or energy malnutrition and inadequate intake.
     b. Inability to tolerate enteral feedings.
     c. Combination of feeding modalities (oral, enteral, IDPN) will meet nutritional needs.
     –For example:

10% amino acid formula	550 cc	55 g protein
+ 50% dextrose	250 cc	125 g carbo-hydrate
+ 20% lipids	200 cc	40 g fat
	1000 cc	1005 kcal

1 mg folic acid, 10 ml multivitamin, 1 ml trace elements can be added

  4. Total parenteral nutrition (TPN):
     –Indicated with inadequate oral intake and inability to use GI tract.
     –Provide standard amino acid solution.

Outcome

- Verbalized knowledge of appropriate food choices

- Improved blood pressure control
- Reduced nitrogenous waste products in blood
- Improved or maintain serum albumin equal to or greater than 4.0 g/dl
- Decreased risk of renal osteodystrophy
- Prevention of hyperkalemia and cardiac arrhythmias
- Decreased risk of cardiovascular disease
- Maintains glucose levels with goals

PERITONEAL DIALYSIS

Description

Peritoneal dialysis is dialysis using the semipermeable membrane of the peritoneum. A catheter is surgically placed into the peritoneal cavity. Highly concentrated dextrose solutions are instilled into the peritoneum. Osmosis and diffusion remove waste products from the blood into the dialysate. The fluid is then removed and discarded. This procedure is usually done 4–5 times per day with continuous ambulatory peritoneal dialysis (CAPD), or throughout the night by a machine called a cycler, with continuous cyclic peritoneal dialysis (CCPD), and nocturnal peritoneal dialysis (NPD). With intermittant peritoneal dialysis (IPD), patients are dialyzed by a cycler for 8–12 hours, three times per week. It is considered less efficient than CCPD or CAPD. Exchanges vary in concentration and volume. The dextrose concentration can be 1.5%, 2.5%, or 4.25% with a volume of 1.0 to 3.0 liter per exchange.

Assessment

Anthropometrics

- Height
- Dry weight
- Percent usual body weight
- Percent standard (NHANES II) weight
- BMI
- MAMC, TSF (less precise)
- DEXA as indicated

Laboratory

- Serum albumin
- Serum prealbumin
- BUN
- Serum creatinine/creatinine index
  1. Directly proportional to muscle mass.
  2. The predialysis serum creatinine level will be proportional to dietary protein intake and the somatic mass, thus a low level (less than 10 mg/dl) suggests decreased skeletal muscle mass and/or decreased protein intake.
  3. A low or declining creatinine index correlates with mortality independent of the cause of death.
- Serum cholesterol, lipid profile
- Serum calcium
- Serum potassium
- Serum phosphorus
- nPNA, if available
- Peritoneal equilibration test (PET), if available

Diet History

- Dietary recall: assess for adequacy and compliance with potassium, phosphorus, protein, sodium, fluid, calories
- Weight changes
- Tolerance to oral diet (taste changes, nausea/vomiting/diarrhea/constipation)
- Vitamin/mineral, herbal, or other supplements
- Nutrient/drug interactions
- Assess knowledge of disease state and diet guidelines

Physical Exam

- Ascites, edema
- Nutritional deficiencies
- Decubitus ulcer(s)
- Muscle/fat stores

Social History

- Assess for financial or psychosocial barriers to adequate intake
- Religious or ethnic beliefs

- Potential risk factors for malnutrition
  1. Lives alone
  2. Inadequate income
  3. Unable to buy own food
  4. Inadequate refrigeration or cooking facilities
  5. Alcohol/drug addiction

SGA Score

Estimation of Glucose Absorption

- Initial dialysate solution contains the following amounts of glucose:

      1.5% — 13.0 g/l
      2.5% — 22.5 g/l
      4.25% — 37.6 g/l

  See Table 3–34 for calculation examples.

Problems

- Hyperlipoproteinemia/hyperlipidemia
  1. Elevated cholesterol, triglycerides, VLDL, LDL, HDL
- Protein-calorie malnutrition
  1. Loss of 9 g protein or more through dialysate
  2. Peritonitis increases protein loss
  3. Early satiety
  4. Increased serum leptin levels
  5. Impaired gastric emptying
  6. Comorbidities/concurrent illnesses
  7. Activation of acute phase response, which in turn may suppress appetite and lead to catabolism of lean body mass
- Renal osteodystrophy
- Weight gain/obesity due to 400–700 calories absorbed daily from dialysate
- Hypotension requiring additional fluid and sodium replacement
- Vitamin deficiency: vitamin D, B vitamins, vitamin C, folic acid

Treatment

- Nutrition counseling should include meeting protein needs, maintenance of desirable weight or weight control, limiting phosphorus, control of edema, and hyperlipidemia

See Table 3–33.
- Protein
  1. 1.2–1.3 g pro/kg/d; at least 50% high biological value
- Energy
  1. Adjusted dietary calorie requirement = dietary calorie requirement − calories from dialysate
  2. 35 kcal/kg/d for those less than age 60 years
  3. 30–35 kcal/kg/d for those greater than age 60 years, due to increased sedentary lifestyle
  4. Adjusted edema-free body weight should be used for dialysis patients who have an edema-free body weight less than 95% or greater than 115% of the median standard weight, as determined from the NHANES II data
  5. Adjusted BW = actual BW + [(SBW − actual BW) × 0.25]
  6. For patients whose weight is between 95% and 115%, use the actual edema-free weight
  7. Other predictive equations have been studied in the inpatient and outpatient setting, including the use of an average/mean weight with the Harris-Benedict equation
  8. There are no validated methods for estimating protein needs in the obese patient with renal failure
  9. Clinical judgement should be used on an individual basis
- Sodium/fluids
  1. Patients with edema, hypertension, and congestive heart failure may require a more restrictive intake of fluids and sodium.
- Phosphorus
  1. 8–12 mg/kg can decrease the risk of severe hyperparathyroidism
- Vitamins/minerals/trace elements
  1. Multivitamins for renal patients, such as *Nephro-Vite Rx* (R & D Laboratories) and *NephroCap* (Fleming), contain water-soluble vitamins and folate.

Table 3–34 Estimation of Glucose Absorption

Examples of several methods available:
1. $y = 11.3 (x) - 10.9$
   $y =$ glucose absorbed/liter of exchange
   $x =$ average initial concentration (gm/liter) of dextrose solution

   For example: 4, 2-liter exchanges in 24 hours
                      2 exchanges 2.5% solution
                      2 exchanges 4.25% solution
      average initial concentration of dextrose:
      2.2 g/dL $\times$ 4 L $=$ 8.8 g dextrose
      3.8 g/dL $\times$ 4 L $=$ 15.2 g dextrose

      24.0 g dextrose

   24.0 g dextrose/ 8 L $=$ 3.0 g/L average
   $y = 11.3 (3.0) - 10.9$
     $=$ 23 g dextrose absorbed/L
   23 g glucose/L $\times$ 8 L $=$ 184 g dextrose absorbed
   220 $\times$ 3.4 kcal/g $=$ approximately 626 kcal absorbed/day
2. Calories from dialysate $=$
   Dextrose concentration [g/L $\times$ 3.4 (kcal/kg) $\times$ 0.8 $\times$ volume (L)]

   For example: (from Equation 1)
   38 g/L $\times$ 3.4 kcal/g $\times$ 0.8 $\times$ 4 L $=$ 413 kcal
   22 g/L $\times$ 3.4 kcal/g $\times$ 0.8 $\times$ 4 L $=$ 239 kcal
   ----
      approximately 652 kcal absorbed/day
3. Glucose (G) $= (1\text{-}D/D_0) \times G_i$
   Where:
        $D_0 =$ Initial dextrose in the dialysate at zero hours (g)
        $D =$ Remaining dextrose in the dialysate after an appropriate dwell time (g)
        $D/D_0 =$ Fraction of dextrose remaining in the dialysate
                (determined after 4 hour dwell from PET)
        $G_i =$ Initial grams dextrose instilled

   Example (from above):
   Initial g instilled $= (4 \text{ L} \times 22 \text{ g/L}) + (4 \text{ L} \times 38 \text{ g/L}) = 240$ g

   D/D_0 from PET $= 0.59$

   Grams of dextrose absorbed $= (1 - 0.59) \times 240 = 98.4$ g

   Calories absorbed $= 98.4 \times 3.4$ kcal/g $= 335$ kcal/d

---

2. 1-25 dihydroxyvitamin D_3 supplement or its analogs may be indicated, as there is a loss through dialysate.
3. Oral iron supplements as needed, taken separately from phosphate binders.
4. Vitamin A should not be supplemented due to risk of toxicity.

- Calcium
  1. The more hypertonic the peritoneal dialysate, the greater the dialysate outflow volume and calcium losses.
  2. Supplements may be needed, but no more than 2000 mg elemental calcium/day.
- Potassium

1. Restriction is not usually needed as peritoneal dialysis is a daily procedure.
2. If elevated, should be restricted to 60–70 mEq/day.
- Early satiety
  1. Drain dialysate prior to mealtime and reinfuse with fresh exchange at the end of the meal.
  2. Small, frequent meals.
  3. Limit fluids at mealtimes.
- Hyperlipidemia/hyperlipoproteinemia
  1. Low cholesterol/low saturated fat diet (NCEP guidelines).
- Diabetes
  1. Follow diet appropriate for diabetes, adjusted to meet protein and calorie needs, control hyperlipidemia and fluid retention; weight reduction as indicated.
  2. Insulin can be added to dialysate, rather than being injected subcutaneously, which results in less fluctuation of plasma glucose levels.
  3. Energy
     –Complex carbohydrates
     –Good glycemic control can reduce triglyceride levels
- Inadequate oral intake
  1. Total calorie intake may be adequate as additional calories are contributed by dialysate, but protein intake may be inadequate.
  2. Liquid nutrition supplements can be used, high in protein.
  3. Modular protein supplements, such as *Promod* (Ross) and *Proteinex* (Llorens Pharmaceuticals), can be added to foods.
  4. Nasogastric or nasoenteric tubes can be used for up to 4 weeks.
  5. Limited literature supporting placement of gastrostomy tubes due to risk of peritonitis.
  6. Total parenteral nutrition (TPN) if inadequate bowel function.
  7. Intraperitoneal amino acids (IPAA) if tube feedings are not used, and patient is unable to consume adequate amounts orally.
     –Two liters of dialysate solution containing 1.1% amino acid infused daily provides a net uptake of about 17 g amino acids

–May benefit from treatment if each of the following are met:
  a. Evidence of protein malnutrition with inadequate intake
  b. Inability to tolerate enteral nutrition
  c. Combination of feeding modalities will meet nutritional needs
–Randomized, controlled trials are needed

Outcome

- Achieved or maintained nitrogen balance
- Prevention of excessive weight gain
- Decreased risk of renal osteodystrophy
- Decreased risk of cardiovascular disease

ACUTE RENAL FAILURE

Description

Acute renal failure is the acute loss of excretory function, it can be reversible. There are three phases. During the oliguric phase, urine volume is decreased, azotemia and acidosis develops; with increased potassium and phosphorus levels, high blood pressure and edema. There are large fluid and electrolyte losses during the diuretic phase. The recovery phase is a gradual return of renal function.

Cause

- Shock
- Sepsis
- Trauma
- Multisystem organ failure
- Obstruction
- Toxins
- Medications (NSAIDs, aminoglycoside antibiotics)
- Certain types of glomerulonephritis
- Rhabdomyolysis

Assessment

Anthropometrics

- Height/weight (without edema; postdialysis)
- BMI

Diet History

- Vitamin/mineral/herbal supplement use
- Weight changes
- GI symptoms (diarrhea/constipation/nausea/vomiting)
- Other medications
- Alcohol or drug abuse
- Chewing/swallowing ability

Medical History

- Condition leading to acute renal failure
- Other disease states (diabetes mellitus, HIV/AIDS)
- Other conditions with potential nutritional implications (mechanical ventilation, surgery, CVA)
- Type of dialysis, if any
- Intake/output

Physical Exam

- Edema
- Cachexia or obesity
- Decreased muscle mass
- Decubitus ulcer(s)
- Skin turgor
- Ascites

Laboratory Values

- GFR
  1. Creatinine clearance is readily calculated and has been used to approximate GFR.

     $-Cl_{creat}$ (ml/min)
     $$= \frac{(140 - age) \times body\ weight}{72 \times serum\ creatinine}$$

     –The value for women is adjusted by multiplying the result by 0.85
     –Abbreviated MDRD Study Equations
       a. $= 186 \times (S_{Cr})^{-1.154} \times (age)^{-0.203} \times$ (0.742 if female) $\times$ (1.210 if African-American)
       b. $= exp(5.228 - 1.154 \times In(S_{Cr}) - 0.20 \times In(age) - (0.299\ if\ female) + (0.192\ if\ African-American)$

- BUN/serum creatinine
- Serum sodium
- Serum potassium
- Serum phosphorus

- Serum calcium
- Serum magnesium
- Serum chloride
- Serum bicarbonate
- Serum glucose
- Serum albumin/prealbumin
  1. Levels will be altered due to non-nutritional factors such as in acute illness, volume overload, liver damage
- Hematocrit/hemoglobin

Determine Appropriate Feeding Route

- Oral
- Enteral nutrition
- TPN
- Combination of above

Problems

- Hypermetabolic/hypercatabolic
- Renal replacement therapy (RRT) (peritoneal dialysis, hemodialysis), or continuous RRT (CRRT), continuous arteriovenous hemofiltration (CAVH), or with hemodiafiltration (CAVHD), continuous venovenous hemofiltration (CVVH) or with hemodiafiltration (CVVHD), or slow continuous ultrafiltration (SCUF) increase protein and water-soluble vitamin losses
- Insulin resistance; hyperglycemia
- Metabolic acidosis
- Affects glucose metabolism by contributing to glucose intolerance
- Altered lipid metabolism
- Electrolyte imbalance (elevated or depleted)
- Decreased PO intake due to nausea/vomiting, confusion

Treatment/Management

Nutrition therapy should consist of control of protein, sodium, potassium, fluids, and calories according to dialysis therapy and needs of the individual

Energy

- Indirect calorimetry (should be done several hours after dialysis)

- Harris-Benedict equation × stress factor only
- 30–40 kcal/kg desirable body weight
- 25–35 kcal/kg/d with CRRT
- Adjust total calories for dextrose absorption, which occurs with CRRT in techniques which use dextrose-containing dialysate solutions.
  1. 1.5% dialysate, assume 43% absorption
  2. 2.5% dialysate, assume 45% absorption

Protein

- 0.8 g/kg/d in unstressed nondialyzed patients
- 1.3–1.5 g/kg/d for catabolic patients
- Up to 2.0 g pro/kg/d with CRRT

Fluids

- Urine output plus 500 ml for insensible loss
- With vomiting, diarrhea, give additional fluid
- Follow daily weights
- Up to 3 liters in diuretic stage

Vitamins/Minerals/Electrolytes

- Vitamin C should be limited to < 100–200 mg/day
- Water-soluble vitamins should be supplemented
- Avoid vitamin A as levels are increased
- Other vitamin/mineral requirements are not well defined
- Electrolytes should be monitored for both dialyzed and nondialyzed patients

Oral Feedings

- High-calorie, and depending on provision of dialysis, high-protein supplements may be needed to meet nutritional needs
- Consistency modifications as indicated

Enteral Nutrition

- Enteral route should be used whenever possible
- For patients undergoing CRRT, calorically-dense, renal-specific, or standard high-protein formulas may be used, depending on electrolyte levels, fluid balance
- Advance rate over 24–48 hours

Parenteral Nutrition

- Balanced solution of macronutrients
- Daily electrolyte monitoring and fluid balance
- Frequent blood glucose monitoring; may need insulin added to TPN
- Trace mineral requirements have not been defined in uremic patients receiving TPN, and are probably not necessary, with the exception of zinc and iron

Outcome

- Decreased protein catabolism and wasting of lean body mass
- Prevented overhydration
- Minimized accumulation of nitrogenous wastes in the blood
- Maintained electrolytes, glucose within goal ranges

NEPHROTIC SYNDROME

Description

Nephrotic syndrome is a complex of symptoms caused by increased glomerular permeability resulting in loss of plasma proteins into the urine. It is characterized by proteinuria (> 3 g/d), lipuria, hypoalbuminemia, hypercholesterolemia, and edema.

Cause

Includes:

- Diabetes mellitus
- Glomerulonephritis
- Renal vein thrombosis

Assessment

Anthropometrics

- Height
- Weight gain or loss
- BMI
- TSF/MAC (without edema)

Laboratory

- Serum albumin
- Serum prealbumin

- Serum cholesterol and lipid profile
- Serum calcium
- Serum phosphorus
- 24-hour urinary protein
- GFR

Diet History

- Assess calorie, protein, sodium, lipid intake
- Dietary recall: assess for adequacy and compliance with protein, sodium, fluid, calories, lipid intake
- Tolerance to oral diet (taste changes, nausea/vomiting/diarrhea/constipation)
- Vitamin/mineral, herbal, or other supplements
- Nutrient/drug interactions
- Assess knowledge of disease state and diet guidelines

Social History

- Assess for financial or psychosocial barriers to adequate intake
- Religious or ethnic beliefs
- Potential risk factors for malnutrition
  1. Lives alone
  2. Inadequate income
  3. Unable to buy own food
  4. Inadequate refrigeration or cooking facilities
  5. Alcohol/drug addiction

Physical Exam

- Edema
- Nutritional deficiencies
- Decubitus ulcer(s)
- Muscle/fat stores

SGA

Problems

- Proteinuria
  1. Average daily losses 6–8 g daily, leads to catabolism of lean body mass
- Dyslipidemia leading to atherosclerosis
  1. Elevated total cholesterol, LDL, VLDL
  2. HDL levels are unaffected or reduced
- Anorexia

- Urinary losses of vitamins and trace elements that are protein bound (Vitamin D, iron, zinc)
- Edema
- Loss of immunglobulin can increase infection risk
- Loss of transferrin can lead to anemia
- Hypocalcemia
- Hypovitaminosis D

Treatment/Management

Nutrition counseling should focus on appropriate protein, calorie, lipid, and sodium intake

Protein

- Diets high in protein increase renal injury
- Protein-restricted diets decrease progression of renal failure
- 0.7–1.0 g protein/kg/day
- Soy protein may be less harmful

Energy

- 35 kcal/kg/day for weight maintenance
- 20–25 kcal/kg/day for weight loss
- 40–50 kcal/kg/day for weight gain

Lipids

- Low cholesterol/low saturated fat diet (NCEP guidelines)

Sodium

- Restrict with edema (60–90 mEq/day)

Vitamins/Minerals

- Supplement vitamin D, zinc, iron, copper, calcium with large amount of proteinuria or with documented deficiency
- Potassium and magnesium may need supplementation with diuretic use

Monitor Weight Daily

Outcome

- Controlled blood pressure
- Minimized edema
- Decreased urinary albumin loss

- Decreased protein malnutrition/prevented muscle catabolism
- Slowed progression of renal disease

KIDNEY STONES

Description

Kidney stones are the concentration of components in the urine reaches a level in which crystallization occurs. Stones that are composed of calcium salts (calcium oxalate and calcium phosphate) are more responsive to dietary modifications, whereas uric acid, cystine, or struvite calculi are less responsive.

Cause

Includes:

- Bowel disease causing malabsorption
- Cysteinuria
- Glucocorticoid excess
- Hyperparathyroidism
- Paget's disease
- Recurrent urinary tract infections

Table 3–35 Nutrition Therapy for Calcium Urolithiasis

Dietary Component	Modification	Rationale
Fluid	3 L taken in divided doses throughout the day; 50% of total volume from water	Ensure minimum urine output of 2 L/day; reduce risk of recurrent urolithiasis
Sodium	100–150 mEq (mmol)/d in presence of hypercalciuria	Promote decrease in urinary calcium excretion; prevent supersaturation of urine with calcium salts
Calcium	800 mg/d (20 mmol/d) in presence of absorptive hypercalciuria; 1200 mg/d (30 mmol/d) in pregnant and lactating women; 1200–1500 mg/d (30–37.4 mmol/d) in post-menopausal women; 1000 mg/d (25 mmol/d) in presence of idiopathic hypercalciuria with normal intestinal absorption of calcium	Decrease urinary calcium excretion; use simultaneously with oxalate restriction to prevent excessive oxalate excretion
Oxalate	50–60 mg/d; limit intake of foods high in bioavailable oxalate; used simultaneously with calcium-restricted regimens (800–1000 mg/d, 20–25 mmol/d)	Prevent hyperoxaluria; decrease supersaturation of urine with calcium oxalate crystals; prevent stimulus of increased oxalate excretion that occurs when calcium intake is restricted
Protein	Moderate intake (0.8–1.0 g/kg/d); encourage consumption of vegetable protein sources; reduce consumption of animal protein sources rich in purines	Prevent increased susceptibility to recurrent calcium urolithiasis; animal protein sources have greater impact on increasing urinary risk factors; decrease urinary acid excretion

© 2000, American Dietetic Association. *Manual of Clinical Dietetics*, 6e. Used with permission.

- Vitamin D intoxication
- Excessive vitamin C ingestion

Assessment

Diet History

- Assess for fluid intake, excess intake of calcium, oxalate, protein, vitamin C

Problems

- Extremely painful when passing through the ureters
- Stone can block urine flow or cause infection or kidney damage

Treatment/Management

See Table 3–35

- Large volume of oral fluid intake, to produce > 2 liters urine per day; the goal is to keep the urine dilute to prevent crystallization
- Avoid excessive doses of vitamin C which metabolizes to oxalate
- There may be benefit in limiting protein intake to RDI

Outcome

- Reduced intake of stone-forming materials
- Decreased recurrence of stones
- Maintained dilute urine

REFERENCES

Alfrey AC, Hammond WS. Renal Iron Handling in the Nephrotic Syndrome. *Kidney Int.* 1990;37:1409–1413.

Allman A, et al. Energy Supplementation and Nutritional Status of Hemodialysis Patients. *Am J Clin Nutr.* 1990; 51:558–562.

Alvestrand A. Protein Metabolism and Nutrition in Hemodialysis. *Contrib Nephrol.* 1990;78:102–118.

American Diabetes Association. Diabetic Nephropathy Position Statement. *Diabetes Care.* 2003;26(supplement 1).

American Dietetic Association. Nutrition Recommendations and Principles for People with Diabetes Mellitus. *J Am Diet Assoc.* 1994;94:504–506.

Ames M, Bayne C, et al. Renal Disease. In: Pemberton CM, Moxness KE, et al., eds. *Mayo Clinic Diet Manual.* 6th ed. Toronto, Ontario: BC Decker, Inc; 1988:212–255.

Askanazi J, Rosenbaum SH, et al. Respiratory Changes Induced By the Large Glucose Loads of Total Parenteral Nutrition. *JAMA.* 1980;243:1444–1447.

Auwerx J, DeKeyser L, et al. Decreased Free 1,25 Dihydroxycholecalciferol Index in Patients with Nephrotic Syndrome. *Nephron.* 1986;42:231–235.

Barak N, Wall-Alonso E, Sitrin MD. Evaluation of stress factors and body weight adjustments currently used to estimate energy expenditure in hospitalized patients. *JPEN.* 2002;26:231–238

Bergstrom J. Nutritional Requirements of Hemodialysis Patients. In: Mitch WE, Klahr S eds. Boston, MA: Little, Brown & Co.; 1993:263–289.

Blake PG, Sombolos K, Abraham G, et al. Lack of Correlation Between Urea Kinetic Indicies and Clinical Outcomes in CAPD Patients. *Kidney Int.* 1991;37:700–706.

Block GA, Hulbert-Shearon TE, Levin NW, et al. Association of Serum Phosphorus and Calcium × Phosphate Product with Mortality Risk in Chronic Hemodialysis Patients: A National Study. *Am J Kid Dis.* 1998;31:607–617.

Blumenkrantz MJ, et al. Methods for Assessing Nutritional Status of Patients with Renal Failure. *Am J Clin Nutr.* 1980;33:1567–1585.

Blumenkrantz MJ, Gahl GM, et al. Protein Losses During Peritoneal Dialysis. *Kidney Int.* 1981;19:593–602.

Blumenkrantz MJ, Kopple JD, et al. Nitrogen Metabolism and Urea Kinetics in Patients Undergoing Continuous Ambulatory Peritoneal Dialysis. *Kidney Int.* 1979;16:882.

Blumenkrantz MJ, Kopple JD, et al. Metabolic Balance Studies and Dietary Protein Requirements in Patients Undergoing Continuous Ambulatory Peritoneal Dialysis. *Kidney Int.* 1982;21:849–861.

Bodnar DM. An Update on Peritoneal Dialysis and Nutrition. *Support Line.* 1993;15:5–8.

Bodnar DM, Busch S, Fuchs J, et al. Estimating Glucose Absorption in Peritoneal Dialysis Using Peritoneal Equilibration Tests. *Adv Peritonal Dial.* 1993;9:114–118.

Bosch JP. Continuous Arteriovenous Hemofiltration: Operational Characteristics and Clinical Use. *AKF Nephrology Letter.* 1986;3:15.

Bostom AG, Shmin D, Verhoef P, et al. Elevated Fasting Total Plasma Homocysteine Levels and Cardiovascular Disease Outcomes in Maintenance Dialysis Patients: A Prospective Study. *Arterioscler Thromb Vasc Biol.* 1997; 17:2554–2558.

Bouffard Y, et al. Energy Expenditure in the Acute Renal Failure Patient Mechanically Ventilated. *Intens Care Med.* 1987;13:401–404.

Brodsky IG, Robbins DC, et al. Effects of Low Protein Diets On Protein Metabolism in Insulin-Dependent Diabetes

Mellitus Patients With Early Nephropathy. *J Clin Endocrinol Metab.* 1992;75:351.

Brown WW, Wolfson M. Diet As Culprit or Therapy; Stone Disease, Chronic Renal Failure, and Nephrotic Syndrome. *Med Clinics NA.* 1993;77:783–794.

Burrows JD, Cockram DB, et al. Cross-sectional Relationship Between Dietary Protein and Energy Intake, Nutritional Status, Functional Status, and Comorbidity in Older versus Younger Hemodialysis Patients. *J Renal Nutrition.* 2002;12(2):87–95.

Burrowes JD, Levin NW. Morbidity and Mortality in Dialysis Patients. *Dietetic Currents.* 1992;19:1–4.

Carvounis CD, et al. Nutritional Status of Maintenance Hemodialysis Patients. *Amer J Clin Nutr.* 1986;43:946–954.

Chan MK, et al. Lipid Abnormalities in Uremia. *Kidney Int.* 1981;19:625–634.

Charney P, Charney D. Nutrition Support in Acute Renal Failure. In: Shikora SA, Martindale RG, Schwaitzberg SD, eds. *Nutritional Considerations in the Intensive Care Unit, Science Rational and Practice.* Dubuque, IA: Kendall/Hunt Publishing Co., 2002:209–217.

Chicago Dietetic Assocation, South Suburban Dietetic Association, Dietitians of Canada. Renal Failure, *Manual of Clinical Dietetics,* 6th ed. Chicago, IL: American Dietetic Association; 2000.

Crockcroft DW, Gault MH. Prediction of Creatinine Clearance from Serum Creatinine. *Nephron.* 1976;16:31–41.

D'Amico G, Remuzzi G, et al. Effect of Dietary Proteins and Lipids in Patients with Membranous Nephropathy and Nephrotic Syndrome. *Clin Nephrology.* 1991; 35:237–242.

Davis SP, Reaveley DA, et al. Amino Acid Clearances and Daily Losses in Patients with Acute Renal Failure Treated by Continuous Arteriovenous Hemofiltration. *Crit Care Med.* 1991;19:1510–1515.

Depner TA, Daugirdas JT: Equations for Normalized Protein Catabolic Rate Based On Two-Point Modeling of Hemodialysis Urea Kinetics. *J Am Soc Nephrol.* 7:780–785. 1996.

Dietch EA, Winterton J, Berg R. The Gut As a Portal of Entry for Bacteremia. *Ann Surg.* 1987;205:681–692.

Druml W. Nutritional Support in Acute Renal Failure. In: Mitch WE, Klahr S, eds. *Nutrition and the Kidney.* 2nd ed. Boston, MA: Little Brown & Co; 1993:314–345.

Dwyer J, Kenler SR. Assessment of Nutritional Status in Renal Disease. In: Mitch WE, Klahr S, eds. *Nutrition and the Kidney.* 2nd ed. Boston, MA: Little Brown & Co; 1993:61–89.

Evanoff G, et al. Prolonged Dietary Protein Restriction in Diabetic Nephropathy. *Arch Intern Med.* 1989; 149:1129–1133.

Feinstein EI, Blumenkrantz MJ, et al. Clinical and Metabolic Responses to Parenteral Nutrition in Acute Renal Failure. *Medicine.* 1981;60:124–137.

Feinstein EI, Kopple JD, et al. Total Parenteral Nutrition with High or Low Nitrogen Intakes in Patients with Acute Renal Failure. *Kidney Int.* 1983;26:S319–S323.

Fleming LW, et al. The Effect of Oral Aluminum Therapy on Plasma Aluminum Levels in Patients with Chronic Renal Failure in an Area with Low Water Aluminum. *Clin Nephrol.* 1982;17:222.

Food and Nutrition Board of the Institutes of Medicine. *Dietary Reference Intakes, 1997, 1998, 2000, 2001.* www.nap.edu.

Foulks CJ. An Evidence-based Evaluation of Intradilytic Parenteral Nutrition. *Am J Kid Dis.* 1999;33:186–192.

Frankenfeld DC, Muth ER, Rowe WA. The Harris-Benedict Studies of Human Basal Metabolism: History and Limitations. *J Am Diet Assoc.* 1998;98:439–445.

Franz MJ, Horton ES, et al. Nutrition Principles for the Management of Diabetes and Related Complications (Technical Review). *Diabetes Care.* 1994;17:490–518.

Gilmore ER, Hartley GH, Goodship THJ. Trace elements and vitamins in renal disease. In: Mitch WE, Klahr S, eds. *Handbook of Nutrition and the Kidney.* 3rd ed. Philadelphia, PA: Lippincott-Raven Publishers; 1998:107–122.

Glynn CC, Greene GW, Winkler MF, Albina JE. Predictive vs. Measure Energy Expenditure Using Limits-of-Agreement Analysis in Hospitalized, Obese Patients. *JPEN.* 1999;23:147–154.

Goldfarb S. Dietary Factors in the Pathogenesis and Prophlaxis of Calcium Nephrolithiasis. *Kidney Int.* 1988;34:544–555.

Golper TA. Continuous Arteriovenous Hemofiltration in Acute Renal Failure. *Am J Kid Dis.* 1985;6:373–386.

Grant A, Dehoog S. History and Anthropometry. In: Grant A, Dehoog S, eds. *Nutrition Assessment and Support.* 3rd ed./rev. Seattle, WA: Anne Grant and Susan Dehoog Publishers; 1985:1–18.

Grodstein GP, Blumenkrantz MJ, et al. Glucose Absorption During Continuous Ambulatory Peritoneal Dialysis. *Kidney Int.* 1981;19:564–567.

Grodstein GP, Kopple JD. Urea Nitrogen Appearance, A Simple and Practical Indicator of Total Nitrogen Output. *Kidney Int.* 1979;16:953.

Holmes J. Intradialytic Parenteral Nutrition. *Contemp Dial and Nephr.* 1990;4:50–53.

Hostetter TH, Mitch WE. Protein Intake and the Prevention of Chronic Renal Disease. In: Schrier RW, Gottschalk CW, eds. *Diseases of the Kidney.* 5th ed. Boston, MA: Little Brown & Co; 1993:3131–3149.

Ireton-Jones CS, Jones JD. Improved Equations for Predicting Energy Expenditure in Patients: The Ireton-Jones Equations. *Nutr Clin Prac.* 2002;17:29–31.

Joven J, Villabona C, et al. Abnormalities of Lipoprotein Metabolism in Patients with Nephrotic Syndrome. *N Engl J Med.* 1990;323:579–584.

Kaysen GA. The Nephrotic Syndrome: Nutritional Consequences and Dietary Management. In: Mitch WE, Klahr S, eds. *Handbook of Nutrition and the Kidney.* 3rd ed. Philadelphia, PA: Lippincott-Raven Publishers; 1998: 201–212.

Kaysen GA, Ganbertoglio J, et al. Effect of Dietary Protein Intake on Albumin Homeostasis in Nephrotic Patients. *Kidney Int.* 1986;29:572–577.

Klahr S, Levey AS, et al. The Effects of Dietary Protein Restriction and Blood Pressure Control on the Progression of Chronic Renal Disease. *N Eng J Med.* 1994; 330:877–884.

Kopple JD. Nutritional Status of Patients with Different Levels of Chronic Renal Failure. *Kidney Int.* 1989; 27:S184–S194.

Kopple JD. Dietary Considerations in Patients with Advanced Chronic Renal Failure, Acute Renal Failure and Transplantation. In: Schrier RW, Gottschalk CW, eds. *Diseases of the Kidney.* 5th ed. Boston, MA: Little Brown & Co; 1993:3167–3210.

Kopple JD. Nutrition, Diet and the Kidney. In: Shils M, Olson J, Shike M, eds. *Modern Nutrition in Health and Disease.* 8th ed. Philadelphia, PA: Lea & Ferbiger; 1994:1110–1134.

Kopple JD, Hirschberg R. Nutrition and Peritoneal Dialysis. In: Mitch WE, Klahr S, eds. *Nutrition and the Kidney.* 2nd ed. Boston, MA: Little Brown & Co; 1993:290–311.

Kopple JD, Monteon FJ, Shaib JK. Effect of Energy Intake on Nitrogen Metabolism in Non-Dialyzed Patients with Chronic Renal Failure. *Kidney Int.* 1986;29:734.

Kopple JD, Swendseid ME. Evidence that Histidine is an Essential Amino Acid in Normal and Chronically Uremic Man. *J Clin Invest.* 1975;55:881.

Krumlovsky, FA. Disorders of Protein and Lipid Metabolism Associated With Chronic Renal Failure and Chronic Dialysis. *Ann Clin Lab Sci.* 1981;11:350–360.

Lau YK, Wasserstein AG, et al. Proximal Tubular Defects in Idiopathic Hypercalcuria: Resistance to Phosphate Administration. *Miner Electrolyte Metab.* 1982;7:f237–249.

Lazarus JM. Recommended Criteria for Initiating and Discontinuing Intradialytic Parenteral Nutrition Therapy. *Am J Kid Dis.* 1999;33:211–216.

Leavey SF, Strawderman RD, Jones CA, Port FK, Held PJ. Simple Nutritional Indicators as Independent Predictors of Mortality in Hemodialysis Patients. *Am J Kid Dis.* 1998;31:997–1006.

Legrain M, Rottembourg J. Peritoneal Dialysis in Diabetics. In: Nolph KD, ed. *Peritoneal Dialysis.* Boston, MA: M. Nijhoff; 1985:506.

Levey AS, Adler S, Caggiula AW, et al. Effects of Dietary Protein Restriction on the Progression of Advanced Renal Disease in the Modifcation of Diet in Renal Disease Study. *Am J Kid Dis.* 1996;27(5):652–663.

Levey AS, Bosch JP, Lewis JB, Greene T, Rogers N, Roth D.: A More Accurate Method to Estimate Glomerular Filtration Rate from Serum Creatinine: A New Prediction Equation. Modification of Diet in Renal Disease Study Group. *Ann Intern Med.* 1999;130:461–470.

Levey AS, Greene T, Kusek JW, Beck GJ. A Simplified Equation to Predict Glomerular Filtration Rate from Serum Creatinine. *J Am Soc Nephrol.* 2000;11:A0828 (abstr).

Libetta C, DeNicola L, Rampino T, et al. Inflammatory Effects of Peritoneal Dialysis: Evidence of Systemic Monocyte Activation. *Kid International.* 1996;49:506–511.

Lowrie EG, Lew NL. Death Risk in Hemodialysis Patients. *Am J Kidney Dis.* 1990;15:458–482.

Macias WL, Alaka KJ, et al. Impact of the Nutritional Regimen on Protein Catabolism and Nitrogen Balance in Patients with Acute Renal Failure. *JPEN.* 1996;20:56–62.

Madigan KM, Olshan A, Yingling DJ. Effectiveness of Intradialytic Parenteral Nutrition in Diabetic Patients With End-Stage Renal Disease. *J Am Diet Assoc.* 1990; 9:861–863.

Mai ML, Emmett M, et al. Calcium Acetate, an Effective Phosphorus Binder in Patients With Renal Failure. *Kidney Int.* 1989;36:690–695.

Makoff R, et al. Folic Acid, Pyridoxine, Cobalmin, and Homocysteine and Their Relationship to Cardiovascular Disease in End-Stage Renal Disease. *J Renal Nutr.* 1996; 6:2–11.

Makoff R, Gonick H. Renal Failure and the Concomitant Derangement of Micronutrient Metabolism. *Nutr Clin Prac.* 1999;14:238–246.

Mansy H, Goodship THJ, et al. Effect of a High Protein Diet in Patients with Nephrotic Syndrome. *Clin Science.* 1989;77:445–451.

Marckmann P. Nutritional Status and Mortality of Patients in Regular Dialysis Therapy. *J Inter Med.* 1989; 26:429–432.

Maroni JB. Requirements for Protein, Calories and Fat in the Predialysis Patient. In: Mitch WE, Klahr S, eds. *Nutrition and the Kidney.* 2nd ed. Boston, MA: Little Brown & Co; 1993:185–212.

Maroni BJ, Mitch WE. Role of Nutrition in Prevention of the Progression of Renal Disease. *Annu Rev Nutr.* 1997; 17:435–455.

Massry SG, Kopple JD. Requirements for Calcium, Phosphorus and Vitamin D. In: Mitch WE, Klahr S, eds. *Nutrition and the Kidney.* 2nd ed. Boston, MA: Little Brown & Co; 1993:96–110.

McCann L. Nutrition Management of the Adult Peritoneal Dialysis Patient. In: Stover J, ed. *A Clinical Guide to Nutrition Care in End-Stage Renal Disease.* 2nd ed. Chicago, IL: American Dietetic Association; 1994:45.

Mitch WE, May RC, et al. Influence of Insulin Resistance and Amino Acid Supply on Muscle Protein Turnover. *Kidney Int.* 1987;32(suppl 22):104–108.

Monson P, Mehta RL. Nutritional Considerations in Continuous Renal Replacement Therapies. *Seminars in Dialysis.* 1996;9:152–160.

Nath KA, Hostetter TH. Nutritional Requirements of Diabetics with Nephropathy. In: Mitch WE, Klahr S, eds. *Nutrition and the Kidney.* 2nd ed. Boston, MA: Little Brown & Co; 1993:152–184.

National Cholesterol Education Program. Executive Summary of the Third Report of the National Cholesterol Education Program (NCEP). Expert Panel on Detection, Evaluation, and Treatment of High Blood Cholesterol in Adults (Adult treatment panel III). *JAMA.* 2001; 285(19):2486–2497.

National Kidney Foundation. Kidney Disease Outcomes Quality Initiative (K/DOQI). 2000. http://www.kidney. org/professionals/doqi/index.cfm.

National Kidney Foundation. K/DOQI Clinical Practice Guidelines for Chronic Kidney Disease: Evaluation, Classification and Stratification. *Am J Kidney Dis.* 2002;39: S1–S000. (suppl 1).

Norwood K. An Expanded Role For the Dietitian in the Treatment of Renal Osteodystrophy and Secondary Hyperparathyroidism. *Contemp Dial and Neph.* 1987; 8:22–26.

Pagenkemper JJ. Attaining Nutritional Goals for Hyperlipidemic and Obese Renal Patients. In: *Renal Nutrition, Report of the Eleventh Ross Roundtable on Medical Issues.* Columbus, OH: Ross Laboratories; 1991:26–33.

Pak CYC, et al. Ambulatory Evaluation of Nephrolithiasis: Classification, Clinical Presentation and Diagnostic Criteria. *Am J Med.* 1980;69:19.

Pak CYC, et al. Evidence Justifying a High Fluid Intake in Treatment of Nephrolithiasis. *Ann Inter Med.* 1989; 93:36–39.

Panzetta G, Maschio G. Dietary Problems of the Dialysis Patient. *Blood Purif.* 1985;3:63–74.

Pecoits-Filho R, Barany P, et al. Interleukin-6 is an Independent Predictor of Mortality in Patients Starting Dialysis Treatment. *Nephrol Dial Transplant.* 2002;17: 1684–2168.

Powers DV. Prolonged Experience with Intradialytic Hyperalimentation in Marasmic Chronic Hemodialysis Patients, An Overview. *Contemp Dial and Nephr.* 1989;5:22–28.

Rocco MV, Makoff R. Approprite vitamin therapy for dialysis patients. *Semin Dial.* 1997;10:272–277.

Sargent J, Gotch F, et al. Urea Kinetics: A Guide to Nutritional Management of Renal Failure. *Am J Clin Nutr.* 1978;31:1696–1702.

Schmitz O. Insulin-Mediated Glucose Uptake in Non-Dialyzed and Dialyzed Uremic Insulin-Dependant Diabetic Subjects. *Diabetes.* 1985;34:1152.

Schneeweiss B, Graininger W, et al. Energy Metabolism in Acute and Chronic Renal Failure. *Am J Clin Nutr.* 1990;52:596.

Schrier RW. Acute Renal Failure. *JAMA.* 1982;247: 2518–2525.

Seidner DL, Mascioli EA, et al. Effect of Long-Chain Triglyceride Emulsions on Reticuloendothelial System Function in Humans. *JPEN.* 1989;6:614–619.

Stec J, Podracka L, et al. Zinc and Copper Metabolism in Nephrotic Syndrome. *Nephron.* 1990;56:186–187.

Warwick GL, Caslake MJ, et al. Low-Density Lipoprotein Metabolism in the Nephrotic Syndrome. *Metabolism.* 1990;39:187–192.

Wiggins KL. *Guidelines for Nutrition Care of Renal Patients.* 3rd ed. Chicago, IL: Renal Dietitans Dietetic Practice Group, American Dietetic Association, 2002.

Wolfson M, Jones MR, Kopple JD. Amino Acid Losses During Hemodialysis with Infusion of Amino Acids and Glucose. *Kidney Int.* 1981;21:500–506.

Zeller K, et al. Effect of Restricting Dietary Protein on the Progression of Renal Failure in Patients with Insulin-Dependant Diabetes Mellitus. *N Eng J Med.* 1991;324: 78–84.

Zeller KR. Low Protein Diets in Renal Disease. *Diabetes Care.* 1991;14:856–866.

Solid Organ Transplantation

Jeanette M. Hasse, PhD, RD, FADA, CNSD

DESCRIPTION

Solid organ transplantation is a viable option for individuals suffering from end-stage organ failure that is refractory to medical or surgical treatment. The majority of donor organs are cadaveric (from a brain-dead donor). However, living donors can donate a kidney, or a portion of his/her lung or liver, to a designated recipient.

Living donors exceeded cadaveric donors for the first time in the year 2002.

TYPES OF ORGAN TRANSPLANTATION

- heart
- kidney
- liver

Table 3–36 Objective Parameters Used to Help Determine Nutritional Status

Parameter	Confounding Factors
Laboratory Measures	
Serum albumin	Hydration; albumin infusion; liver function; administration of corticosteroids; renal insufficiency; zinc deficiency; burn; loss through skin, GI tract, or wound; blood loss
Serum transferrin	Hydration, liver function, iron deficiency or overload, zinc deficiency, increased excretion such as burns or nephrotic syndrome
Serum thyroxine-binding prealbumin	Hydration, liver function, renal function, infection
Serum retinol-binding protein	Hydration, renal failure, vitamin A supplementation or deficiency, hyperthyroidism, cystic fibrosis
Total lymphocyte count	Immunosuppressive medication, infection, cancer, liver disease, kidney failure, trauma
Glycosylated hemoglobin	Uremia, aspirin intake, alcoholism, anemia
Anthropometric Measures	
Body weight	Hydration
Tricep skinfolds	Hydration, age, evaluator's technique, insensitive measurement (i.e., small changes over a short period of time are difficult to detect)
Midarm circumference	Hydration, evaluator's technique, insensitive measurement (i.e., small changes over a short period of time are difficult to detect)
Other Objective Measures	
Skin antigen testing	Immunosuppressive medication
Creatinine-height index	Liver and renal function, aging, protein intake
Nitrogen balance	Renal function, protein intake, other sites of losses (e.g., ostomy, chest tubes)
3-methylhistidine excretion	Age, gender, protein intake, renal function, infection
Indirect calorimetry	Measurement will vary with changes in patient condition

- lung
- pancreas (and islet cells)
- small bowel

NUTRITIONAL ASSESSMENT

Objective Nutritional Assessment Parameters

Many objective parameters can be affected by symptoms of organ failure (e.g., fluid retention) or by organ failure itself (e.g., inability of the liver to synthesize serum proteins during failure). Table 3–36 shows factors that must be taken into consideration if objective parameters are used to help determine nutritional status.

Subjective Nutritional Assessment Parameters

Evaluating subjective parameters of nutritional status is vital to assess transplant patients. A patient's nutritional status usually can be determined using a combination of appropriate objective parameters and the Subjective Global Assessment technique. The evaluator should focus especially on persistent or recurring symptoms and findings of the physical examination. The primary confounding factors for obtaining subjective history is the ability of the patient to recall the information and the ability of the evaluator to do a brief physical assessment. The following areas should be covered:

- weight history (ask about weight changes due to fluid fluctuations)
- appetite history
- dietary history (current and recent dietary intake compared to estimated needs)
- gastrointestinal (GI) symptoms (duration and severity of nausea, vomiting, diarrhea, steatorrhea, constipation)
- ability to chew and swallow
- current diet restrictions
- use of dietary and/or vitamin and mineral supplements
- use of tube feeding or parenteral nutrition
- diabetes history
- alcohol usage

- social history
- coexisting diseases
- current medications
- physical exam (muscle, fat, edema, ascites)
- current physical functional capacity

PRETRANSPLANT PROBLEMS AND TREATMENT

See sections on organ failure: "Cardiology," "Gastroenterology," "Pulmonary Conditions," "Diabetes," and "Renal Conditions."

POSTTRANSPLANT PROBLEMS

Common nutritional problems during the short-term posttransplant phase (usually up to 2 months posttransplant) include:

- depressed appetite
- early satiety
- taste changes
- GI problems (nausea, vomiting, diarrhea, constipation)
- preexisting malnutrition

Common nutritional problems during the long-term posttransplant phase (usually more than 2 months posttransplant) include:

- increased appetite
- excessive weight gain
- hyperlipidemia
- hypertension
- diabetes
- osteoporosis

Medical complications can occur postoperatively. These complications influence nutrient needs and delivery. Complications include:

- Infection
  1. Nutrient needs may increase.
  2. Treatment with medications can cause anorexia, nausea, vomiting, or diarrhea.
- Rejection
  1. Treatment often involves administering additional corticosteroids which can cause hyperglycemia and increase nitrogen loss.

2. Persistent rejection may require the use of monoclonal antibodies (OKT3) or antithymocyte globulin, which can cause anorexia, nausea, vomiting, or diarrhea.

- Technical problems (e.g., bleeding, anastomotic leakages)
  1. If surgery is required to treat the problem, the patient may require a period of NPO status.
  2. If a patient is significantly malnourished, nutritional support should be considered.
- Renal insufficiency
  1. It may be necessary to restrict sodium, fluid, phosphorus, or potassium
  2. If dialysis is initiated, diet goals need to be adjusted
- Organ failure
  1. Refer to material on organ failure for review of nutritional needs during organ dysfunction.

Specific needs related to islet cell transplantation have not been elucidated. There are special nutritional considerations unique to small bowel transplant patients:

- Transit time
  1. Transit time can vary from 30 minutes to 5 hours (mean = 2 hours).
  2. A sudden change in transit time may suggest infection or rejection.
  3. Some transplant teams use paregoric, loperamide, pectin, or somatostatin to increase transit time after rejection is excluded.
- Malabsorption
  1. Lacteals and lymphatics are severed during transplant, resulting in malabsorption.
  2. Some carbohydrate enzymes are deficient in the early posttransplant phase.
  3. A lactose- and fat-restricted diet is better tolerated early posttransplant than a full liquid diet.
- Ostomy output
  1. Output can be as high as > 4 L/day.
  2. Fluid and electrolytes need to be replenished daily.
  3. Metabolic acidosis may occur and require treatment with sodium bicarbonate.

4. Zinc supplementation may be required with increased ostomy output.

Drug–Nutrient Interactions

Transplant recipients must take immunosuppressive medications to prevent rejection of their new organs. These drugs have multiple nutrient side effects (Table 3–37).

Table 3–37 Drug Side Effects

Drug	Common Side Effects
Antithymocyte globulin	Nausea, vomiting
Azathioprine	Nausea, vomiting, sore throat, anorexia Altered taste acuity
Basiliximab	No nutrition symptom known
Cyclosporine	Hyperlipidemia Hyperglycemia Hypomagnesemia Hyperkalemia
Daclizumab	No nutrition symptom known
Deoxyspergualin	GI symptoms
Glucocorticoids	Catabolism/impaired wound healing Hyperlipidemia Hyperglycemia Sodium retention Hyperphagia Increased calciuria
Muromonab CD3	Nausea, vomiting, diarrhea, anorexia
Mycophenolate mofetil	Diarrhea
Sirolimus	Hyperlipidemia Impaired wound healing
Tacrolimus	Hyperglycemia Hyperkalemia Nausea and vomiting

TREATMENT/MANAGEMENT

Short-Term Nutritional Management

Tube Feeding

Tube feeding is indicated when patients cannot eat adequately. Consider immediate postoperative tube feeding for liver transplant recipients.

- The feeding tube usually should be placed in the small bowel; patients are more likely to have delayed emptying from the stomach soon after the transplant.
- Nasointestinal tubes are appropriate when tube feeding is for a short duration.
- Tube feeding can be started within 12 hours after transplant (except in the case of small-bowel transplant).
- Tube feeding should be initiated at a low rate and increased gradually.
- Small-bowel transplant recipients may receive enteral feedings when signs of bowel function are present (output via terminal ileostomy), usually at 1–2 weeks posttransplant. Starting enteral feedings too early may contribute to ischemic necrosis of the graft.
- Ideal tube-feeding formulas should be isotonic with a high protein content. Concentrated formulas are available if fluid restriction is necessary. Low-potassium, low-phosphorus formulas are available if serum levels of these nutrients are elevated. An ideal formula for feeding small-bowel transplant recipients would be of low osmolality, with small peptides, glutamine, and medium-chain triglycerides.

Total Parenteral Nutrition (TPN)

- TPN is required initially for small-bowel transplant recipients; as enteral feedings are tolerated, TPN can be weaned.
- When rejection or infection is present in small-bowel transplant recipients, gut function tends to be decreased, and TPN may be required.
- For other types of organ transplant, TPN is reserved for malnourished patients without functioning GI tracts who will require nutrition support for at least 5 days.
- A TPN formula should be individualized based on macro- and micronutrient requirements as well as fluid needs.

Oral Feeding

- Small meals with snacks and/or supplements help patients achieve caloric and protein goals.
- Oral feedings may start as early as 12 hours posttransplant (kidney transplant); oral diets usually are allowed when patients are passing flatus and/or having bowel movements.
- Acceptance of oral diets may be poor in small-bowel transplant patients who have been TPN dependent for a long time.

Suggested Treatments for Nutritional Problems

- Decreased appetite, taste changes, early satiety
  1. Offer small, frequent meals and snacks.
  2. Offer alternative foods.
  3. Consider tube feeding.
- Diarrhea/constipation
  1. Rule out infectious causes of diarrhea. Rule out mechanical problems causing constipation.
  2. Review medications as a cause of GI disturbance.
  3. If possible, change drug.
  4. Adjust fiber and fluid intake.
- Nausea/vomiting
  1. Review medications as a cause of GI disturbance.
  2. Offer small, frequent meals and snacks.
  3. Offer alternative foods.
  4. Consider tube feeding.
- Increased loss of nitrogen secondary to corticosteroids
  1. Offer high-protein snacks, supplements.
  2. Use high-nitrogen tube-feeding formula.
- Renal insufficiency
  1. Adjust sodium, potassium, phosphorus, and fluid intake as needed.

Specific Guidelines for Short-Term Nutrient Goals

- *Calories:* 1.3–1.5 × basal energy expenditure (BEE) depending on goals (weight maintenance vs. weight gain)
- *Protein:* 1.5– 2.0 g/kg dry weight; requirement increases when corticosteroid dose is increased
- *Carbohydrate:* ∼ 50% of nonprotein calories
- *Fat:* ∼ 30% of nonprotein calories
- *Vitamins:* supplement to recommended dietary allowance (RDA); supplement those likely to be depleted due to preexisting disease
- *Minerals/electrolytes:* restrict sodium if edema or ascites is present; monitor serum potassium level and treat with restriction or supplementation if indicated; magnesium and phosphorus deplete rapidly; consider zinc losses via wounds, drains, or ostomy
- *Fluid:* monitor intake and output

Long-Term Nutritional Management

Weight Management

- Patients with a previous history of obesity are at highest risk of excessive weight gain.
- Counsel on appropriate caloric intake to achieve/maintain desirable body weight.
- Encourage regular aerobic exercise.
- Consider long-term behavioral and nutritional counseling when excess weight gain is expected to be a problem.

Hyperlipidemia

- Encourage a low-fat diet (less than 30% of calories as fat).
- Encourage the intake of monounsaturated oils and avoidance of trans fatty acids.
- Stress weight maintenance.
- Limit alcohol and simple sugars when serum triglyceride level is elevated.
- Encourage a high fiber intake (25–30 g fiber) including sources of soluble fiber.
- Consider use of medications (such as HMG-CoA reductase inhibitors) to treat hyperlipidemia.

- Hyperhomocysteinemia correlates with renal function and folate, vitamin B_6, and vitamin B_{12} status in kidney transplant recipients. Hyperhomocysteinemia may be an additional risk factor for arteriosclerosis in these patients.

Hypertension

- Stress weight maintenance.
- Impose moderate sodium restriction.
- Encourage calcium intake (1000–1500 mg/day).

Diabetes

- Instruct patients on an individualized carbohydrate-controlled diet.
- Stress weight maintenance.
- Encourage regular aerobic exercise.
- Instruct patients on self-monitoring of glucose and administration of medication.

Osteoporosis

- Encourage calcium intake of 1500 mg/day; supplement as needed.
- Consider hormone replacement for women past menopause.
- Encourage regular aerobic exercise.
- Discourage smoking.
- Consider use of bone-rebuilding medications such as alendronate sodium.

Specific Guidelines for Nutrient Goals

- *Calories:* 1.2–1.3 × BEE for maintenance; subtract calories for weight loss
- *Protein:* 0.8–1.0 g/kg
- *Carbohydrate:* 50% calories; carbohydrate-controlled diet for diabetes mellitus
- *Fat:* 25%–35% calories; less than 7%–10% calories as saturated fat; less than 300 mg cholesterol/day
- *Vitamins:* supplement to RDA with consideration to vitamins that may have been deficient prior to transplantation due to original disease.
- *Minerals/electrolytes:* supplement to RDA with consideration to calcium, magnesium,

phosphorus; hyperkalemia occurs 15%–30% of the time and may require a potassium-restricted diet.

- *Fluid:* moderate sodium restriction, adjust based on major shifts in fluid output.

PRECAUTION

Because all transplant patients are immuno-suppressed, they should avoid uncooked or undercooked meats and wash raw fruits and vegetables well. Grapefruit and grapefruit juice should be avoided. Naringin and aglycone naringenen are flavonoids in grapefruit. They inhibit cytochrome P450 enzymes and increase serum concentrations of cyclosporine and tacrolimus.

REFERENCES

Abbott WJ, Thomson A, Steadman C, et al. Child-Pugh class, nutritional indicators, and early liver transplant outcomes. *Hepato-Gastroenterology.* 2001;48:823–827.

Abu-Elmagd K, Reyes J, Bond G, et al. Clinical transplantation: A decade of experience at a single center. *Ann Surg.* 2001;234(3):404–417.

Arnadottir M, Hultberg B, Vladov V, et al. Hyperhomocysteinemia in cyclosporine-treated renal transplant recipients. *Transplantation.* 1996;61(3):509–512.

Arnadottir M, Hultberg B, Wahlberg J, et al. Serum total homocysteine concentration before and after renal transplantation. *Kidney Int.* 1998;54(4):1380–1384.

Baid S, Cosimi AB, Larrell ML, et al. Posttransplant diabetes mellitus in liver transplant recipients: Risk factors, temporal relationship with hepatitis C virus allograft hepatitis, and impact on mortality. *Transplantation.* 2001;72(6):1066–1072.

Bartucci MR, Hricik DE. Kidney transplantation. In: Cupples SA, Ohler L, eds. *Solid Organ Transplantation: A Handbook for Primary Health Care Providers.* New York: Springer; 2002:189–222.

Blue LS. Adult kidney transplantation. Overview and immunosuppression. In: Hasse JM, Blue LS, eds. *Comprehensive Guide to Transplant Nutrition.* Chicago, IL: American Dietetic Association; 2002:44–57.

Bostom AG, Gohh RY, Beaulieu AJ, et al. Treatment of hyperhomocysteinemia in renal transplant recipients: A randomized placebo-controlled trial. *Ann Intern Med.* 1997;127:1089–1092.

Caillard S, Leray C, Kunz K, et al. Effects of cerivastatin on lipid profiles, lipid peroxidation and platelet and endothelial activation in renal transplant recipients. *Transplant Proc.* 2000;32:2787–2788.

Canzanello VJ, Schwartz L, Taler SJ, et al. Evolution of cardiovascular risk after liver transplantation: A comparison of cyclosporine A and tacrolimus (FK506). *Liver Transpl Surg.* 1997;3(1):1–9.

DiCecco SR, Francisco-Ziller N, Moore D. Overview and immunosuppression. In: Hasse JM, Blue LS, eds. *Comprehensive Guide to Transplant Nutrition.* Chicago, IL: American Dietetic Association; 2002:1–30.

DiCecco S, Wieners EJ, Wiesner RH, et al. Assessment of nutritional status of patients with end-stage liver disease undergoing liver transplantation. *Mayo Clin Proc.* 1989;64:95–102.

Downey P, Maiz A, Vaccarezza A, et al. Renal transplantation and dyslipidemia: Characterization of a population and treatment with diet and low dose lovastatin. *Transplant Proc.* 1995;27(2):1803–1805.

Epstein S, Shane E, Bilezikian J. Organ transplantation and osteoprosis. *Current Opinions in Rheumatology.* 1995;7:255–261.

Everhardt J, Lonbardero M, Lake J, et al. Weight changes and obesity after liver transplantation: Incidence and risk factors. *Liver Transpl Surg.* 1998;4:285–296.

Fan SL, Almond MK, Ball E, et al. Pamidronate therapy as prevention of bone loss following renal transplantation. *Kidney Int.* 2000;57(2):684–690.

Fernández-Miranda C, de la Calle A, Morales JM, et al. Lipoprotein abnormalities in long-term stable liver and renal transplanted patients. A comparative study. *Clin Transplant.* 1998;12:136–141.

Figueiredo F, Dickson ER, Pasha T, et al. Impact of nutritional status on outcomes after liver transplantation. *Transplantation.* 2000;70(9):1347–1352.

Filler G, Neuschulz I, Vollmer I, et al. Tacrolimus reversibly reduces insulin secretion in pediatric renal transplant recipients. *Nephrology Dialysis Transplantation.* 2000;15:867–871.

Hasse J. Nutritional issues in adult solid organ transplantation. In: Cupples SA, Ohler L, eds. *Solid Organ Transplantation: A Handbook for Primary Health Care Providers.* New York: Springer; 2002:64–87.

Hasse JM. Adult liver transplantation. In: Hasse JM, Blue LS, eds. *Comprehensive Guide to Transplant Nutrition.* Chicago, IL: American Dietetic Association; 2002: 58–89.

Hasse JM. Nutrition assessment and support of organ transplant recipients. *JPEN.* 2001;25(3):120–131.

Hasse JM, Blue LS, Liepa GU, et al. Early enteral nutrition support in patients undergoing liver transplantation. *JPEN.* 1995;19:437–443.

Huh W, Kim B, Kim SJ, et al. Changes of fasting plasma total homocysteine in the early phase of renal transplantation. *Transplant Proc.* 2000;32:2811–2813.

Imagawa DK, Dawson S, Holt CD, et al. Hyperlipidemia after liver transplantation: Natural history and treatment with the hydroxy-methylglutaryl-coenzyme A reductase inhibitor pravastatin. *Transplantation.* 1996;62:934–942.

Janes S, Beath SV, Jones R, et al. Enteral feeding after intestinal transplantation: The Birmingham experience. *Transplant Proc.* 1997;29:1855–1856.

Jawad F, Rizvi SAH. Posttransplant diabetes mellitus in live-related renal transplantation. *Transplant Proc.* 2000:32:1888.

Jindal RM, Sidner RA, Hughes D, et al. Metabolic problems in recipients of liver transplants. *Clinical Transplant.* 1996;10:213–217.

Jindal RM, Sidner RA, Milgrom ML. Post-transplant diabetes mellitus: The role of immunosuppression. *Drug Safety.* 1997;16(4):242–257.

Katz IA, Epstein S. Posttransplant bone disease. *J Bone Min Res.* 1992;7:123–126.

Keogh JB, Tsalamandris C, Sewell RB, et al. Bone loss at the proximal femur and reduced lean mass following liver transplantation: A longitudinal study. *Nutrition.* 1999; 15:661–664.

Kim SI, Yoo TH, Song HY, et al. Hyperhomocysteinemia in renal transplant recipients with cyclosporine. *Transplant Proc.* 2000;32:1878–1879.

Knoll GA, Bell RC. Tacrolimus versus cyclosporine for immunosuppression in renal transplantation: Meta-analysis of randomized trials. *Br Med J.* 1999;318:1104–1107.

Kobashigawa JA, Kasiske BL. Hyperlipidemia in solid organ transplantation. *Transplantation.* 1997;63:331–338.

Leidig-Bruckner G, Hosch S, Dodidou P, et al. Frequency and predictors of osteoporotic fractures after cardiac or liver transplantation: A follow-up study. *Lancet.* 2001; 357(9253):342–347.

Ligtenberg G, Hene RJ, Blankestijn PJ, et al. Cardiovascular risk factors in renal transplant patients: Cyclosporine A versus tacrolimus. *J Am Soc Nephrol.* 2001;12(2): 368–373.

Lopes IM, Martín M, Errasti P, Martínez JA. Benefits of a dietary intervention on weight loss, body composition, and lipid profile after renal transplantation. *Nutrition.* 1999;15:7–10.

Lorenzetti M, Giannarelli R, Paleologo G, et al. Risk factors for cardiovascular disease in patients with functioning kidney grafts. *Transplant Proc.* 1998;30:2047.

MacDonald AS. Impact of immunosuppressive therapy on hypertension. *Transplantation.* 2000;70(11):SS70–SS76.

Malyszko JS, Malyszko J, Mysliwiec M. Serum lipids and hemostasis in kidney allograft recipients treated with fluvastatin (Lescol) for 3 months. *Transplant Proc.* 2000;32:1344–1346.

Martínez-Castelao A, Grinyó JM, Fiol C, et al. Fluvastatin and low-density lipoprotein oxidation in hypercholesterolemic renal transplant patients. *Kid Int.* 1999; 56(Suppl 71):S231–S234.

Martins L, Queirós J, Ferreira A, et al. Renal osteodistrophy: Histologic evaluation after renal transplantation. *Transplant Proc.* 2000;32:2599–2601.

McCune TR, Thacker LR, Peters TG, et al. Effects of tacrolimus on hyperlipidemia after successful renal transplantation. *Transplantation.* 1998;65(1):87–92.

Mehta PL, Alaka KJ, Filo RS, et al. Nutrition support following liver transplantation: A comparison of jejunal versus parenteral routes. *Clin Transplant.* 1995;344: 837–840.

Merritt WT. Metabolism and liver transplantation: Review of perioperative issues. *Liver Transplantation.* 2000;6(4, Suppl 1):S76–S84.

Mor E, Facklam D, Hasse J, et al. Weight gain and lipid profile changes in liver transplant recipients: Long-term results of the American FK506 multicenter study. *Transplant Proc.* 1995;27(1):1126.

Morena M, Vela C, Garrigue V, et al. Low-density lipoprotein composition and oxidation are not influenced by calcineurin inhibitors in renal transplant patients. *Transplant Proc.* 2000;32:2785–2786.

Nam J-H, Moon JI, Chung S-S, et al. Pamidronate and calcitriol trial for the prevention of early bone loss after renal transplantation. *Transplant Proc.* 2000;32:1876.

Navasa M, Bustamante J, Marroni C, et al. Diabetes mellitus after liver transplantation: Prevalence and predictive factors. *J Hepatol.* 1996;25:64–71.

Nisbeth U, Lindh E, Ljunghall S, et al. Increased fracture rate in diabetes mellitus and females after renal transplantation. *Transplantation.* 1999; 67(9):1218–1222.

Niv Y, Mor E, Tzakis AG. Small bowel transplantation: A clinical review. *Am J Gastroenterol.* 1999;94(11): 3126–3130.

Obayashi PA. Adult pancreas transplantation. In: Hasse JM, Blue LS, eds. *Comprehensive Guide to Transplant Nutrition.* Chicago, IL: American Dietetic Association; 2002: 90–105.

Pahwa N, Hedberg A. Adult heart and lung transplantation. In: Hasse JM, Blue LS, eds. *Comprehensive Guide to Transplant Nutrition.* Chicago, IL: American Dietetic Association; 2002:31–43.

Patel MG. The effect of dietary intervention on weight gains after renal transplantation. *J Renal Nutr.* 1998;8(3): 137–141.

Pescovitz MD, Mehta PL, Leapman SB, et al. Tube jejunostomy in liver transplant recipients. *Surgery.* 1995;117: 642–647.

Pikul J, Sharpe MD, Lowndes R, et al. Degree of preoperative malnutrition is predictive of postoperative morbidity and mortality in liver transplant recipients. *Transplantation.* 1994;57:469–472.

Plevak DJ, DiCecco SR, Wiesner RH, et al. Nutritional support for liver transplantation: Identifying caloric and protein requirements. *Mayo Clin Proc.* 1994;69:225–230.

Porayko MK, DiCecco S, O'Keefe SJ. Impact of malnutrition and its therapy on liver transplantation. *Semin Liv Dis.* 1991;11:305–314.

Porayko MK, Wiesner RH, Hay J, et al. Bone disease in liver transplant recipients: Incidence, timing, and risk factors. *Transplant Proc.* 1991;23:1462–1465.

Rayes N, Seehofer D, Hansen S, et al. Early enteral supply of lactobacillus and fiber versus selective bowel decontamination: A controlled trial in liver transplant recipients. *Transplantation.* 2002;74(1):123–127.

Reilly J, Mehta R, Teperman L, et al. Nutritional support after liver transplantation: A randomized prospective study. *JPEN.* 1990;14:386–391.

Riordan SM, Williams R. Nutrition and liver transplantation. *J Hepatol.* 1999;31:955–962.

Romero R, Calviño J, Rodriguez J, et al. Short-term effect of atorvastatin in hypercholesterolaemic renal-transplant patients unresponsive to other statins. *Nephrol Dial Transplant.* 2000;15:1446–1449.

Rovera GM, Graham TO, Hutson WR, et al. Nutritional management of intestinal allograft recipients. *Transplant Proc.* 1998;30:2517–2518.

Silva F, Queirós J, Vargas G, et al. Risk factors for posttransplant diabetes mellitus and impact of this complication after renal transplantation. *Transplant Proc.* 2000;32:2609–2610.

Stegall MD, Everson GT, Schroter G, et al. Prednisone withdrawal late after adult liver transplantation reduces diabetes, hypertension and hypercholesterolemia without causing graft loss. *Hepatology.* 1997;25:173–177.

Stein G, Muller A, Busch M, et al. Homocysteine, its metabolites, and B-group vitamins in renal transplant patients. *Kidney Int.* 2001;59(Suppl 78):262–265.

Strohm SL, Koehler AN, Mazariegos GV, et al. Nutrition management in pediatric small bowel transplant. *Nutr Clin Prac.* 1999;14:58–63.

Sudan DL, Iverson A, Weseman RA, et al. Assessment of function, growth and development, and long-term quality of life after small bowel transplantation. *Transplant Proc.* 2000;32:1211–1212.

Trautwein C, Possienke M, Schlitt H-J, et al. Bone density and metabolism in patients with viral hepatitis and cholestatic liver diseases before and after liver transplantation. *Am J Gastroenterol.* 2000;95:2343–2351.

Van Cleemput J, Daenen W, Nijs J, et al. Timing and quantification of bone loss in cardiac transplant recipients. *Transpl Int.* 1995;8:196–200.

Vedi S, Greer S, Skingle SJ, et al. Mechanism of bone loss after liver transplantation: A histomorphometric analysis. *J Bone Min Res.* 1999;14(2):281–287.

Weseman RA. Adult small bowel transplantation. In: Hasse JM, Blue LS, eds. *Comprehensive Guide to Transplant Nutrition.* Chicago, IL: American Dietetic Association; 2002:106–122.

Westeel FP, Mazouz K, Ezaitouni F, Hottelart C, et al. Cyclosporine bone remodeling effect prevents steroid osteopenia after kidney transplantation. *Kidney Int.* 2000;58:1788–1796.

Wheeler DC, Steiger J. Evolution and etiology of cardiovascular diseases in renal transplant recipients. *Transplantation.* 2000;70(11 Suppl):S541–S545.

Wicks C, Somasundaram S, Buarnason I, et al. Comparison of enteral feeding and total parenteral nutrition after liver transplantation. *Lancet.* 1994;344:837–840.

Wissing KM, Abramowicz D, Broeders N, et al. Hypercholestolemia is associated with increased kidney loss caused by chronic rejection in male patients with previous acute rejection. *Transplantation.* 2000;70(3):464–472.

Yagi M, Sakamoto K, Inoue T, et al. Effect of a glutamine-enriched elemental diet on regeneration of the small bowel mucosa following isotransplantation of small intestine. *Transplant Proc.* 1994;26:2297–2298.

CHAPTER 4

Nutrition Support

- Enteral Nutrition
- Parenteral Nutrition
- Transitional Feeding

Enteral Nutrition

Elizabeth A. Lennon, MS, RD, LD, CNSD, PA-S
and Laura E. Matarese, MS, RD

DESCRIPTION

Enteral nutrition (EN) is the delivery of nutrients through the gastrointestinal (GI) tract.

RATIONALE/BENEFITS

- Absorption of nutrients through the GI tract, with subsequent delivery to the liver, may better support hepatic transport protein synthesis, regulation of metabolic processes, and enhancement of immune competence.
- Enteral nutrition prevents intestinal atrophy.
- Delivery of nutrients through the GI tract may prevent the translocation of bacteria into systemic circulation.
- Although EN is not without potential complications, it is generally considered to be safer than parenteral nutrition.
- EN is generally more convenient than parenteral nutrition (PN).
- EN is less expensive than PN.

INDICATIONS

- The GI tract must be functional, accessible, and safe to use as indicated by

1. a normal abdominal exam (i.e., abdomen is soft, nontender, and nondistended)
2. normal upper-GI and small-bowel X-rays.
3. presence of flatus or bowel movement
4. presence of bowel sounds
5. hunger
6. absence of vomiting or uncontrolled diarrhea
- The individual is adequately nourished, with anticipation of nil per os (NPO) or inadequate intake greater than 7–9 days
- The individual is malnourished, with anticipation of NPO or inadequate intake greater than 5–7 days.

CONTRAINDICATIONS/RELATIVE CONTRAINDICATIONS

- Nonfunctioning GI tract
- Mechanical obstruction of the GI tract
- Prolonged ileus
- Intractable vomiting or diarrhea
- Upper-GI hemorrhage
- Requirement for bowel rest
- High risk for aspiration or severe GERD
- Adequate oral intake
- High output proximal fistula

ENTERAL ROUTE

- The route of administration is determined by GI anatomy and function, risk of aspiration, and anticipated duration of therapy.
- Nasoenteric tubes are used for short-term therapy, generally 4–6 weeks.
  1. Nasogastric tubes are indicated for patients with an intact gag reflex and normal gastric emptying.
  2. Nasoduodenal or nasojejunal tubes are used for patients at risk for aspiration or with impaired gastric emptying.
- Percutaneous or surgically placed feeding tubes are indicated for long-term therapy since they are more comfortable and less conspicious. Types include
  1. percutaneous endoscopic gastrostomy (PEG)
  2. percutaneous endoscopic jejunostomy (PEJ)
  3. direct endoscopic jejunostomy (DEJ)
  4. surgical gastrostomy
  5. surgical jejunostomy
  6. needle catheter jejunostomy

ENTERAL FORMULAS

Enteral formulas are generally classified according to their composition and use (Table 4–1):

- *Polymeric formulas,* containing intact nutrients
- *Predigested formulas,* containing partially or completely hydrolyzed nutrients
- *Condition-specific formulas,* for use in organ dysfunction or specific metabolic conditions
- *Modular formulas,* for supplemental use or to create a formula for specific use

In selecting a formula, consider:

- limiting factors such as digestive or absorptive capabilities
- fluid requirements
- nutrient requirements
- whether fiber-containing formula is indicated
- the presence of metabolic abnormalities that necessitate the use of a specialized or modified formula
- route of administration
- formula availability and cost

ADMINISTRATION TECHNIQUES

- *Bolus:* Rapid delivery by syringe or feeding reservoir; 240–400 ml of formula is given every 4–8 hours.
- *Timed intermittent:* 100–400 ml of formula administered over 20–40 minutes every 2–4 hours.
- *Continuous:* Formula is delivered by infusion pump or gravity drip over 16–24 hours.
- *Cyclic:* Formula is infused over 8–16 hours, usually overnight by infusion pump, then discontinued in the morning.

MANAGEMENT OF COMPLICATIONS

Infectious

Pulmonary Aspiration

- Verify the location of the feeding tube tip by x ray before initiation of feedings.
- Elevate head of bed greater than 30–45 degrees.
- Use of measured gastric residual volume (GRV) alone is not adequate to assess risk of aspiration. Clinical assessment needs to accompany monitoring of GRVs. EN should be immediately stopped for overt regurgitation/aspiration or GRV of greater than 500 ml. EN may be continued with residuals less than 500 ml with close clinical monitoring and maintenance of aspiration precautions.
- Consider changing feeding schedule from bolus or intermittent to continuous feedings
- Consider prokinetic agents.
- Optimize oral hygiene
- Reassess the need for and dosage of sedating medications.
- Blue food coloring should not be added to EN formulas as a means to detect aspiration because of low sensitivity of this method and potential toxic effects, particularly in critically ill patients.

Table 4–1 Comparison of Enteral Feeding Formulas

Type	Description	Indications for Use	Advantages	Disadvantages
Standard	Nutritionally complete; low residue; lactose free; isotonic; 1.0 kcal/ml 80%–85% water	EN needs of most adults; supplement inadequate oral intake	Inexpensive; readily available	Requires normal digestion and absorption
Fiber-supplemented	Nutritionally complete; lactose free; fiber source mainly soy polysaccharide; contains 5–14 g fiber/1000 ml	Normalize bowel function; long-term feeding	May improve glycemic control	Adequate water needed to minimize gastrointestinal side effects
High nitrogen	Nutritionally complete; lactose free; low residue; protein > 15% total calories; 1.0 kcal/ml	Increased protein requirements	Increased protein content without increased caloric level	Increased renal solute load may increase water requirements
Concentrated	Nutritionally complete; lactose free; low residue; 1.2–2.0 kcal/ml 70%–80% water	Fluid restrictions; limited formula volume tolerance	Allows provision of energy and nutrient needs in a limited volume of formula	Hypertonic; lower percentage water may increase risk of dehydration; well tolerated in most patients
Condition-specific	Specific organ dysfunction and/or hypercatabolism	Renal failure; diabetes; respiratory failure; stress/trauma; hepatic failure; immune-enhancing	Alteration of macro- and micronutrients for clients with specific diseases	Higher cost; controversial efficacy
Predigested	Nutritionally complete; low residue; peptide and/or amino acid-based; very low fat content (1%–15% of calories); osmolality of 450–700 mOsm/kg of water; low in fat or fat mainly in form of MCT	Malabsorption; maldigestion transition from TPN to enteral nutrition	Easily digested and absorbed	Higher cost; less palatable; hypertonic
Modular	Single or multiple nutrients; carbohydrate, fat, or protein modules	Highly specialized nutrient requirements or specific intolerances; supplement to commercial enteral formulas	Can be tailored to individual client requirements	Increased risk of contamination; requires expertise in enteral feeding; increased labor costs; must add micronutrient preparation

- Consider small-bowel enteral feedings with simultaneous decompression of gastric contents.

Formula Contamination

- Use commercially prepared sterile formulas.
- Use clean technique.
- Hang feedings for no longer than 8 hours unless using a closed feeding system.
- Change administration container and tubing every 24 hours.
- Refrigerate open formula and use within 24 hours.

Gastrointestinal

Diarrhea

- Evaluate for causes other than the feeding formula such as medications or underlying physiology.
- Evaluate for *Clostridium difficile.*
- Consider composition and osmolality of enteral formula. Formulas should be lactose free. Consider changing to a low-fat, predigested, or fiber-containing formula.
- Decrease the rate and/or extend the infusion time.
- To minimize bacterial contamination, use clean technique and hang formulas for no longer than 8 hours unless using a closed feeding system.
- Consider use of antidiarrheal agents.
- If diarrhea persists despite the measures above, evaluate for a resolving ileus or impaction.

Nausea and Vomiting

- Evaluate for causes other than the feeding such as underlying physiology or medications.
- Nausea and vomiting can result from gastric retention, rapid infusion of feeding, high-fat formulas, or the odor of the formula (particularly predigested formulas).
- Use an isotonic, lower-fat formula when possible.
- Consider prokinetic medications and/or small-bowel feedings.

- Feedings should be at room temperature, initiated slowly, and advanced as tolerated
- Switch from bolus/intermittent to continuous feedings.
- Feeding tube placement should be reconfirmed in patients with severe vomiting.

Abdominal Distention, Cramps, Flatulence

- This can be caused by rapid delivery of cold formula, delayed gastric emptying, malabsorption, or lactose intolerance.
- Feedings should be administered slowly and at room temperature.
- The feeding formula may need to be changed to low fat, predigested, or fiber free if symptoms persist or the patient has malabsorption.

Constipation

- The patient may require more free water or fiber.
- Encourage ambulation if possible.
- May be a sign of GI obstruction or fecal impaction.

Metabolic

Refeeding Syndrome

- Fluid and electrolyte shifts resulting in hypophosphatemia, hypokalemia, and/or hypomagnesemia may occur if enteral feedings are initiated too rapidly in malnourished patients.
- If possible, correct electrolyte abnormalities before initiating enteral nutrition. Start with hypocaloric feedings and gradually increase to caloric goal. Monitor glucose and electrolytes closely, particularly serum potassium, phosphorus, and magnesium.

Dehydration

- Results from inadequate fluid intake or excessive losses and /or administration of hypertonic, concentrated formulas.
- Provide adequate free water; monitor daily weights, intake and output records, serum electrolytes and clinical manifestations of dehydration.

Overhydration

- May result from excessive fluid intake or rapid infusion of enteral feeding, especially for patients with cardiac, renal, or hepatic insufficiency.
- Administer feedings slowly; monitor daily weights, intake and output records, serum electrolytes, and clinical manifestations of overhydration.
- May be necessary to restrict volume by use of a calorically dense formula and minimize additional sources of fluid such as flushes, PO intake, medications, and IV fluids.
- Institute diuretic therapy as appropriate.

Hypernatremia

- Results from inadequate water intake or excessive water losses or excessive sodium intake.
- Monitor daily weights, intake and output records, serum electrolytes, and clinical manifestations of dehydration.
- Replace fluid as additional free water as feeding tube flushes or as intravenous fluids.

Hyponatremia

- May be caused by excess fluid intake, fluid overload, syndrome of inappropriate antidiuretic hormone (SIADH), or excessive GI losses.
- Monitor daily weights, intake and output records, serum electrolytes, and clinical manifestations of overhydration.
- Restrict fluid intake; use calorically dense enteral formula; institue diuretic therapy as necessary. Sodium is generally restricted in order to decrease fluid retention; supplement sodium intake only if necessary.

Hyperkalemia

- Occurs in metabolic acidosis, cardiac or renal disease, or excessive potassium intake.
- Monitor serum potassium levels; assess all sources of potassium intake such as diet, EN, IV fluids, and medications.

- Decrease potassium intake; may need to administer Kayexelate or glucose infusion with insulin therapy.
- Evaluate for potential changes in cardiac status; order EKG as needed.

Hypokalemia

- May occur as a consequence of refeeding syndrome, diuretic or insulin therapy, or metabolic alkalosis.
- Monitor serum potassium levels; supplement potassium enterally or intravenously.
- Avoid overzealous refeeding of malnourished patients. Advance calories slowly and maintain hypocaloric feedings until potassium levels are normalized.

Hyperphosphatemia

- Occurs with renal insufficiency, excessive phosphorus intake (diet or phosphorus-containing antacids), or increased endogenous phosphorus load (extracellular shift or cellular destruction).
- Monitor serum phosphorus levels; use phosphate binders as needed; use a low phosphorus formula; change antacids.

Hypophosphatemia

- Occurs in refeeding syndrome, with insulin therapy, or with excessive use of phosphorus-binding antacids.
- Monitor serum phosphorus levels; correct hypophosphatemia prior to initiating EN if possible; severe hypophosphatemia may require intravenous repletion; change antacids.

Hypercapnia

- May occur with excessive calorie and/or carbohydrate administration, especially among patients with respiratory compromise.
- Estimate caloric requirements carefully or use indirect calorimetry to avoid overfeeding; use an enteral formula with a balanced distribution of carbohydrate, protein, and fat.

Hyperglycemia

- Less likely with EN than PN; usually can be explained by underlying physiology or disease state (i.e., diabetes mellitus or metabolic stress) or medications (i.e., steroids).
- Optimize medical management with oral hypoglycemic agents or insulin therapy and reduce or omit medications that precipitate hyperglycemia.
- Normalization of blood glucose levels appears to reduce complications, morbidity, and mortality among patients, particularly those who are critically ill.
- Avoid overfeeding of calories and carbohydrate by carefully estimating caloric needs and utilizing an enteral formula with a balanced distribution of carbohydrate, protein, fat, and added fiber.
- Consider a hypocaloric, high-protein enteral feeding regime for obese, insulin-resistant patients. Closely monitor clinical status and response to therapy, weight, serum glucose levels, and nutritional status.

Mechanical

Tube Occlusion

- Irrigate feeding tube frequently with water.
- Minimize use of the feeding tube as a means to administer medications.
- Flush with water before and after aspirating from the tube.
- If an occlusion occurs, use irrigants such as warm water, a sodium bicarbonate/pancrealipase mixture, meat tenderizer, or commercially prepared formulations.
- Mechanical methods for clearing occluded tubes, such as use of a commercial declogging device or small catheter, should only be used by an experienced practitioner.

Nasopharyngeal/Nasolabial Irritation

- Results from prolonged use of large-bore nasogastric feeding tubes, especially those made from vinyl, rubber, or polyvinylchloride.

- Use small-bore tubes made from polyurethane or silicone.
- Tape tubes securely and avoid putting pressure on the nares.

Acute Otitis Media/Acute Sinusitis

- Acute otitis media may result from pressure of a nasoenteric feeding tube at the opening of the eustachian tube.
- Acute sinusitis may occur when a nasoenteric feeding tube occludes the sinus tract.
- Use small-bore feeding tubes made of polyurethane or silicone.

REFERENCES

American Society for Parenteral and Enteral Nutrition, Board of Directors and Clinical Guidelines Task Force. Guidelines for the use of parenteral and enteral nutrition in adult and pediatric patients. *JPEN*. 2002; 26(no 1, suppl):18SA–20SA, 33SA–35SA, 38SA–41SA.

Beyer PL. Complications of enteral nutrition. In: Matarese LE, Gottschlich MM, eds. *Contemporary Nutrition Support Practice, A Clinical Guide*. New York, NY: Saunders; 2003:201–214.

Choban PS, Burge JC, Flancbaum L. Nutrition support of obese hospitalized patients. *NCP*. 1997;12:149–154.

DeChicco RS, Matarese LE. Determining the nutrition support regime. In: Matarese LE, Gottschlich MM, eds. *Contemporary Nutrition Support Practice, A Clinical Guide*. New York, NY: Saunders; 2003:181–187.

Franzi LR, Seidner DL. Enteral nutrition. In: Parekh NP, Dechicco RS, eds. *The Cleveland Clinic Foundation Nutrition Support Handbook*. Cleveland, OH: The Cleveland Clinic Foundation; 2003.

McClave SA, DeMeo MT, DeLegge MH, et al. North American summit on aspiration in the critically ill patient: A consensus statement. *JPEN*. 2002;26 (no 6, suppl): S80–S85.

Russell M, Cromer M, Grant J. Complications of enteral nutrition therapy. In: Gottschlich MM, ed. *The Science and Practice of Nutrition Support. A Case-Based Core Curriculum*. Dubuque, IA: Kendall/Hunt; 2001:189–210.

Van Den Berghe G, Wouters P, Verwaest C, et al. Intensive insulin therapy in critically ill patients. *NEJM*. 2001; 345:1359–1367.

Parenteral Nutrition

By Neha Parekh, RD and Jo Ann McCrae, MS, RD

DESCRIPTION

Parenteral nutrition (PN) is the intravenous provision of macronutrients and micronutrients to patients whose gastrointestinal (GI) tract is nonfunctional, inaccessible, or unsafe to use.

Total Parenteral Nutrition (TPN)

The administration of PN through a large-diameter central vein is known as total parenteral nutrition, or TPN. TPN allows for the use of a highly concentrated, hypertonic solution which can be tailored to meet the macronutrient and fluid requirements of individual patients. It may be used indefinitely, especially if a tunneled vascular access is used.

Vascular Access Devices for TPN

- Temporary central venous catheter
- Long-term central venous catheter
  1. Tunneled central venous catheter
  2. Implanted port
  3. Peripherally inserted central catheter (PICC). Considerations for using PICC include:
     –lower cost of placement
     –less risk of insertion complications
     –higher rate of catheter malfunction
     –difficult for the patient to care for alone

Peripheral Parenteral Nutrition (PPN)

PPN avoids the use of a central vein and the complications that can arise from its use. Because it is administered by a peripheral vein, the osmolarity of a PPN solution should be < 900 mOsm/l to prevent vein damage and thrombophlebitis. As a result, PPN solutions are generally lipid based and will provide less total calories, protein, and electrolytes per liter than hypertonic TPN solutions. PPN is therefore not intended to meet or exceed nutrient requirements in hypermetabolic, severely malnourished, or fluid-restricted individuals. It is more suitable for the mild to moderately malnourished patient unable to ingest and utilize adequate amounts of nutrients orally or enterally, or for those for whom central access for TPN is not feasible. The duration of PPN is usually limited to < 2 weeks because of potential injury to the peripheral veins and the frequent need to change the infusion site.

INDICATIONS FOR PN

PN should be used

- in patients unable to absorb nutrients via the GI tract due to
  1. massive small-bowel resection
  2. severe malabsorption
  3. intractable vomiting or diarrhea (as frequently seen with high-dose chemotherapy, radiation, or bone marrow transplant therapy)
  4. radiation enteritis
  5. persistent GI bleeding
  6. high output fistula
- in moderately to severely malnourished patients with a GI tract expected to be inaccessible or nonfunctional for > 5–7 days due to
  1. small- or large-bowel obstruction awaiting spontaneous or surgical resolution
  2. bowel ischemia awaiting surgical resolution
  3. severe pancreatitis
  4. prolonged small-bowel ileus or colonic inertia
  5. repeated failure of enteral feeding or failure to maintain enteral access

PN is of limited use

- in well-nourished patients whose GI tract may be used within 10 days
- in immediately postoperative patients
- in patients undergoing minimal stress

PN should not be used

- in patients with a functional GI tract
- when PN is needed for less than 5 days
- when an urgent operation would have to be delayed for administration of PN
- when PN is not desired by the patient/ guardian and when the patient's/guardian's wishes are in accordance with hospital policy and existing law
- when prognosis does not warrant aggressive therapy
- when risks exceed potential benefits

COMPONENTS OF PN SOLUTIONS

PN solutions are routinely made up of carbo-hydrate, protein, electrolytes, vitamins, miner-als, trace metals, medications, and sterile water. Fat may be added daily to the PN solution to form a total nutrient admixture (TNA), or may be administered separately.

Carbohydrates

Considerations

- Carbohydrate is the primary energy substrate of the brain. The average adult requires about 100 g of carbohydrate per day to meet mini-mum requirements for central nervous system function. The maximum amount of tolerable carbohydrate infusion is ∼ 5–7 mg/kg/min.
- Carbohydrate is provided in the form of dex-trose (3.4 kcal/g) in PN solutions.
- Dextrose concentration ranges from 5%–70% (2.38 kcal/cc). Higher dextrose concentrations are used to decrease total volume in cases of fluid restriction.
- In calculating osmolarity of PPN solutions, dextrose contributes approximately 5 mOsm/g.

Precautions

- Excess carbohydrate infusion may lead to lipid synthesis, fatty liver, and elevations in liver function tests.
- Glucose oxidation causes an increase in car-bon dioxide production, which may be clini-cally significant in patients with respiratory insufficiency. Therefore, it is important to avoid overfeeding of both carbohydrate and total calories in this patient population.
- High carbohydrate doses may cause hyper-glycemia.
  1. Glucose intolerance is commonly seen with diabetes mellitus, infection, trauma, pancreatitis, steroid therapy, chromium de-ficiency, or postoperative stress.
  2. Hyperglycemia can be managed by admin-istering exogenous insulin or by adding regular insulin directly to the PN bag.
  3. To prevent hyperglycemia, advance dextrose infusions slowly, starting with 150–200 g/day. A mixture of carbohydrate and lipid calories may be used to decrease dextrose load in cases of glucose intolerance.

Lipids

Considerations

- Lipids are a concentrated source of energy (9 kcal/g). They are a structural component of cell membranes, precursors for prostaglandin synthesis, and they serve to prevent essential fatty acid deficiency.
- Lipid emulsions are isotonic and are com-posed of soybean oil or soybean/safflower oil long-chain triglycerides.
- Lipid emulsions are available in 10% (1.1 kcal/cc), 20% (2 kcal/cc), and 30% (3 kcal/cc) concentrations.
- Approximately 4% of calories must be pro-vided as essential fatty acids to prevent a defi-ciency. This requirement may be met through the administration of 500 cc of 20% intra-venous (IV) lipid emulsion once per week. Al-ternately, 500 cc of 10% IV lipid or 250 cc of 20% IV lipid may be given 3 times per week.

Precautions

- Rapid infusion of IV lipids has been associ-ated with reduced lipid clearance, immuno-suppression, and dysfunction of the reticuloendothelial system.

1. Provision of $< 30\%$ of total calories as lipids and infusion of lipids at a rate < 1.0 g/kg/day is recommended to reduce adverse reactions.
2. Potential adverse reactions include respiratory difficulties, fever, chills, headache, back or chest pain, nausea, and vomiting.

- Hypertriglyceridemia can also occur with excess lipid administration or rapid infusion.
  1. In cases of suspected altered lipid metabolism, as seen in pancreatitis, familial hyperlipidemia, severe stress, and moderate to severe liver disease, serum triglycerides should be monitored closely when initiating PN.
  2. Lipid clearance is evaluated by measuring serum triglyceride concentration preinfusion and 6 hours postinfusion.
  3. Lipid administration should be held when serum triglyceride levels exceed 400 mg/dl with no other suspected cause.
- Allergic reactions to IV lipids are rare and are usually a result of an allergy to the egg phospholipid used as an emulsifier in IV lipid solutions. In instances of confirmed egg/IV lipid allergy, it may be necessary to cutaneously apply or orally ingest oils to prevent essential fatty acid deficiency.
- Structured lipid emulsions are a mixture of medium- and long-chain triglycerides.
  1. Available only for research purposes in the United States.
  2. Administration may result in decreased bacterial sequestration in the lung and improved reticuloendothelial system (RES) function.

Amino Acids

Considerations

- Amino acids (4 kcal/g) are required for cell structure and skeletal muscle. The requirement for healthy adults is 0.8 g/kg/day. There is 0.16 g nitrogen per g protein (6.25 g protein per g nitrogen).
- Protein needs depend on age, nutritional status, physical activity, metabolism and stress, and renal and hepatic function.

1. Critical illness: 1.2–1.5 g protein/kg/day.
2. Trauma: > 1.5 g protein/kg/day.
3. Renal and hepatic disease may require a protein restriction.

- Standard amino acid solutions are composed of essential, semiessential, and nonessential amino acids.
- Standard amino acid solutions are available in 3.5% (35 g/l) to 15% (150 g/l) concentrations.
- Parenteral formula for stable patients: 300 nonprotein calories per gram nitrogen.
- Parenteral formula for patients under stress: 100–150 nonprotein calories per gram nitrogen.
- In calculating osmolarity of PPN solutions, dextrose contributes approximately 5 mOsm/g.
- Solutions elevated in branched-chain amino acid (BCAA) have been used in cases of hepatic encephalopathy refractory to medical treatment and in severe stress or critical illness.
  1. BCAAs (leucine, isoleucine, and valine) are oxidized primarily in muscle whereas aromatic amino acids (AAAs) are metabolized by the liver and accumulate in liver failure.
  2. AAAs function as precursors to neurotransmitters in the brain and may lead to hepatic encephalopathy.
  3. Indications for use of this specialized amino acid formula are controversial and efficacy with morbidity and mortality has not been proven in comparison to standard amino acid solutions.
- Essential amino acid (EAA) solutions may be used for a period up to 2 weeks in acute renal failure when dialysis is not possible.

Vitamins

- See Appendix G for guidelines on usual parenteral daily intake of vitamins for adults.
- Commercially available as injectable multivitamin infusions (MVI) or single-vitamin products (with the exception of biotin, pantothenic acid, riboflavin, vitamin A, and vitamin E).

- Stability is affected by light, temperature, pH, storage time, and solution.
- Should be added on a daily basis prior to infusion.
- Vitamin K is added separately as a daily or weekly dose unless contained in the MVI solution.

Trace Elements

- Refer to guidelines on usual parenteral daily intake of trace elements for adults.
- Commercially available in various injectable combinations or as single-element products.
- Additional chromium or zinc supplementation may be needed in cases of excess GI or urinary losses.
- *CAUTION:* Parenteral iron supplementation has been associated with anaphylaxis and death. Test doses are required before administration. Iron cannot be added to a lipid-based PN solution because it will destabilize the formula.

Electrolytes

- Standard electrolyte doses are used in the majority of patients.
- Electrolyte disorders secondary to disease, organ dysfunction, GI losses, and medical or drug therapy can be treated not only by attention to possible causes, but also by adjustment of the parenteral solution followed by careful monitoring (see Table 4–2).
- Increased losses via the GI tract may be due to vomiting, diarrhea, ostomies, fistulas, and nasogastric suctioning.
- Excess calcium and phosphorus supplementation may cause crystalline precipitation, which can cause catheter occlusion and death. Strict adherence to pharmacy guidelines is needed.
- Usual daily adult electrolyte requirements are:
    Calcium: 10–15 mEq
    Phosphorus: 20–40 mM
    Potassium: 1–2 mEq/kg
    Sodium: 1–2 mEq/kg
    Magnesium: 8–20 mEq

Fluids

- Estimation of fluid requirements:
    1. ~ 1cc/kcal/day
    2. 30–35 cc/kg body weight
    3. Daily measured output (allowing 1.5 to 2 L per day for urine) plus 500 cc for insensible losses; minus any fluid intake from sources other than PN.
- Needs are increased with renal, GI (fistulas, drainage tubes, diarrhea, nasogastric suction, and ostomies), respiratory, and skin losses.
- Needs are decreased with renal, hepatic, or cardiac failure.
- Monitoring of intake and output records, laboratory values (sodium, chloride, blood urea nitrogen, creatinine, and albumin), weight changes, and physical signs of hydration status is important to adjust fluid provisions as needed.

TOTAL NUTRIENT ADMIXTURES (TNA)

TNA is a combination of glucose, amino acids, and lipids in a single container for intravenous administration. The use of TNAs may decrease risk of external contamination, decrease nursing and pharmacy time, and improve patient compliance. However, the TNA medium provides increased opportunity for the growth of bacteria. A larger filter must also be used with the addition of lipid to the PN solution, which is less effective at removing potential contaminants.

- Compatibility of a TNA solution is of major concern.
    1. Refer to your pharmacy for compatible ranges of amino acids, dextrose, and fat to guarantee 24-hour stability of a TNA solution.
    2. If the emulsion breaks or cracks, discard the formula. Report to pharmacy when oil globules on the surface of a creamed emulsion coalesce.
- Instability of a TNA solution may also result from the addition of iron.
    1. The iron cation has the potential of decreasing the surface charge of lipid particles to thereby destabilize the lipid emulsion.

Table 4–2 Electrolyte Disorders: Etiology and Treatment by Adjustment of PN

Electrolyte Disorder	Possible Etiology	Treatment
Hypercalcemia	Renal failure	Decrease calcium administration
	Bone cancer	Isotonic saline
	Immobilization, stress	Phosphorus supplementation
	Excess vitamin D administration	
Hypocalcemia	Low vitamin D intake	Calcium supplementation if
	Hypoalbuminemia	ionized calcium is low
	Hypoparathyroidism	Correct magnesium deficiency
	Hypomagnesemia, hyperphosphatemia	
	Malabsorption, inadequate Ca in TPN	
Hyperphosphatemia	Renal failure	Phosphate binders
	Excess phosphate administration	Decrease phosphorus administration
Hypophosphatemia	Refeeding syndrome	Phosphorus supplementation
	Exogenous insulin	Check on antacids
	Phosphate-binding antacids	
	Alcoholism	
	Diabetic ketoacidosis	
Hypermagnesemia	Renal failure	Decrease Mg administration
	Excess Mg administration	
Hypomagnesemia	Refeeding syndrome	Magnesium supplementation
	Chemotherapy	
	Alcoholism	
	Diuretics	
	Medications (cisplatin, amphotericin B)	
	GI losses	
Hyperkalemia	Renal failure	Decrease potassium administration
	Metabolic acidosis	Potassium binders
	Excess potassium administration	
	Medications	
	Catabolism	
Hypokalemia	Refeeding syndrome	Potassium supplementation
	Medications	
	Inadequate potassium intake	
	Excess losses (GI drainage, ostomies, fistulas, diarrhea, diuretics)	
Hypernatremia	Dehydration, excess water losses	Fluid replacement if dehydrated
	Excess sodium intake	Decrease sodium administration
	Osmotic diuresis secondary to hyperglycemia	
Hyponatremia	Excess water intake	Decrease fluid intake
	Cirrhosis	Increase sodium in PN if appropriate
	Congestive heart failure	
	SIADH	
	Excessive losses	

Table 4–3 Monitoring of Laboratory Values During PN Administration

Laboratory Value	Frequency of Monitoring
Serum glucose	Monitor daily until stable, then 2–3 times per week
Blood urea nitrogen/creatinine	Monitor daily until stable, then 2–3 times per week
Major serum electrolytes (potassium, sodium)	Monitor daily until stable, then 2-3 times per week
Serum calcium, phosphorus, and magnesium	Monitor daily until stable, then weekly
Serum triglycerides	Take baseline and pre- and post-infusion levels initially in patients with suspected lipid intolerance (i.e., pancreatitis)
Liver function tests (AST, alkaline phosphatase, bilirubin)	Take initially and then weekly
Visceral proteins (albumin, transferrin, prealbumin)	Monitor weekly
Prothrombin levels (PT, PTT, INR)	Monitor weekly
Complete blood count (CBC) with differential and platelets (white blood cells, hemoglobin, hematocrit)	Monitor weekly

2. The administration of iron dextran with PN should be reserved for solutions containing only dextrose and protein (i.e., 2-in-1 solutions).

MONITORING

Monitoring of PN should include the following:

- Daily weights
- Daily intake and output (including nutrient intake records if eating by mouth)
- Urinary or finger glucose
- Changing of tubing, bag, and filter according to policy (not to exceed 48 hours)
- Laboratory values (see Table 4–3)
- Changes in clinical status including acid-base balance, medical therapy, drug–nutrient interactions, GI function and losses, major organ function, and fever
- Progress toward attaining goals of nutrition therapy

This chapter is dedicated to my dear friend and colleague, Joann Davey McCrae, MS, RD—one of our country's first nutrition support dietitians, and one of our finest—who recently passed away from ovarian cancer.

REFERENCES

ASPEN Board of Directors and The Clinical Guidelines Task Force. Guidelines for the use of parenteral and enteral nutrition in adult and pediatric patients. *JPEN.* 2002; 26(1 suppl):1SA–138SA.

Barber JR, Miller SJ, Sacks GS. Parenteral feeding formulations. In: Gottschlich MM, ed. *The Science and Practice of Nutrition Support. A Case-Based Core Curriculum.* Dubuque, IA: Kendall/Hunt; 2001:251–268.

Bellantone R, Bossola M, Carriero C, et al. Structured versus long-chain triglycerides: A safety, tolerance, and efficacy randomized study in colorectal surgical patients. *JPEN.* 1999;23:123–127.

Benotti PN, Bistrian B. Metabolic and nutritional aspects of weaning from mechanical ventilation. *Crit Care Med.* 1989; 17:181–185.

Driscoll DF, Newton DW, Bistrian BR. Precipitation of calcium phosphate from parenteral nutrition fluids. *Am J Hosp Pharm.* 1994;51:2834–2836.

Fischer J. Branched-chain-enriched amino acid solution in patients with liver failure: An early example of nutritional pharmacology. *JPEN.* 1990;14:249S–256S.

Fuhrman MP. Complication management in parenteral nutrition. In: Matarese LE, Gottschlich MM, eds. *Contem-*

porary Nutrition Support Practice. 2nd ed. Philadelphia, PA: WB Saunders; 2003:242–262.

Jensen GL, Biakley J. Clinical manifestation of nutrient deficiency. *JPEN.* 2002;26:S29–S33.

Kelly DG. Guidelines and available products for parenteral vitamins and trace elements. *JPEN.* 2002;26:S34–S36.

Lennon EA, Speerhas R. Parenteral nutrition. In: Parekh NR, DeChicco RS, eds. *The Cleveland Clinic Foundation Nutrition Support Handbook.* Cleveland, OH: The Cleveland Clinic Foundation; 2003.

Lowry SF, Brennan MF. Abnormal liver function during parenteral nutrition: Relation to infusion excess. *J Surg Res.* 1979;26:300–307.

Matarese LE. Metabolic complications of parenteral nutrition therapy. In: Gottschlich MM, ed. *The Science and Practice of Nutrition Support. A Case-Based Core Curriculum.* Dubuque, IA: Kendall/Hunt; 2001:269–286.

Mirtallo JM. Introduction to parenteral nutrition. In: Gottschlich MM, ed. *The Science and Practice of Nutrition Support. A Case-Based Core Curriculum.* Dubuque, IA: Kendall/Hunt; 2001:211–223.

Parekh NR, Seidner DL. Disease specific nutrition. In: Irwin RS, Rippe JM, eds. *Irwin and Rippe's Intensive Care Medicine.* 5th ed. Philadelphia, PA: Lippincott, Williams and Wilkins; 2003:2069–2080.

Rosemarin DK, Wardlaw GM, Mirtallo JM. Hyperglycemia associated with high, continuous infusion rates of total parenteral nutrition dextrose. *Nutr Clin Pract.* 1996; 11:151–156.

Seidner DL, Masscioli EA, Istfan NW, et al. Effects of long-chain triglyceride emulsions on reticuloendothelial system function in humans. *JPEN.* 1989;13:614–619.

Skipper A. Parenteral nutrition. In: Matarese LE, Gottschlich MM, eds. *Contemporary Nutrition Support Practice.* 2nd ed. Philadelphia, PA: WB Saunders; 2003:227–241.

Veterans Affairs Total Parenteral Nutrition Cooperative Study Group. Perioperative total parenteral nutrition in surgical patients. *N Engl J Med.* 1991;325:525–532.

Wolfe RR, O'Donnell TF Jr, Stone MD. Investigation of factors determining the optimal glucose infusion rate in total parenteral nutrition. *Metabolism.* 1980;29:892–900.

Transitional Feeding

Marion F. Winkler, MS, RD, LDN, CNSD

DESCRIPTION

Transitional feeding is the period of time during the progression from parenteral nutrition support to enteral tube feeding or oral diet, or from enteral tube feeding to oral diet. The overlapping of one regimen with another is essential for successful transitioning and allows for maintenance of nutrient intake.

CAUSE

Readiness to make the transition from one form of nutrition support to another is related to gastrointestinal function; adequacy of fluid, nutrient, and caloric intake; and availability of an access route. Transitional feeding can occur over a short period of time in an acute care setting, or over a longer period of time in the home environment. Patients with short-bowel syn-

drome have greatly reduced small-bowel surface area and the need for parenteral nutrition varies depending on the presence or absence of the ileocecal valve, jejunum, and colon. Treatment goals should emphasize early transition to enteral or oral nutrition with the understanding that a prolonged transitional feeding period may be required as gut adaptation occurs.

ASSESSMENT

- Evaluate gastrointestinal function and ability to tolerate enteral or oral nutrients. Tests for malabsorption and a gastrointestinal workup may be necessary. For patients with massive small-bowel resection, it is helpful to determine the amount of residual intestine; small bowel length of 100 cm or less usually requires long-term parenteral nutrition or intravenous fluid therapy.

- Evaluate potential enteral access sites if the transition is from a parenteral to an enteral route. Feeding tube placement is related to the patient's overall condition and anticipated duration of nutrition support therapy.
- Note any change in the patient's ability to feed dependently or independently.
- Assess adequacy of intake for fluids, nutrients, and calories during the transitional feeding period.

PROBLEMS

- Children who receive parenteral or enteral nutrition in infancy and early childhood may require special attention with oral feeding techniques and behavior as oral intake increases. A four-step process to ensure a smooth transition to oral feeding has been promoted. This program includes:
  1. promoting a positive feeding relationship between the child and caregiver
  2. determining readiness to feed
  3. normalizing feeding, including oral stimulation, eating-related behaviors, environment, and regulation
  4. initiating a behavioral feeding plan.
- Inability to tolerate enteral or oral feedings due to impaired digestion or absorption.
- Inability to maintain weight, hydration status, electrolyte balance, and/or nutritional parameters without parenteral nutrition or intravenous fluid support.
- Rebound hypoglycemia due to sudden cessation of parenteral nutrition feedings.
- Discontinuation of nutrition support despite inadequate oral intake.

TREATMENT/MANAGEMENT

- Anticipate long-term needs for nutrition support; recommend placement of percutaneous endoscopic feeding tubes or postpyloric feeding tubes at the time of endoscopy or gastrointestinal workup; recommend placement

of gastrostomy or jejunostomy tube at the time of other operative procedures.
- Recommend simultaneous decrease in parenteral nutrition support as enteral tube feeding or oral intake improves, or recommend decrease in enteral nutrition as improvement in oral diet is noted; take into account total calories, nutrients, and fluid intake.
- The selection of enteral tube-feeding product is based on digestive and absorptive capacity, disease state, organ function, and overall clinical status. Progression to oral diet is typically advancement from clear liquids to full liquids to soft or regular diet, with modifications made on the basis of digestive and absorptive function, disease state, overall clinical status, and the ability to chew and swallow. Oral nutritional or between-meal supplements should be used to augment caloric intake if necessary. Parenteral and enteral nutrition have not been shown to effect appetite; patients typically increase oral intake spontaneously when they feel better.
- Weaning can occur by decreasing the total volume of formula, changing the concentration or caloric density of the formula, decreasing the number of hours of infusion, or decreasing the number of days/nights of infusion.
- Cyclic infusions of parenteral or enteral nutrition support or intermittent enteral tube feedings are useful during the transition to oral diet and allow the patient the freedom to eat meals during the day while receiving supplemental nutrition overnight. In the case of weaning from enteral tube feeding to oral diet, tube feedings can be temporarily stopped for 1 hour before and after meals.
- Parenteral nutrition should be tapered cautiously to avoid rebound hypoglycemia. Intravenous solutions of 5% or 10% dextrose can be used upon discontinuation of total parenteral nutrition (TPN) if the patient is not receiving tube feedings or a meal.

- Caloric counts or food diaries should be kept during the period of transitional feeding.
- Document tolerance and achievement of at least 50% of required fluid, nutrient, and caloric goals for 3 consecutive days before completely discontinuing parenteral or enteral nutrition support.
- Document improvement in nutritional status (change in or maintenance of plasma proteins and weight and change in functional ability), growth and development in children, and achievement of nutritional goals.
- Pharmacologic treatment and the use of specific nutrients (glutamine) and growth factors (growth hormone, glucagon-like peptide-2, insulin-like growth factor I) have been used to stimulate intestinal absorption and adaptation in patients with short-bowel syndrome. Intestinal rehabilitation and/or transplant may be a treatment option for some patients.

EXAMPLE

A 30-year-old male suffered pancreatic injuries and a transected colon in a motor vehicle accident. He underwent multiple operative procedures for pancreatic debridement, bowel resection, and creation of an ileostomy. His postoperative course was complicated by multiple abdominal abscesses that required drainage. He remained in the surgical intensive care unit, was sedated, and was on mechanical ventilation. TPN was begun on postoperative day 2 and was advanced over several days to provide 2500 kcal and 120 g of protein to meet measured energy expenditure and 1.5 g protein/kg. When his condition stabilized and his ileostomy began to function, a nasoduodenal tube was placed under fluoroscopy for enteral feedings. A low-fat, elemental diet was selected because of presumed maldigestion and malabsorption secondary to pancreatic insufficiency. Tube feedings were initiated at 40 ml/hr and were advanced slowly. Parenteral nutrition was simultaneously tapered as tube feedings were increased, as indicated:

Enteral Intake	
0	
1000 kcal	40 g protein
1500 kcal	60 g protein
2000 kcal	75 g protein
2500 kcal	100 g protein

Parenteral Intake	
2500 kcal	120 g protein
2000 kcal	100 g protein
1500 kcal	75 g protein
1000 kcal	50 g protein
0	

The patient tolerated tube feedings for 7 days before a trial with a polymeric diet was attempted, in an effort to increase caloric density and achieve adequate protein intake. TPN was maintained until tolerance to the tube-feeding formula was demonstrated and goals were achieved. The volume, consistency, and color of the ileostomy output were monitored. The patient experienced no increase or change in ileostomy output with transition to the polymeric diet. Parenteral nutrition was then discontinued, as the patient was tolerating 2500 kcal and 100 g of protein via the nasoduodenal feeding.

REFERENCES

American Society for Parenteral and Enteral Nutrition Board of Directors. Guidelines for the use of parenteral and enteral nutrition in adult and pediatric patients. *J Parenter Enteral Nutr.* 2002;26(suppl).

Dell'Olio J, Hollenstein J, Dwyer J. Noah grows up: Transitioning problems from special feeding routes to oral intake. *Nutr Rev.* 2000;58:118–128.

Jeppesen PB, Mortensen PB. Enhancing bowel adaptation in short bowel syndrome. *Curr Gastroenterol Rep.* 2002; 4:338–347.

Piazza-Barnett R. Combined and transitional feeding modalities. In: Matarese LE, Gottschlich MM, eds. *Contemporary Nutrition Support Practice.* Philadelphia, PA: Saunders/Elsevier Science; 2003:290–300.

Schauster H, Dwyer J. Transition from tube feedings to feedings by mouth in children: Preventing eating dysfunction. *J Am Diet Assoc.* 1996;96:277–281.

Stratton RJ, Elia M. The effects of enteral tube feeding and parenteral nutrition on appetite sensations and food intake in health and disease. *Clin Nutr.* 1999;18:63–70.

Sundaram A, Koutkia P, Apovian CM. Nutritional management of short bowel syndrome in adults. *J Clin Gastroenterol.* 2002;34:207–220.

Ukleja A, Scolapio JS, Buchman AL. Nutritional management of short bowel syndrome. *Semin Gastrointest Dis.* 2002;13:161–168.

Winkler MF, Pomp A, Caldwell MD, Albina JE. Transitional feeding: The relationship between nutritional intake and plasma protein concentrations. *J Am Diet Assoc.* 1989; 89:969–970.

Winkler MF, Watkins CK, Albina JE. Adequacy of TPN intake: An indicator quality nutrition care. *J Am Diet Assoc.* 1991;91(Suppl):A–50. Abstract.

CHAPTER 5

Hospital Discharge Planning: The Role of the Dietitian

Karen Masino, RD, RN

DESCRIPTION

Length of hospital stay continues to decrease, leaving increasingly complex and malnourished patients to be cared for in the outpatient setting. To provide a smooth transition from the hospital to the home care setting in patients requiring continued nutrition support, an interdisciplinary approach to discharge planning is necessary. It is essential for the dietitian to collaborate with other members of the health care team, including the physician, nurse, pharmacist, social worker, hospital case manager, and discharge planner. The dietitian must communicate with home care and durable medical equipment (DME) companies to process certification of medical necessity and treatment authorization request forms to negotiate reimbursement for nutritional therapies at home. It is imperative that he or she assess the postacute nutritional needs of the patient and develop a plan to address these needs prior to discharge. An appropriate nutrition plan of care with pertinent documentation must be developed to meet requirements to justify reimbursement. Early and effective hospital discharge planning will facilitate the patient's transition between the hospital and the home, skilled nursing facility, or rehabilitation center.

PREDISCHARGE NUTRITION CARE PLAN

Nutrition History

Evaluate the following:

- Demographic information.
- Medical–surgical history.
- Current medical management, including recent diagnostic tests and procedures.
- Clinical variables affecting food intake, digestion, or absorption, such as malabsorption, maldigestion, and mastication difficulties or swallowing dysfunction.
- Changes in appetite, intake, and food intolerances.
- Previous diet history for food habits and eating patterns, food allergies.
- Appetite changes, anorexia, dysphagia, nausea, vomiting, diarrhea, or constipation and mastication difficulties.
- Current or previous therapeutic diets, nutritional supplement use, and preferences and use of vitamins, minerals, and herbs.
- Previous or current use of enteral or parenteral nutrition.
- Social data including support system, financial limitations, and barriers to implementing a nutrition plan of care.

- Education needs and barriers to learning.
- Weight history including usual weight, weight changes, and ideal body weight.
- Nutrient deficiencies.
- Medications.
- Laboratory data.
  1. chemistries including blood glucose, hemoglobin A1C, blood urea nitrogen, electrolytes, measures of protein status, lipid profile, CBC

Nutrition Assessment

- Review and update previously collected nutrition assessment information. See Chapter 1, Screening and Assessment, for further information on completing a nutrition assessment.
- Analyze diet history for adequacy based on food groups or nutrient composition tables.
- assess nutrient needs:
  1. Daily calorie/protein goal (kcal/day, kcal/kg) (protein g/day, protein g/kg).
  2. Fluid requirements (ml/day, ml/kg).
  3. See sections on Specific Medical Conditions in Chapter 3, for determination of nutrient needs.
- Evaluate appropriateness of current diet order and appropriate discharge diet prescription.
- Assess adequacy of current nutrition support regimens in relation to goals of nutrition therapy and need for supplementation:
  1. Evaluate patient's ability to purchase products in the outpatient setting.

Nutrition Plan of Care

- determine appropriate nutrition prescription
- provide appropriate nutrition education

Nutrition Education

Nutrition education and diet counseling are provided to patients who require dietary modification to prevent disease or to treat a preexisting condition. For a complete overview of meal plans and dietary modifications, indications for use of therapeutic diets, and the nutritional adequacy of various diets, refer to Chapter 3 on Nutrition Management in Specific Medical Conditions.

Barriers to Learning

Any barriers that may impact ability to educate the patient and/or caregiver need to be addressed such as: language, cognitive and/or memory deficits, cultural and religious considerations.

Basic Principles in Nutrition Education

- Keep it simple.
- Write everything down.
- Use terms patient and caregivers can understand.
- Identify the primary caregiver and include him or her in all education.
- Encourage the patient to discuss eating problems with the dietitian.
- Review good nutrition principles and the link between proper nutrition and health.
  1. Identify diet prescription and explain rationale.
  2. Educate on nutrient needs for protein/calories (kcal/day) for maintenance, repletion, or restriction as appropriate.
  3. Educate on restrictions; fluid, electrolytes, minerals as appropriate.
  4. Educate on vitamin/mineral requirements and recommend supplementation as appropriate.
- Assist in developing a meal plan consistent with the prescribed diet.
  1. Review daily intake (servings per day) from the food groups.
  2. Recommend a meal pattern for the patient to follow.
- Review prescribed or restricted food lists/food groups.
  1. Instruct on acceptable foods and amount/serving.
  2. If restrictions are indicated, provide a list of foods to avoid as appropriate.
  3. Provide a list of alternatives to substitute for items restricted.
- Offer the following general advice for post-discharge meal preparation and consumption:
  1. Make use of timesavers such as prepared foods.

2. Make use of resources, for example, a home meal delivery program such as "Meals on Wheels"and other community resources such as home health aides, relatives, friends, and neighbors.
3. The hospital discharge planner or social worker can assist in providing community resources for patients requiring assistance with meal preparation by
   –making appropriate referrals to the social worker for patients identified in the hospital setting that have difficulties with meal preparation or shopping.
4. Preparing menus to assist the patient with grocery shopping.
5. Suggesting a pleasant mealtime atmosphere, which encourages food intake.
6. Recommending that the patient avoid foods that are unappealing.

- Specific eating problems may require additional instruction, the use of oral supplements, and follow-up by a dietetics professional or home health nurse:
  1. Anorexia (small frequent feedings with nutrient dense foods will optimize intake).
  2. Nausea and vomiting (small frequent feedings, use of antiemetic medications as prescribed, and low-fat nonodorous foods may be better tolerated).
  3. Chewing and swallowing difficulties (modifications of food consistency and liquids may be necessary).
  4. Medically prescribed diets with multiple restrictions.

DISCHARGE PLANNING

The following data should be collected for use in coordinating the discharge planning process for patients requiring follow-up on the nutrition plan of care in the home setting.

- Patient name/address, and phone number
- Primary caregiver name, address, and phone number
- Referring primary care physician name, address, and phone/fax number

- Home care agency/DME company, address, and phone/fax number
- Home care nurse or home care dietitian contact information
- Health care benefits: Medicaid, Medicare, insurance, insurance benefits contact persons
- Hospital nutrition plan of care
- Home storage capabilities; an additional small refrigerator or closet may be necessary to store all supplies related to feeding

HOME PARENTERAL AND ENTERAL NUTRITION (HPEN)

Planning for HPEN needs to begin in the hospital. The dietetics professional should be involved in determining the appropriateness of enteral therapy, enteral access, the appropriate enteral regimen, and the process of implementation of the enteral nutrition plan in the home. The dietetics professional should also be involved in documentation of the rationale for parenteral nutrition, appropriate formulation, and nutrient needs of the patient.

Reimbursement for home enteral nutrition may vary based on the insurance carrier. For patients requiring home parenteral nutrition, most commercial insurance carriers and Medicaid will reimburse if deemed necessary by a physician. However, Medicare has strict criteria for reimbursement of HPEN and some commercial insurance carriers will abide by Medicare rules to determine eligibility for reimbursement. It is imperative that the dietetics professional communicate with the discharge planner in evaluating reimbursement eligibility to assure that there is appropriate documentation or that an alternative plan using less expensive options can be developed if the patient has limited or no coverage for the intended nutritional therapy. (See Table 5–1 on Medicare reimbursement criteria.)

Evaluate patient eligibility for home enteral nutrition using preestablished criteria for patient selection:

- Gastrointestinal (GI) tract is functional and nutrient absorption is adequate.

Table 5–1 Medicare Criteria for Reimbursement for HPEN

Medicare provides reimbursement for formula and equipment for home enteral nutrition under Part B if documentation includes:
- condition is permanent with a duration of at least 3 months
- enteral nutrition must be the sole source of nutrition and feeding must continue for a minimum of 3 months
- there is a functional impairment to obtaining oral nutrition and enteral nutrition is the sole source of nutrition
- specialty or disease-specific formulas require additional documentation for enteral formulas within the following categories
  1. Category IB—intact protein/protein isolates commonly known as blenderized nutrients —additional documentation must provide sufficient information that the patient has an intolerance or allergic reaction to nutritionally equivalent (semisynthetic) products; or requires a blenderized formula to alleviate adverse symptoms expected to be of permanent duration with continued use of semisynthetic products.
  2. Category III—hydrolyzed protein/amino acids
  3. Category IV—defined formula diets for special metabolic needs
  4. Category V—standardized nutrients
  5. Category VI—modular components
- Enteral feeding pumps require documentation of intolerance to bolus feeding, such as vomiting, diarrhea, abdominal distention, or cramping

Medicare provides reimbursement for parenteral nutrition under Part B if documentation includes:
- clinical conditions exist precluding the ability to maintain nutritional status via PO intake or enteral feeding
  1. small-bowel resection with less than 5 feet of remaining small bowel
- diet modification and pharmacological intervention have been unsuccessful in maintaining nutritional status
  1. short-bowel syndrome with 2.5 to 3 liters of oral intake and enteral losses greater than 50% of intake and urine output less than 1 liter
  2. significant malnutrition* with intestinal motility disorder unresponsive to prokinetic agents
- significant malnutrition* with a fecal fat concentration of 50% per 72-hour fecal fat collection
- complete mechanical small-bowel resection not amenable to surgery
- bowel rest of 3 months or greater is indicated due to pancreatitis, regional enteritis, or enterocutaneous fistula with a feeding tube distal to the fistula not possible
- significant malnutrition* with failure of a tube feeding trial including pharmacological interventions (e.g., anticholinergics, pancreatic enzymes, bile salts, prokinetic agents)

*Significant malnutrition (10% or greater weight loss over 3 months or less and serum albumin less than 3.4 g/dl)

- Patient is unable to meet nutrient needs by oral route alone.
- Patient has stable clinical and hydration status.
- Calorie, protein, and fluid (free water) needs are achievable by tube feeding.
- Calories should be provided in the range of 20–35 kcal/kg.
- Patient and/or caregivers are willing to comply with home feedings and are physically, psychologically, and cognitively prepared to administer the home enteral feeding regimen.

- Tolerance to enteral nutrition has been established.
- Home environment is safe and affords necessary facilities including running water, refrigeration, and temperature-controlled dry storage.
- Financial responsibilities and insurance arrangements have been considered.
- Follow-up care for monitoring and tube feeding-related problems is available.

Evaluate patient eligibility for home parenteral nutrition using preestablished criteria for patient selection:

- Gastrointestinal (GI) tract function is severely diminished with either impaired absorption of nutrients or inability of nutrients to be transported via the GI tract, with documentation that nutritional status cannot be maintained by oral intake or enteral nutrition.
- GI tract function is compromised so that only partial nutritional needs can be met with oral intake alone due to a permanent abnormality of the GI tract.
- Nutrients must be provided within the following ranges: 20–35 kcal/kg/day total calorie intake and 0.8–1.5 g/kg/day protein intake.
- Final dextrose concentration not less than 10%, and lipids of 15 units of 20% emulsion or 30 units of 500 ml 10% emulsion monthly.
- Patient with stable clinical and hydration status.
- Calorie, protein, and fluid (free water) needs are achievable with parenteral nutrition.
- Patient and/or caregivers are willing to comply with parenteral feeding regimen and are physically, psychologically, and cognitively prepared to administer the home parenteral feeding regimen.
- Anticipated duration of parenteral nutrition is sufficient for insurance reimbursement and sufficient to meet nutrition goals.
- Tolerance to parenteral nutrition has been demonstrated.
- Home environment is safe and affords necessary facilities including running water, refrigeration, and temperature-controlled dry

storage. (See Table 5–2 on home assessment criteria.)
- Financial responsibilities and insurance arrangements have been considered.
- Follow-up care for monitoring and parenteral nutrition-related problems is available.

Selection of access route, formula and administration schedule of HPEN:

- See section on enteral nutrition in Chapter 4 for a comprehensive review of feeding tube placement, formula selection, and feeding progression.
- Consider patient's/caregiver's lifestyle and scheduled activities in determining feeding regimen.
- Only permanent feeding ostomy tubes are recommended for home enteral nutrition.
- In general, standard polymeric or regular nutrient-dense formulas will meet the needs of most patients. The use of specialty formulas for specific disease states or elemental, defined formula diets will require additional documentation to justify their use.
- Intermittent feedings via gravity generally are recommended for ease of administration in home setting and more physiologically consistent with normal eating patterns.
- Access devices for home parenteral nutrition are usually implantable ports, Hickman catheters, or peripherally inserted central catheters (PICC).
- Parenteral infusions are generally cycled to a 12-hour or 14-hour infusion regimen.
- If other parenteral infusions need to be given, these must be coordinated with the nutrition regimen since not all IV products are compatible with parenteral nutrition solutions.

Discharge Prescription/Documentation

- Document the formula name, administration method, quantity of each feeding and rate, water flush, and type of feeding tube for enteral nutrition.
- Document concentration and volume of dextrose/amino acids/lipids, schedule, and rate for parenteral formulas.

Table 5–2 Home Assessment Criteria

Electricity
Is electricity available in the home and is outlet compatible/grounded with the use of an infusion pump?
Is there frequent interruption of the electrical service that would warrant the use of a backup pump?
Does the infusion pump have sufficient battery backup?
Has the electric company been notified about the presence of medical equipment in the home?

Refrigeration
Is a refrigerator available for storage of the PN solutions and if so, can it accommodate 1 to 2 weeks
  of PN and related supplies, or is an additional refrigerator required?

Telephone
Is a telephone available for emergency calls to the nursing agency or ambulance service?
Has a list of emergency numbers been prepared for the patient?

Water
Is water available for cleaning of preparation areas and for handwashing?

General cleanliness
Is home free of insects and rodents?
Is there an area that can be used for supply storage that is secure from pets and children?

Safety issues
How difficult is it for the patient to get from the bedroom to the bathroom?
Can an IV pole and pump be maneuvered into the bathroom or does the patient need a bedside
  commode?
Are there stairs that need to be negotiated during the infusion period?
Do area rugs pose a safety hazard?
Is there an area for sharps disposal that can be secured and out of the reach of small children and
  pets?

*Adapted from Ireton-Jones, C., DeLegge, M., Epperson, L., & Alexander, J. Management of the home parenteral
nutrition patient. *Nutrition in Clinical Practice.* 2003;18(4):310–317.

- Document diagnosis and any clinical factors necessitating the intended nutritional therapy such as weight loss and depleted protein stores, and any supporting tests such as a d-xylose absorption or fecal fat test, and pharmacologic and surgical interventions attempted to provide oral or enteral feeding.
- Certificate of medical necessity (CMN) is required for all new HPEN patients and must be complete and accurate to assure reimbursement.

Factors to consider when selecting a home care company:

- *Staff:* availability of interdidisciplinary team members skilled in providing nutrition support including a nurse, dietitian, and pharmacist; physician availability
- *Equipment and supplies:* types available, method and frequency of delivery, inventory and rotation of stock in home, availability of 24/7 home delivery, maintenance capabilities
- *Services:* evaluation of the home environment, home visitation policies, instruction materials, geographic service area, feedback referral, provision of laboratory services, processing and reporting results, medication availability, disaster plan
- *Financial policies:* billing systems and reimbursement assistance, creative payment plans

for clients, process of application for medical assistance
- *Quality management procedures:* written protocols and procedures for assessment and monitoring of professional services, patient satisfaction surveys, patient grievance resolution plan, outcome analysis, criteria for subcontracting
- *Communication:* provision of written reports on all home visits, written incident reports, and written confirmation of all verbal orders to the primary physician
- *Note:* Many patients will be directed to use specific home care equipment companies and home care agencies as determined by their insurance/HMO/PPO providers. In these cases, there will not be a choice as to the selection of the home supporting agency.

The following are strategies for negotiating with insurance companies and case managers:

- Document rationale for placement of tube enterostomy and the need for enteral nutrition support (e.g., s/p neck dissection, dysphagia, promotion of wound healing).
- Document that enteral feeding is the patient's sole source of both hydration and nutrition.
- If a specialty or disease-specific formula is indicated, document rationale for its use and the modifications in nutrient content in relation to the disease state.
- Bill as a prescription for medical nutrition therapy—*not food.*
- Have prescription signed by the attending Medicare-certified physician.
- Discuss dietitian involvement postdischarge.
  1. Dietitian will see patient at clinic visits.
  2. Frequent telephone conversations with patient, caregiver, and home care nurse.
  3. Dietitian will monitor laboratory data.
  4. Dietitian will document patient's progress and inform the case manager.
- Be flexible when negotiating payment options, per diem, and separate billing for durable medical equipment.

Home Tube-Feeding Instruction

The following techniques of home enteral feeding should be reviewed with the patient and caregiver prior to discharge. In some institutions, the dietitian and the primary nurse share the responsibility for home tube-feeding education. When more than one health care professional is responsible for home tube-feeding education, a checklist should be used to ensure that all necessary information is reviewed prior to discharge. (See sample interdisciplinary home enteral nutrition education checklist [Appendix 20].) Any education not completed prior to discharge should be communicated to the home health care team so that a smooth transition into the home setting can be accomplished.

General Nutrition Information

- Educate the patient on the need for good nutrition for complete recovery from illness.
- Describe the general content of the tube feeding formula: calories for energy (carbohydrate and fat), protein for building and maintaining muscle mass and other body tissues, vitamins and minerals to help the body use the calories and protein, and water to maintain hydration status.
- If the patient is taking an oral diet, review dietary requirements and/or modifications and adjustments in the tube feeding volume based on oral intake as appropriate.
- Review the procedure for ordering supplies.

Feeding Catheter

- Identify the tube by its name.
- Identify entrance (insertion) site and location of tip.

Formula

- Identify each product included in the diet prescription.
- Specify amount needed per day and per week so that patient can anticipate storage needs.
- Substitutions should not be considered without approval from the health care team.

- Review the following precautions concerning formula storage:
  1. Unopened cans, bottles, packets, or envelopes are sterile and should be stored in a dry, cool location.
  2. Check expiration dates on product containers and on each case of formula.
  3. Product should not be used after the expiration date.
  4. Opened cans or bottles or prepared formulas should be stored covered, labeled, and refrigerated for up to 24 hours.
  5. Discard unused opened formula after 24 hours.
- If a concentrated formula is used, be sure to specify additional free water needed since the formula may provide significantly less free water for the volume of tube feeding formula that is being given, and dehydration may occur.
- Procedure for supply ordering.

Formula Preparation

- Emphasize that preparation area should be clean.
- Review proper handwashing technique prior to handling formula.
- Ready-to-use formula should be shaken and top of container cleaned prior to opening.
- Educate on proper procedure for mixing powder formulas or mixing products together.
- When additives are part of the formulation, supply a list of items, the amounts to be added per feeding, and explain rationale for their use.
- Review procedure for measuring in common household or metric measures.

Enteral Feeding Equipment

- formula
- feeding bags
- pump (optional)
- large piston syringe at least 50 ml
- 4 × 4 split gauze sponges
- tape
- feeding pole or wall hook
- measuring utensils

Tube Feeding Administration Schedule

- Indicate if feeding is to be intermittent, bolus, continuous, pump, or gravity.
- Provide schedule of times of feedings, volume of each feeding, and length of time for each feeding to infuse.
- Indicate volume of flush either in household measures or in terms of the amount of the syringe (e.g., one full syringe, ½ syringe) or in metric measurements as indicated on syringe.
- Tube should be flushed at least after each feeding.
- Additional flush may be indicated to provide adequate fluid.
  1. Recommend use of household measures as much as possible, or indicate in cans the amount to be given since patients are more familiar with these measurements than metric measurements.
- If patient is discharged on less than goal volume of feeding, it will be necessary to advance feeding in home setting; provide clear instructions on how the feeding will be increased.
- If feeding infusing via pump, specify rate and length of time feeding to infuse and demonstrate use of pump.
- If feeding via gravity, demonstrate how to adjust rate of feeding by adjusting roller clamp on tubing attached to bag, or how to instill feeding using barrel of a syringe.
- Tubing attached to bag of formula should be primed (completely filled) with formula prior to attaching to feeding catheter to prevent boluses of air entering GI tract.
- As a general rule, medications should not be added to tube feeding formula. Before adding medications, the tube should be flushed with a minimum of 5–10 ml of water, the medication thoroughly crushed and mixed with appropriate diluent, flushed into tube, and followed by another flush of water. If possible, medications should be converted to a liquid formulation. Crushing of medications and mixing with diluent needs to be carefully demonstrated by the hospital or home health nurse to assure the medication is appropriate for crush-

ing, is thoroughly pulverized, and the tube is properly cleared after administration.

- Educate patient on clamping the feeding tube prior to opening it to flush or instill tube feeding formula to prevent leakage of gastric contents.
  1. Many standard gastrostomy and jejunostomy tubes have a clamp attached to them.
- Evaluate sanitation in home to determine length of use of the feeding equipment; however, follow manufacturer guidelines for maximum amount of time feeding bags and tubing should be changed.
  1. Some systems can be used for 2–3 days if equipment is thoroughly rinsed and allowed to air dry.

Confirming Tube Position

- Nasogastric feeding tubes are not recommended routes for home enteral feeding due to the ease with which these tubes can become dislodged and the increased risk for aspiration. However, occasionally patients will be discharged with nasogastric tubes that have been sutured in place for short-term tube feeding (less than 2 weeks). To verify placement, the patient should be taught to measure the length of the feeding tube that is visible outside of the nares.
  1. If length changes or a suture breaks, patient's primary health care provider or home health nurse should be contacted prior to administering anything into the feeding catheter.
  2. Patients/caregivers can also be taught to evaluate position by auscultation of air into the stomach with a syringe, but reliability is not confirmed by study.
- Permanent feeding catheters, such as gastrostomy and jejunostomy feeding tubes, may have numbered lines on catheter to help verify position within the gut. If a standard gastrostomy or jejunostomy feeding tube designed for other purposes (such as a Foley catheter) has been used instead of a catheter:
  1. For standard feeding catheters, patient should be instructed on checking the num-

bered line placement on feeding tube to verify that the tube has not migrated.
  2. These tubes have a bumper on the outside that is designed to help anchor the tube to maintain placement. This minimizes friction to the stoma from a loose feeding catheter that is constantly moving within the stoma opening.
     –If the bumper is mobile, it should be kept close to the stoma opening.
  3. If the length of tubing on the outside of the stoma opening has changed from its original length, the home health nurse or primary care provider should be contacted prior to administering anything into the feeding catheter.
- Nonstandard gastrostomy or jejunostomy feeding tubes.
  1. The length of tubing outside of the stoma opening should be measured with the same measuring tape to verify position.
  2. If the length of tubing on the outside of the stoma opening has changed from its original length, the home health nurse or primary care provider should be contacted prior to administering anything into the feeding catheter.

Gastric Residuals

- There are no definitive guidelines on use of gastric residuals in evaluating tolerance or risk for aspiration.
- They are not indicated to evaluate on a routine basis in the home setting.
- Evaluation of gastric residual may be indicated in the following clinical situations:
  1. New or worsening abdominal distention.
  2. Patient complaints of nausea, vomiting.
- Clogged tubes.
  1. Commercial declogging products or pancreatic enzymes can be used.
  2. Contact home health nurse or primary health care provider.
- Educate patient that certain nutrition information will continue to be required to monitor patient progress on enteral nutrition.

1. Record weight as determined by the home care provider protocol.
2. laboratory evaluation:
   –Based on disease protocol and metabolic stability.
   –Laboratory evaluations will be included as part of the assessment process when indicated, such as for complications that may alter electrolyte balance or when infection may be a concern.
3. Ongoing physical assessment to monitor enteral stoma site, and to monitor for adequate hydration.

Home Parenteral Nutrition Instruction

Patients discharged with parenteral nutrition therapy require intensive education by trained nutrition support practitioners. Education is very complex and consists of multiple learning tasks that require training over an extended period of time. A teaching flowsheet is recommended to assure that appropriate education is provided. A teaching plan flowsheet (Exhibit 5–1) is included in this chapter. Education of the patient and/or caregiver should include:

- Rationale for therapy
- Measures to control infection, including proper aseptic technique and handwashing
- Proper flushing technique
- Proper care of access site
- Priming IV tubing and filter
- Evaluation of IV solutions prior to use
- Use of infusion pump with proper technique for initiating and discontinuing infusion

Exhibit 5–1 Teaching Plan Flowsheet

Teaching Checklist						
_____Date/Initials				Teaching Content		Teaching goal met
Identify purpose and goals of home TPN				TPN education packet Review teaching plan		Date_____ Initial_____
Describe basic TPN components/additives				Additives		Date_____ Initial_____
Demonstrate proper storage/disposal of TPN and associated supplies				TPN refrigerated Supply area kept clean and safe from children/pets		Date_____ Initial_____
Describe type and location of VAD				Review VAD written instructions		Date_____ Initial_____
State schedule				Write out schedule		Date_____ Initial_____
Verbalize rationale for laboratory studies, glucose monitoring and weights				Write on calendar Explain rationale Provide log for recording		Date_____ Initial_____
Demonstrate proper handwashing				Proper handwash and dry hands with paper towel		Date_____ Initial_____
Demonstrate aseptic technique				Review aseptic technique		Date_____ Initial_____

Exhibit 5–1 continued

Teaching Checklist							
_____Date/Initials					Teaching Content	Teaching goal met	
Prepare TPN solution					Mixing additives with aseptic technique/correct solution	Date_____ Initial_____	
Prime tubing					How to prime tubing	Date_____ Initial_____	
Demonstrates use of infusion pump					How to read settings/alarms on pump	Date_____ Initial_____	
Initiate/discontinue infusion					Review aseptic technique Setting up pump–connecting/ disconnecting infusion from line	Date_____ Initial_____	
Flush VAD					Review aseptic technique Drawing up flush	Date_____ Initial_____	
Date/Initials					Teaching content	Teaching goal met	
Perform VAD care					Site care/dressing change	Date_____ Initial_____	
Describe any activity limitations d/t VAD					Dressing/bathing safely Threading tubing through clothing Carrying/wearing pump	Date_____ Initial_____	
State complications and appropriate actions					Infection/occlusion/catheter Damage/hypo or hyperglycemia	Date_____ Initial_____	
Identify emergency contacts and contacts for supplies							
Identify support groups					Oley foundation Local support groups	Date_____ Initial_____	

Signatures/Title: _____

_____

Adapted from Gorski, L.A. In TPN update: Making each visit count. *Home Healthcare Nurse.* 2001;19:15–21. Reprinted with permission.

- Mixing additives into primary infusion bag
- Infusion rate and schedule
- Ongoing monitoring, including blood glucose and other laboratory values, weight, and temperature
- Storage of parenteral nutrition products
- Safety issues, including disposal of sharps and checking expiration dates of nutritional products
- Complications (infection/catheter occlusion/malfunction/fluid volume excess or deficit/hypo or hyperglycemia)
- Emergency contacts

Complications of HPEN

Refer to the sections on enteral and parenteral nutrition in Chapter 3, Nutrition Management of the Patient Outside the Hospital Setting, for a thorough review of complications and their management. Patients should be instructed to contact their primary health care provider or home health nurse if complications develop.

Care and Maintenance Issues in HPEN

- Oral care
  1. Mouth care, including brushing, flossing, and rinsing of teeth and gums should continue even if there is no oral intake.
- Enteral feeding tube maintenance
  1. Catheter site should be gently cleaned daily with soap and water unless instructed otherwise.

     –Patients with new gastrostomy and jejunostomy feeding tubes may be instructed to use a cleansing agent or diluted peroxide/water followed by an antibiotic ointment for the first 72 hours following tube insertion.
- A clean dressing should be applied around the stoma site and secured in place with tape.

  –When healed, a dressing may no longer be necessary.
- If purulent drainage, redness, tenderness, or leakage around the stoma site is noted the home health nurse or primary care provider should be notified.
- Parenteral access site maintenance.
  1. Type of access site will determine the appropriate maintenance.
  2. Site should be kept clean and dry and covered with an appropriate dressing.
  3. Continuously monitor for signs of infection and catheter malfunction.

     –Home health nurse should be involved in ongoing monitoring of the access site.
- Resource support groups:
  1. **Horizon Health Care Home Services**
     http://www.horizonhealthcareservices.com/resources/enteral_therapy_tube.htm

Description: Step-by-step instructions for care of the feeding tube, care of the tube site, mouth care, proper tube positioning, and when to notify your home health nurse of problems.

2. **The State University of New York: SUNY Upstate Medical University Hospital**
   http://www.upstate.edu/uhpated/pdf/peds/gastrogravitysyringe.pdf
   Description: Three pages of instructions in a downloadable pdf format for the care and use of the gastrostomy feedings–gravity drip or syringe method of feeding a child.
3. **The Oley Foundation**
   http://www.wizvax.net/oleyfdn
   Description: Support for home tube feeding and for TPN patients and families.

REFERENCES

ASPEN Board of Directors. Standards for Home Nutrition Support. *Nutrition in Clinical Practice.* 1999;13:157–166.

ASPEN Board of Directors. Standards of Practice for Nutrition Support Dietitians. *JADA.* 2001;101:827–832.

Buzby, K., & Ulrich, J. Hospital Discharge Planning: The Role of the Dietitian. In Lysen, L. *Quick Reference to Clinical Dietetics.* Aspen Publishers. Gaithersburg, MD: 1997;191–197.

Capoza, C. Reimbursement and Medicare Standards. *Support Line.* 1996;18:6–8.

Centers for Medicare and Medicaid website. http://www.cms.hhs.gov/manuals. Accessed 2/2004.

Edwards, S., & Metheny, N. Measurement of Gastric Residual Volume: State of the Science. *Medsurg Nursing.* 2000; 9:125–128.

Estoup, M. Approaches and Limitations of Medication Delivery in Patients with Enteral Feeding Tubes. *Critical Care Nurse.* 1994;68–81.

Gorski, LA. TPN Update: Making Each Visit Count. *Home Healthcare Nurse.* 2001;19:15–21.

Grant, J. Recognition, Prevention, and Treatment of Home Total Parenteral Nutrition Central Venous Access Complications. *JPEN.* 2002; 26:S21–S28.

Hammond, K., Szeszycki, E., & Pfister, D. Transitioning to Home and Other Alternate Sites. In Gottschlich, M., Fuhrman, P., Hammond, K., Holcombe, B., & Seidner, D. (eds). *The Science and Practice of Nutrition Support: A*

Case-Based Core Curriculum. Kendall/Hunt, Dubuque, IA: 2001.

Ireton-Jones, C., DeLegge, M., Epperson, L., & Alexander, J. Management of the Home Parenteral Nutrition Patient. *Nutrition in Clinical Practice.* 2003;18(4):310–317.

Kovacevich, D., Canada, T., & Lown, D. Monitoring Home and Other Alternate Site Nutrition Support. In *The Science and Practice of Nutrition Support: A Case-Based Core Curriculum.* 2001.

Marcuard, S., & Stegall, K. Unclogging Feeding Tubes with Pancreatic Enzyme. *JPEN.* 1990;14:198–200.

McClave, S., Snider, H., Lowen, C., McLaughlin, A., Greene, L., McCombs, R. et al. Use of Residual Volume as a Marker for Enteral Feeding Intolerance: Prospective Blinded Comparison with Physical Examination and Radiographic Findings. *JPEN.* 1992;16:99–105

McClave, S., & Snider, H. Clinical Use of Gastric Residual Volumes As a Monitor for Patients on Enteral Tube Feeding. *JPEN.* 2002;26:S43–S50.

Mueller, C., & Shronts, E. Position of the American Dietetic Association: The role of Registered Dietitians in Enteral and Parenteral Nutrition Support. *JADA.* 1997;97: 302–304.

Romano, M. Home Enteral Nutrition: What the Hospital-Based Dietitian Needs to Know. *Support Line.* 2003; 25:17–19.

Sceery, N. Managing Nutrition Support in the Home: Integrating Hospital and Home Care Services. *Support Line.* 2002;24:9–13,16.

Speerhaus, R. Administering Medications with Enteral Feedings. *Support Line.* 1994;16:1–4.

CHAPTER 6

Nutrition Management of the Patient Outside the Hospital Setting

- Home Care
- Long-Term Care
- Functional Foods
- An Alternative Option to Weight Loss

- The Zone Diet
- Complementary and Alternative Medicine (CAM)
- Reimbursement for Medical Nutrition Therapy

Home Care

Carol S. Ireton-Jones, PhD, RD, LD, CNSD, FACN

HOME CARE

Home care is defined as provision of services and/or simple to complex medical therapies in the home when a person prefers to stay at home but needs ongoing care that cannot easily or effectively be provided solely by family and friends.

Who receives home care?

- Patients of all ages
- Disabled patients
- Patients recuperating from acute illness
- Chronically ill infants, children, or adults
- Adults and children diagnosed with terminal illness
- Patients requiring short-term, long-term, or lifetime therapy

Therapies/services provided in the home:

- Home infusion therapies (including home parenteral and enteral nutrition)
- Home health nursing
- Nurses' aides
- Durable medical equipment

Who provides home health care? Depending on the therapy needed, care can be provided by:

- Durable Medical Equipment (DME) companies—can provide anything from supplies such as beds and wheelchairs to enteral nutrition formulas and supplies
- Home Health Agencies—usually provide nursing, nurse aides, and potentially other services such as physical or occupational therapy
- Home Infusion Agencies—may provide nursing but are usually focused on providing home infusion therapies through pharmacies

NUTRITION CARE PROVIDED BY DIETITIANS IN HOME CARE

- Dietitians and Dietetic Technicians—may be employed in home care through home care agencies, DME companies, and home infusion agencies
- Dietitians and Dietetic Technicians—may provide Medical Nutrition Therapy for patients receiving home care. They may also provide:
  1. nutrition screening
  2. nutrition assessment
  3. clinical monitoring, including participation in Clinical Pathways for Home Care

Medical Nutrition Therapy

- Medical Nutrition Therapy (MNT) is an essential component of comprehensive health care services, including home health care.
- People with a variety of conditions and illnesses receiving home health care can improve their health and quality of life by receiving MNT.
- MNT includes a complete assessment of overall nutritional status, medical information, and history of dietary habits, followed by development of and instruction in a personalized treatment plan.

Nutrition Screening

- Nutrition screening is defined as the process of identifying characteristics known to be associated with nutrition problems.
- It is a cost-effective method of ensuring early, cost-effective MNT interventions.
- The purpose is to identify individuals who are at nutritional risk or are malnourished so that further intervention, if needed, can occur.
- It is particularly useful for identifying patients at risk for malnutrition who are receiving all types of therapies in the home (not just those who are receiving home nutrition support.)
- Patients within certain age groups should always receive a nutrition screening—including the very young and the elderly and certain disease categories such as cancer, human immunodeficiency virus (HIV), diabetes, renal disease, and cardiovascular disease.

When the nutrition screening parameters indicate the need for further intervention, a nutrition assessment may be warranted.

Nutrition Assessment

Nutrition assessment provides a comprehensive approach to defining a patient's nutritional status. The assessment includes the organization/evaluation of information to declare a professional judgment.

A nutrition assessment includes:
- Medical, nutrition, and medication histories

- Physical examination
  1. A review of systems approach to the evaluation of physical signs and symptoms of nutritional status.
  2. It is extremely important to complete in home care, as biochemical and other laboratory measures may not be available.
- Anthropometric measurements
  1. In home care, anthropometeric measurements most readily available will be height, weight, and body mass index (BMI).
- Laboratory data
  1. An analysis of serum protein status is a standard component of an in-depth nutrition assessment. The serum protein most often measured in home care and long-term care is serum albumin because of the long half-life of 21 days.
  2. Vitamin status is rarely determined in acute or chronic care due to the expense, long time in turnaround of results, and lack of standards for repletion for most vitamins. A physical assessment may identify signs of nutrient deficiency that warrant laboratory assessment of a vitamin or vitamins. Also, the disease process or symptoms of the disease may warrant the evaluation of a specific vitamin or mineral to avoid deficiency or toxicity. Presence of anemia may be assessed by hematological indices.

A nutrition assessment may be done from a telephone conversation with the patient or caregiver. This type of assessment is most closely related to a technique called Subjective Global Assessment (SGA). SGA uses less extensive measures of nutritional status, which evaluate:

- Nutritional history for weight, appetite, and dietary intake changes
- Presence or history of GI symptoms/problems
- Functional capacity—bedridden to full activity
- Physical symptoms of nutritional deficiency, such as a wasted appearance or ascites

These data are compiled to provide a rating of well-nourished, moderately malnourished, or severely malnourished.

Malnutrition may be categorized by degree:

- *Mild:* Normal to 90% of normal standard
- *Moderate:* 80%–89% of normal standard
- *Severe:* < 79% of normal standard

Nutrition Care Plan

- A nutrition care plan should be developed to address nutritional deficiencies—be it from individual nutrients or from overall malnutrition.
- The nutrition care plan should address nutrient requirements and nutrient delivery.
- Caloric and protein needs should be determined based on the patient's clinical and nutritional status. For patients who are recently discharged from the hospital, caloric and protein needs may be elevated. Careful attention should be paid to assuring that caloric and protein needs are met, and increased or decreased over time as necessary based on monitoring.
- To determine caloric needs:
  1. Standard formulae can be used to determine caloric requirements for home care patients.
  2. Disease process and activity level should be included in the calculation of total caloric need.
  3. Patients on long-term therapies—or those who require only minimal home care therapies—will most likely have "normal" caloric requirements.
  4. For patients receiving home enteral or parenteral nutrition, care should be taken, through careful monitoring and follow-up, to assure that patients are neither over- nor underfed.
  5. Indirect calorimetry (measurement of energy expenditure/caloric requirements) has been unwieldy in the home care setting until recently. A small, easily portable indirect calorimeter can be used for spontaneously-breathing patients in home care or outpatient settings. This allows the clinician to be more exact in determining an individual patient's caloric needs.

- To determine protein needs:
  1. Protein requirements are usually based on the RDA (Recommended Dietary Allowance).
  2. For adults with normal protein requirements, 0.8–1.0 g of protein/kg body weight is acceptable. If the person is obese or extremely underweight, the protein g/kg of body weight should be modified to avoid overfeeding of protein.
  3. For the ill or stressed patient, the protein goal should be to supply adequate protein to promote anabolism.
  4. Protein requirements are often calculated on the basis of g/kg of body weight or "ideal" body weight, which are graduated upward to account for degree of stress or malnutrition.
  5. A rule of thumb for amount of protein to be given to patients with varying degrees of malnutrition or stress is:
     –Mild stress or malnutrition: 0.8–1.0 g/kg/day
     –Moderate stress or malnutrition: 1.0–1.3 g/kg/day
     –Severe stress of malnutrition: ~1.5 g/kg/day
     –Providing levels of protein in excess of 2 g/kg/day may be excessive, especially in patients with compromised renal function.

Monitoring

- Timing and frequency of monitoring a patient who is receiving home care will vary.
- For patients receiving MNT for diet changes, no follow-up may be necessary.
- For patients receiving home nutrition support, the timing and frequency of monitoring will be based on the mode of therapy (enteral or parenteral nutrition), disease state, and status of the patient, and the management plan developed by the nutrition support/home health care team, including the patient's case manager.
- Generally, the patient receiving home enteral (tube feeding) nutrition (HEN) is followed at

less frequent intervals than the patient receiving home parenteral nutrition (HPN).

- For the patient in transition from one feeding technique to another (HEN to HPN or HPN to HEN or oral), follow-up and monitoring may be required more often to ensure a smooth and successful therapy transition and to assure that adequate micronutrients (vitamins and minerals) are provided.
- Patient monitoring may be accomplished by a home visit or by telephone contact. Chart review to monitor weight and laboratory changes may provide the impetus for modifying the monitoring regimen.
- The patient receiving long-term therapy at home will require less frequent therapy changes; however, monitoring should continue to occur at regular intervals.
- It is important to involve the patient's case manager in the development of a monitoring plan for any patient receiving home nutrition support.
- It is also extremely important to involve the patient in all decisions regarding their therapy and allow them to participate in the development of the monitoring plan.

The American Dietetic Association has developed disease-specific protocols for MNT. These are in the process of being revised using the ADA's evidence analysis process.

The current protocols include:

- weight management (adult)
- pediatric failure to thrive
- anorexia and bulimia nervosa (pediatric, adolescent, adult)
- congestive heart failure (adult)
- pressure ulcer management (older adult)
- weight loss (older adult)
- hyperemesis gravidarum (adult)
- enteral (adult)
- parenteral (adult)
- guidelines for type 1 and type 2 diabetes mellitus
- gestational diabetes mellitus
- hyperlipidemia
- chronic kidney disease

Clinical pathways typically used in the hospital may be useful in home care.

CLINICAL PATHWAYS

A clinical pathway (also called *critical pathway, care map,* or *care path*) is an optimal sequencing or timing of interventions by physicians, nurses, and other staff members for a particular diagnosis or procedure. It is designed to utilize resources better, maximize quality of care, and minimize delays. Clinical pathways were first used in hospital reimbursement systems in the 1980s and have been implemented in many hospitals since the 1990s.

Clinical pathways are implemented in hospital and home care patients' management systems to organize information related to patient outcomes and to review diagnostic categories that represented high cost, high risk, and high variability in order to provide a quality outcome to a particular patient population.

Clinical pathways are currently used in health care to define processes in disease state management in order to

- reduce length of stay
- reduce costs associated with specific diagnoses and procedures
- eliminate variances in treatment protocols
- enhance patient outcomes

Clinical pathways should be effective for about 80% of patients placed on them. The pathways should have validity, reliability/reproducibility, clinical applicability, clinical flexibility, and clarity, and should be regularly reviewed.

The components of clinical pathways are

- condition identification
- scope
- categories of action
- documentation

Development of clinical pathways involves

- selection of diagnosis
- utilization of the multidisciplinary team
- identification of characteristics

- statement of current versus ideal care process
- clinical validation and revision

Benefits to using clinical pathways are

- a multidisciplinary plan of care
- enhanced planning and coordination of care
- standardization of care and reduction of variance
- comprehensive education for patients, caregivers, and staff
- cost control and management
- effective communication tool
- potential reduction in litigation

Dietitians can contribute to clinical pathway processes by

- determining if clinical pathways, whether disease-specific (e.g., diabetes, cardiovascular disease) or episode-specific (hip fracture/replacement), are currently in use or are being developed and requesting to be a committee member or tot review current clinical pathways
- providing input as a committee member
- participating in outcome data collection as a part of the formal process, or as ancillary assistance through clinical management

Other Nutrition Services Provided in the Home by Registered Dietitians

- MNT: Diet counseling/diet instructions
- Food preparation and safety instructions
- Diabetic teaching and if the dietitian is a certified diabetes educator (CDE), all aspects of diabetic care
- Metabolic measurement of energy expenditure, using indirect calorimetry
- Teaching and evaluation of enteral feeding techniques and patient care techniques
- Evaluation of intravenous line site status and care technique
- Grocery shopping educational tours
- Determination of accessibility and availability of community or home feeding programs
- Assistance with communication with other health care professionals
- Coordination of all aspects of home care, including but not limited to nutrition support

- In-services for health care professionals on nutrition and on enteral and parenteral products and services
- Hospice care
- Coordination of patient care from physician office to home

REIMBURSEMENT

- Reimbursement for the services of registered dietitians in home care is not guaranteed.
- As of January 1, 2002 Medical Nutrition Therapy became a Medicare Part B benefit covering MNT services when provided by registered dietitians and nutrition professionals to Medicare Part B beneficiaries with diabetes or renal disease.
- Some insurance companies reimburse MNT services provided by registered dietitians. If an insurance company does not cover nutrition services, the patient can call or write a letter to the benefits department to request coverage for nutrition services from a dietitian.
- Patients seen individually for MNT can self-pay for MNT services.
- Dietitians may bill the home health, home care, or home infusion agency when seeing patients referred from one of these agencies.
- Dietitians or dietetic technicians may be full-time, part-time, or per-diem employees of a home health, home care, or home infusion agency.

Getting Started in Home Care

- Determine the services a dietitian can bring to a home care agency.
- Find out what types of services are currently being provided.
- Provide a cost-benefit approach to the marketing of the services to be provided.
- Negotiate a salary or hourly/visit rate that takes into consideration the type of expertise required and the time involved.
- Know the standards and guidelines of the home care, home infusion, and home nutrition support industry.

- Be creative and innovative.
- Be self-motivated and self-sufficient.
- Be knowledgeable and resourceful.
- Have your own diet instruction materials for oral, enteral, and parenteral nutrition, if necessary.

REFERENCES

ADA's definitions for nutrition screening and assessment. *Journal of the American Dietetic Association* 1994;94(6): 664–666.

Anthony PS, Ireton-Jones CS. Dietitians in home care: A new challenge. *Support Line.* 1994;16(6): 1–8.

Baker JP, Detsky AS, Wesson DE, et al. Nutritional assessment: A comparison of clinical judgment and objective measurements. *New England Journal of Medicine.* 1982; 306:969–974.

Coffey RJ, Richards JS, Remmert CS, et al. An introduction to clinical paths. *Quality Manage Health Care.* 1992;I: 45–54.

Detsky AS, McLaughlin JR, Baker JP, et al. What is subjective global assessment of nutritional status? *Journal of Parenteral and Enteral Nutrition.* 1987;11:8–12.

Guidelines for the Use of Parenteral and Enteral Nutrition in Adult and Pediatric Patients. ASPEN Board of Directors. *JPEN.* 2002;26(1):8SA.

Ireton-Jones CS. The home nutrition support team: Case management of the future. *Infusion.* 1998:4(7):16–18.

Ireton-Jones CS. Home Care. In: Matarese L & Gottschlich M (eds): *Contemporary Nutrition Support Practice.* 2nd ed. Philadelphia, PA: WB Saunders; 2002, 301–313.

Ireton-Jones CS. Home enteral nutrition from the provider's perspective. *JPEN.* 2002;26(5):S8–9.

Ireton-Jones CS, DeLegge M, Epperson L, Alexander J. Management of the home parenteral nutrition patient. *Nutrition in Clinical Practice.* 2003;18:310–317.

Ireton-Jones CS, Hasse J. Comprehensive nutritional assessment: The dietitian's contribution to the team effort. *Nutrition.* 1992;8(2):75–81.

Ireton-Jones CS, Hennessy KA, Howard D, Orr ME. Multidisciplinary care of the home parenteral nutrition support patient. *Infusion.* 1995;1(8):21–30.

Ireton-Jones CS, Orr M, Hennessy KA. Clinical pathways in home nutrition support. *JADA.* 1997;97(9):1003–1007.

Lykins TC. Nutrition support clinical pathways. *Nutrition in Clinical Practice.* 1996;11:16–20.

Nagel MR. Nutrition screening: Identifying patients at risk. *Nutrition in Clinical Practice.* 1993;8:171–175.

Sceery NL. Managing nutrition support in the home: Integrating hospital and home care services. *Support Line.* 2002;24(5):9–16.

Sexton-Hamilton K, Newton A, Ireton-Jones C. Home nutrition support team advanced nutrition management outcomes for home parenteral nutrition patients (abstract). *Nutrition in Clinical Practice.* 2003;18(2):186.

Recommended Dietary Allowances, 10th ed. Washington, DC; National Academy Press, 1989.

Viall CD, Crocker KS, Hennessy KA, et al. High tech home care: Surviving and prospering in a changing environment. *Nutrition in Clinical Practice.* 1995;10:32–36.

Long-Term Care

Janice L. Raymond, MS, RD, CNSD

Long-term care covers a diverse array of services provided over a sustained period of time to people of all ages with chronic conditions and functional limitations. The services provided range from minimal assistance with basic activities of life to total care resembling a hospital.

Home- and community-based care is a catchall phrase that refers to a wide variety of noninstitutional long-term care settings. These are congregate living facilities that resemble a home and are known by several names:

- Adult Family Home
- Board and Care Home
- Adult Foster Home
- Assisted Living.

These facilities are not required to use the services of registered dietitians despite the fact that residents of these facilities may need special diets or even tube feedings.

In contrast, nursing homes or nursing facilities, as they are referred to by Medicare/Medicaid, are licensed and regulated by the federal government and state and local jurisdictions and are required to employ the services of a registered dietitian. Nursing facilities represent the major institutional setting for long-term care in the United States. In 1996 there were 16,706 certified nursing facilities in the United States, with an estimated 1.8 million beds.

Skilled Nursing Facilities (SNF) provide for round-the-clock care supervised by registered nurses. Most SNFs have specific beds or a designated unit for Medicare patients. The Medicare program requires specific space allocation, staffing, and documentation (see discussion of OBRA below). SNFs can have subacute units for those residents requiring high-tech care including intravenous therapies, tube feedings, and even ventilator support. Large SNFs can employ full-time dietitians.

ROLES AND RESPONSIBILITIES OF DIETITIANS IN SKILLED NURSING FACILITIES

- Participate in menu development—regulation states that a registered dietitian must approve both regular and therapeutic menus.
- Nutrition assessment—regulation states that care plans must be done upon admission and reviewed every 14 days or as status changes dictate. Residents at high nutrition risk, such as those on tube feedings or with major weight loss, must be assessed by the dietitian monthly.
- Provide in-service training for staff—education is required on a monthly basis and specific education must be provided annually, which includes nutrition and subjects related to nutrition and food service, such as skin care and infection control. (See Table 6–1.)
- Mentoring, and sometimes supervision, of the Dietary Manager—SNFs employ Dietary Managers, who are credentialed through their national professional organization, and they are responsible for the day-to-day nutrition care of residents.

Dietitians can also assist in the collection of information for the Minimum Data Set (MDS)

Table 6–1 Recommended Staff Education Relating to Nutrition and Food Service

---

Nutrition Screening and Assessment
Nutrition and Skin Care
Fluid Needs/Hydration
Infection Control
Feeding Techniques and Assistive Equipment
Activities (food is often incorporated)
Nutritional Interpretation of Laboratory
  Parameters
Tube-Feeding Policies and Procedures
Nutritional Needs for Specific Populations
  (e.g., the elderly)

---

and in the creation of Resident Assessment Protocols (RAPS), which are required under the Omnibus Reconciliation Act of 1987 (OBRA). OBRA was intended to standardize the quality of care provided in nursing facilities nationwide. Dietitians working in long-term care should be familiar with the issues surrounding OBRA.

Nutrition Assessment

A comprehensive nutrition assessment should be completed by the dietitian within 14 days of admission. The initial nutrition assessment should include

- diagnosis, diet order
- mental status, medical history, psychosocial history
- appetite
- allergies, intolerances, likes/dislikes
- medications and nutrient drug interactions
- conditions affecting food intake or nutrient needs
- alcohol intake and history of alcohol or drug abuse
- assessment of intake, both past and present
- height, weight, weight history
- pertinent laboratory data

- summary of resident's nutritional status, evaluation of oral intake, nutrient requirements, and need for assistance with eating
- prioritization of problems relative to nutrition and a plan of action to meet specific goals
- list of specific recommendations
- plan for follow-up
- communication with other facility personnel in regard to meeting nutrition goals

Ongoing Nutritional Evaluation

- Residents should be monitored at least quarterly.
- The dietitian must document nutrition status at least annually and after any readmission.
- High-risk residents must be identified and monitored monthly. (See Table 6–2.)
- A procedure should exist that alerts the dietitian to any change of condition, particularly in the case of unplanned weight loss or decrease in food intake.

REIMBURSEMENT FOR NUTRITION SERVICES IN LONG-TERM CARE

Dietitian services are not reimbursed directly by Medicare/Medicaid. Large facilities employ dietitians as part-time or even full-time employees, but more commonly dietitians are on contract with a facility for a specific number of hours per week or per month. It is prudent to contract for hours based on the acuity of the residents.

Meals are part of a daily rate and are inclusive of any oral supplements provided. Oral supplements are not reimbursable by Medicare. Medicaid reimbursement differs by state, but in general does not provide for reimbursement of oral nutrition of any kind.

Tube feedings are reimbursable by Medicare through the Part B program if the resident meets specific criteria. (See Table 6–3.) Tube feeding and parenteral nutrition are reimbursed under the prosthetic benefit. In the case of tube feeding, the prosthesis is considered to be the feeding tube when someone cannot swallow. If a tube feeding is being provided for any other reason than dysphagia it is not *likely* to be reimbursed. In the case of parenteral nutrition the resident must have a nonfunctioning gastrointestinal tract to be considered reimbursable.

CONCLUSION

The incidence of malnutrition in the U.S. population over 65 years old has been reported to be 25%. In long-term care, the published incidence in one study was as high as 85%. Institutionalization itself does not necessarily lead to

---

Table 6–2 Factors Associated with High Risk for Malnutrition

Under 85% of desirable weight for height
Unplanned weight loss of 5% of body weight over 1 month, 7.5% over 3 months, or 10% over 6 months
Serum albumin less than 3.5 mg/dl or prealbumin less than 18 mg/dl
Serum cholesterol less than 140 mg/dl
Eating less than 75% of food served
Stage II or greater pressure ulcer
Poorly controlled diabetes
Acute illness
Age over 80 years
Blended/pureed food
Chewing/swallowing problems
Depression

Table 6–3 Considerations for Reimbursement of Nutrition Through Medicare Part B

Tube feeding must be necessary for 100% of nutrition needs
Recipient of tube feeding must have dysphagia
When providing more than 30 kcal/kg of body weight, extra documentation justifying high kcal needs
   may be required
Specialty feedings, such as those used for residents with malabsorption, require extra documentation
   to justify reimbursement
Dual feedings (parenteral and enteral) will not be fully reimbursed

malnutrition. A large study in 15 long-term care facilities in the Boston area found that intakes of residents were comparable to those in the free-living population. The malnutrition is likely a result of disease or depression. This population is clearly at nutritional risk and requires the services of a registered dietitian familiar with age-specific nutritional needs and diet therapy and who understands federal, state, and local regulations related to long-term care.

REFERENCES

American Dietetic Association, Consultant Dietitian Practice Group. *Pocket Resource for Nutrition Assessment.* Chicago, IL: American Dietetic Association; 1994.

ASPEN Reference Group. *Long Term Care Administration.* Silver Spring, MD: American Society for Parenteral and Enteral Nutrition; 1995.

Harris, NG. Nutrition in Aging. In: Mahan LK and Escott-Stump S, eds. *Food, Nutrition and Diet Therapy,* 10th ed. Philadelphia, PA: WB Saunders; 2000:285–303.

National Academy of Sciences, Institute of Medicine Executive Summary. *Improving Quality of Long-Term Care.* Washington, DC: National Academy Press; 2001.

Raymond JL. Assessment and nutrition management of the older adult. In: Winkler MF, Lysen LK, eds. *Suggested Guidelines for Nutrition and Metabolic Management of Adult Patients Receiving Nutrition Support.* Chicago, IL: American Dietetic Association; 1993:42–52.

Washington Administration Code. Chapter 97: Nursing Homes, 1994.

Functional Foods: An Overview

P. K. Newby, ScD, MPH, MS

DESCRIPTION

The notion that certain foods have health promoting properties has been around for millennia[1] and, in the broadest context, all foods must be considered "functional."[2] In the past several decades, however, advances in modern nutritional science have provided us with the research tools and methods to recognize that some foods may be particularly beneficial for health and to define this concept as "functional foods." The concept was first developed in Japan in the 1980s, although there is currently no universally accepted definition of functional foods and functional foods are not a legally recognized food category in the United States. Along with many individual authors, several organizations have created their own definitions, several of which are shown below.

- Foods that provide functional benefits beyond basic nutrition[3]
- Foods that, by virtue of physiologically active food components, provide a health benefit beyond basic nutrition[4]
- Foods in which the concentrations of one or more ingredients have been manipulated or modified to enhance their contributions to a healthful diet[5]

Although most organizations generally agree that functional foods are foods and not pills, controversy remains as to what types of foods are considered "functional" and whether or not functional foods are synonymous with "designer foods," "pharmafoods," and "nutraceuticals." One author maintains that nutraceuticals are not functional foods, but supplements in a nonfood matrix (e.g., pill) that are used to enhance health and contain dosages higher than those usually found in foods[6]; many authors use all of these terms interchangeably.

The preceding definitions reflect that functional foods refer to a concept rather than to a specific food, food category, or food component per se. Nonetheless, most definitions reflect that functional foods share several common aspects[7]:

- a functional food is a food, rather than a pill, capsule, or another form of dietary supplement
- effects of functional foods are scientifically accepted
- functional foods provide a beneficial effect on body functions, beyond adequate nutritional effects, that are relevant to an improved state of health and well-being and/or reduction of risk (not prevention) of disease
- functional foods are consumed as part of a normal food pattern.

FUNCTIONAL FOOD CHARACTERISTICS

As suggested by the definitions above, the concept of functional foods spans many differ-

ent types of foodstuffs. Likewise, functional foods that have been modified span many different types of technology. That is, functional foods are end products and are independent of the technology that may have been used in their creation. For example, genetic engineering or traditional fortification may be used to create a functional food.

Roberfroid[7,8] summarized that functional foods share several common characteristics:

- a natural food with benefits beyond basic nutritional value
- a food to which a component has been added that is not normally present in the food and may be a macronutrient, a micronutrient, or a nonnutrient
- a food from which a component has been removed because the component is known to cause a deleterious effect when consumed
- a food where the nature of one of more components has been modified or replaced because the component is known to cause a deleterious effect when consumed
- a food in which the bioavailability of one of more components has been increased
- a food in which the concentration of a naturally occurring component is increased
- any combination of the above.

The above represents just one type of categorization scheme, and controversy remains over what foods are defined or characterized as functional. For example, "natural" (i.e., whole) foods are consider functional by some[7] but not all[5] definitions.

BIOACTIVE COMPONENTS OF FUNCTIONAL FOODS

The definitions of functional foods and their characteristics discussed above suggest that a wide range of foods is considered functional. In fact, an estimated 25,000 different chemicals from plants (phytochemicals) exist in nature[9], and the majority of functional food components are in fact derived from plant foods, including fruits, vegetables, and grains. A number of functional foods are also derived from biologically active chemicals found in animals (zoochemicals). As noted above, however, functional foods include more than natural foods, including processed foods that have been fortified or enriched with phyto- or zoochemicals, as well as foods that have been genetically modified to improve nutritional composition. Perhaps not surprisingly, there is a long and varied list of functional foods with biologically active components that confer a health benefit or reduce risk of disease. The list of functional foods and bioactive food components will continue to grow as new functional chemicals are discovered and rigorous research is conducted that demonstrates a clear health benefit from their consumption.

Because functional foods are not legally defined, there is not one list of functional foods on which there is scientific agreement. Some different types of functional food (groups) and their bioactive components are summarized in Table 6–4. This table mainly includes natural foods, but also includes some foods that have been fortified or modified to improve nutritional content. It is important to remember that many foods contain multiple bioactive chemicals, only one or two of which are mentioned in the table. Likewise, many foods have more than one beneficial health effect, and only one or two health benefits are mentioned in the table. In addition, there are a plethora of nutritional bars and shakes that have been modified to increase vitamins and/or minerals, or provide a specific macronutrient composition, or both. These bars and shakes are included in the table only once, although their composition and functionality may vary. Certain foods are not included in this table, including snack foods with echinacea, gum with phosphatidyl serine, candies with antioxidants or vegetable/fruit extracts, and beverages with herbal additives[13]. Recalling that many foods are fortified, including flour and cereals with B vitamins and iron, snack foods made from fortified grains could therefore theoretically be considered functional but are not included in the table. In addition, foods that have

been genetically modified to improve nutritional composition, such as golden rice, are also not included.

For the reader who is not familiar with some or all of the biologically active components listed in the table, information on the functionality of some of the major zoo- and phytochemicals[10,12] is summarized below. There are many chemicals in plants and animals that play an important biological function in human health, but only a few examples are listed below. It should be remembered that for many of the bioactive components found in functional foods there is currently not enough scientific evidence to conclude which mechanism(s) are responsible for the beneficial health effects that have been observed.

Zoochemicals

- *Conjugated linoleic acid (CLA):* A mixture of structurally similar forms of linoleic acid (*cis*-9, trans-11, octadecadienoic acid) found primarily in ruminant animals that have been shown to inhibit mammary carcinogenesis in animals. Limited evidence suggests it may also decrease body fat, increase muscle mass, and increase bone density.
- *N-3 fatty acids:* Omega-3 fatty acids. The primary n-3 fatty acids are eicosapentanoic acid (EPA; 20:5) and docosahexanoic acid (DHA; 22:6). Both n-3 fatty acids are essential components of the phospholipids of cell membranes, especially in the brain and retina of the eye (DHA). EPA and DHA are predominantly found in fish. Consumption of less saturated, shorter chain polyunsaturated acids (PUFAs) can be converted in vivo to the more unsaturated, longer chain, n-3 fatty acids, although conversion is inefficient.
- *Prebiotics:* Nondigestible food components that, when fermented, stimulate the growth of beneficial microflora already residing in the colon and enhance intestinal-cell differential.[14] Examples: insulin, fructo-oligosaccharides, lignan, resistant starch.
- *Probiotics:* Exogenous live microorganisms that protect the colon from undesirable micro-

Table 6–4 Examples of Functional Foods with Their Biologically Active Component(s) and Health Benefits[3,10–12]

Functional Food or Food Group	Bioactive Component(s)	Health Benefit or Effect
Carrots	β-carotene	Reduce risk of cancer
Citrus fruits	Limonoids, flavanones	Support general and cardiovascular health
Cocoa, chocolate	Catechins, epicatechins, procyanidins	Support cardiovascular health
Cranberry juice	Proanthocyanidins	Reduce urinary tract infections
Cruciferous vegetables	Glucosinolates, indoles, sulforaphane	Reduce risk of cancer
Eggs with n-3 fatty acids	n-3 fatty acids	Reduce total and LDL cholesterol
Fatty fish (tuna, salmon, mackerel, sardines) or fish oil	n-3 fatty acids	Reduce TG and risk of CHD, cardiac death, fatal and nonfatal myocardial infarction
Fermented dairy products (e.g., yogurt)	Probiotics	Support GI health and boost immunity
Flaxseed	Polyunsaturated fatty acids, lignans	Reduce risk of CHD and support healthy mental and visual function
Foods replacing sugars with sugar alcohols	Sugar alcohols	Reduce risk of dental caries
Fortified cereals and grains with folic acid	Folic acid	Reduce risk of neural tube defects
Fortified energy bars and sports drinks	Many vitamins and minerals	Support and improve athletic performance
Fortified foods with calcium	Calcium	Reduce risk of osteoporosis
Fortified foods or beverages with antioxidants	Antioxidants (vitamin E, C, β-carotene)	Support general and cardiovascular health
Fortified margarine with plant sterol or stanol esters	Plant sterol and stanol esters	Reduce total and LDL cholesterol
Grapes/grape juice, berries, cherries, red wine	Phenols, resveratrol, anthocyanidins	Support cardiovascular health
Garlic, onions, leeks, scallions	Organosulfur compounds	Support cardiovascular healthy and boost immunity
		May reduce total and LDL cholesterol and inhibit tumorigenesis (garlic)
Green tea	Catechins	Reduce risk of certain cancers
Jerusalem artichokes, chicory root, bananas, garlic	Prebiotics (e.g., fructo-oligosaccharides)	Support GI health
Lamb, beef, turkey, some dairy (e.g., cheese)	Conjugated linoleic acid (CLA)	Reduce risk of breast cancer
Low-fat foods (as part of a low-fat diet)	Low in total or saturated fat	Reduce risk of CHD and certain cancers

continues

Table 6–4 continued

Functional Food or Food Group	Bioactive Component(s)	Health Benefit or Effect
Milk, low-fat	Calcium	Reduce risk of osteoporosis
Nutritional bars or beverages	Many vitamins and minerals	Support general health
Psyllium-containing products (e.g., pasta, bread, snack foods)	Soluble fiber	Reduce total and LDL cholesterol
Soy foods	Soy protein, phenols, saponins, isoflavones	Reduce total and LDL cholesterol May reduce estrogen-dependent cancers
Spinach, kale, collard greens	Lutein and zeaxanthin	Reduce risk of age-related macular degeneration
Tomatoes and tomato products	Lycopene	Reduce risk of prostate cancer
Tree nuts (e.g., almonds)	Monounsaturated fatty acids	Reduce risk of CHD
Walnuts	Polyunsaturated fatty acids	Reduce risk of CHD and support mental and visual health
Wheat bran	Insoluble fiber	Support GI health
Whole oats, oatmeal, oat bran, oat products	β-glucan soluble fiber	Reduce total and LDL cholesterol
Whole grain breads/high-fiber foods	Fiber, inulin, fructo-oligosaccharides	Reduce risk of CHD and certain cancers and support GI health
Vegetables and fruits	Many vitamins and phytochemicals, fiber	Reduce risk of heart disease and cancer

CHD: coronary heart disease; GI: gastrointestinal; LDL: Low density lipoprotein cholesterol; TG: triglyceride

bial species and may improve immune function.[14–16] May also reduce cholesterol, alleviate constipation, vaginitis, and lactose intolerance.[12] Examples: *Lactobacilli, Bifidobacteria.*

- *Synbiotics:* Probiotic and prebiotic components are combined in the same food product.

Phytochemicals

- *Fibers:* Includes all chemical remains of plant cells that are not hydrolyzed and not absorbed in humans. Different types of fibers have different physiological effects and health benefits. Examples: insoluble fiber, soluble fiber, nondigestible oligosaccharides (inulin, fructo-oligosaccharides), β-glucan.

- *Glucosinolates:* A group of glycosides stored within cell vacuoles of all cruciferous vegetables that are hydrolyzed to isothiocyanates and indoles. Example: sulfuraphane (a potent inducer of Phase II detoxifying enzymes in the liver, this isothiocyanate speeds the inactivation and elimination of toxic substances from the body).

- *Isoflavones:* An example of a flavonoid and structurally similar to estrogens, isoflavones are heterocyclic phenols that are weak estrogens and may act as antiestrogens by competing with endogenous estrogens. Examples: genistein, daidzein.

- *Lignans:* Structurally similar to estrogens, lignans are weak estrogens found in plants (phytoestrogens) that may act as antiestrogens by competing with endogenous estrogens. Examples: enterodiol, enterolactone, secoisolariciresinol diglucoside.

- *Limonoids:* May inhibit tumorigenesis. Example: limonene.
- *Lutein:* A carotenoid that is the main pigment in the macula of the eye; able to neutralize free radicals and prevent photo-oxidation.
- *Lycopene:* A nonprovitamin A carotenoid that acts as an antioxidant and may selectively accumulate in the prostate gland.
- *Organosulfur compounds:* May inhibit the activity of *Heliobacter pylori* and cholesterol metabolism. Examples: allicin, allylic sulfides.
- *Polyphenols:* A general category of antioxidants that reduce platelet aggregation. Example: catechins.
- *Proanthocyanidins (tannins):* Prevents *E. coli* from adhering to the epithelial cells lining the urinary tract.
- *Procyanidins:* May reduce oxidative stress on LDL cholesterol.
- *Sterols/stanols:* Analogous to the function of cholesterol in mammals, sterols (phytosterols) are produced by plants and are an essential constituent of cell membranes; stanol derivatives are saturated. Sterols/stanols are usually esterified to form unsaturated fatty acids (creating sterol/stanol esters) to increase lipid solubility. Not synthesized and poorly absorbed in humans, sterols/stanols lower plasma cholesterol by inhibiting cholesterol absorption. Examples: sitosterol, campesterol, stigmasterol, sitostanol, campestanol.

FUNCTIONAL FOODS IN HEALTH AND DISEASE

Functional foods are generally directed at increasing and improving healthy body functions and decreasing long-term disease risk among healthy individuals, and are not generally designed to treat disease among sick individuals,[1] although they can be used to treat disease in some cases (e.g., treating obesity by promoting weight loss). The most popular functional foods are energy/sports drinks, probiotic dairy products, heart health spreads, and ready-to-eat cereals.[1] There are many functional foods currently on the market, and the number of products will continue to increase over time. Growth in the functional food market will be seen in three general sectors:

1. Products making claims for improved heart health and weight management.
2. Products that enhance physical and mental performance.
3. Products that have general health benefits.[1]

In an attempt to better categorize functional foods, the International Life Science Institute proposed six general areas of biological and physiological systems where functional foods can play a role:

1. Growth, development, and differentiation.
2. Substrate metabolism.
3. Defense against reactive oxidative species.
4. Cardiovascular system.
5. Gastrointestinal physiology.
6. Behavior and psychology.[17]

Additional areas where functional foods may play a role include fetal development and xenobiotic metabolism.[8]

The biological impact of all functional foods begins in the gastrointestinal tract (GIT), since all foods must be metabolized and absorbed (or not absorbed, as is the case with certain functional foods). There are three perspectives that are important to understanding the gastrointestinal (GI) response to foods and meals, hence the metabolic effects of functional foods:

1. Meal-induced responses in the GIT caused by factors in foods that may result in longer-term adaptive changes.
2. The ability of foods or meals to alter the digestive and absorptive functions of the GIT in a manner that influences metabolism.
3. The impact that the GIT, through its adaptation to diet, has on risk factors for disease.[18]

Therefore, many of the benefits of functional foods may occur through their effects on the

GIT. For example, the macronutrients have different effects on the release of peptides from the GIT (e.g., cholecystokinin), which may impact satiety, hence control energy intake. On the other hand, the consumption of pre- and probiotics may directly impact the microflora in the gut, especially in the colon, thereby having a positive impact both on GI health in general as well as reducing the risk of GI tumors and cancers.

Postdigestive and postabsorptive effects of functional foods obviously vary, since phyto- and zoochemicals can play roles in one or more of the aformentioned physiological systems (see Table 6–4). Some functional food components have very specific biological effects, such as the role of plant sterols and stanols in reducing total and LDL cholesterol by inhibiting cholesterol absorption. On the other hand, many functional food components have multiple physiological effects. For example, insulin and fructo-oligosaccharides impact lipid metabolism, strengthen immune function, restore or stabilize colonic microflora by acting as prebiotics, and improve bioavailability of nutrients which may, in turn, have other beneficial health effects.[19] Likewise, soy products may contain multiple bioactive components that impact both cholesterol and estrogen metabolism, for example, which may reduce risk of cardiovascular diseases and estrogen-dependent cancers, respectively.

Functional foods therefore play a role in promoting health and reducing the risk of disease through multiple biological mechanisms and physiological systems. A complete discussion of each physiological system and each disease state is beyond the scope of this chapter but the overview on functional foods, their bioactive components, and their health effects discussed here should provide the necessary background for the reader to understand overall health effects. Specific information on the roles of functional foods in athletic performance,[20] cognition and mood,[21] cancer,[12] the immune system,[16] osteoporosis,[22] and obesity and diabetes[23] are available elsewhere. Because of the high prevalence of overweight and obesity and the large market of weight-maintenance and weight-loss

products, only the example of the roles of functional foods in obesity is discussed below.

Although ultimately due to positive energy balance resulting from caloric imbalance, the development of obesity is multifactorial and a functional food approach can target multiple aspects of the energy balance system, including food intake, energy expenditure, and energy storage.[23] Even within each of these three areas there are many ways functional foods can play a role in preventing weight gain or reducing overweight. For example, functional foods can be used to reduce energy intake by increasing satiation and satiety, thereby reducing total energy intake. The three most promising areas to increase satiation and satiety are to:

1. Modify the energy density of the diet.
2. Modify the macronutrient composition of the diet.
3. Modify the glycemic load of the diet.[23]

There is limited scientific evidence to suggest that caffeine, calcium, and catechins may have modest increases on metabolic rate; therefore, consuming foods with these components may increase energy expenditure. In addition, functional foods may affect energy storage and nutrient partitioning by blocking absorption of carbohydrate of fats.[23] A snack product containing olestra, a sucrose polyester, could therefore be considered a functional food if it reduced energy intake and produced weight loss (or prevented weight gain). Also, given that obesity often precedes Type 2 diabetes, any functional food used in the prevention or treatment of obesity would also be effective in reducing the disease burden of diabetes. Obesity and diabetes are, therefore, two disease states for which functional foods can be used for both risk reduction, and for disease treatment itself.

POSITION OF THE AMERICAN DIETETIC ASSOCIATION (ADA)

The ADA states that all foods are functional at some physiological level[11] and has, in the past several years, developed two position statements on functional foods.[11,13] The most recent statement of the ADA follows:

> It is the position of the ADA that functional foods, including whole foods and fortified, enriched, or enhanced foods, have a potentially beneficial effect on health when consumed as part of a varied diet on a regular basis, at effective levels. The Association supports research to further define the health benefits and risks of individual functional foods and their physiologically active components. Dietetics professionals will continue to work with the food industry, government, the scientific, community, and the media to ensure that the public has accurate information regarding this emerging area of food and nutrition science.[11]

In its position papers, the ADA also points out that no foods should be considered good or bad; an optimal diet is a varied diet that is rich in plant foods, and the biological benefits that are gained from consuming a plant-rich diet may not be replicated through a supplement form, so whole foods should be encouraged.[13]

REGULATION OF FUNCTIONAL FOODS

Although definitions of functional foods remain ambiguous and controversial, whether a food is perceived as functional or not by the consumer is in part determined by whether and how it is labeled. A discussion of functional foods would therefore be incomplete without a brief discussion of the regulations of functional foods, including food labeling and health claims.

The Food and Drug Administration (FDA) is the main body responsible for the regulation of food labeling, but responsibilities are also shared by the food manufacturer as well as the Federal Trade Commission, depending on the type of label used. Currently, the regulation of functional foods is not straightforward and can

occur through several mechanisms, depending on the intended use of the food and whether or not a health claim is used in conjunction with the food. Because functional foods are not a legally defined food category, they must be regulated through extant legally defined food categories (i.e., as a conventional food, food additive, dietary supplement, medical food, or food for special dietary use).[11] Importantly, functional foods (and all foods, in fact) are distinctly different from a drug. The Federal Food, Drug, and Cosmetic Act (FFDCA, 1938) defines food as "articles used for food or drink or components of any such article"[24] and food was further defined by the FDA as "articles used for food or drink for man or other animals, chewing gum, and articles used for components of any such article." Through case law, food was also defined as ". . . articles used primarily for taste, aroma, or nutritive value"[25] (as summarized by Ross[26]). Drugs, however, are ". . . intended for use in the diagnosis, cure, mitigation, treatment or prevention of disease. . . ."[24]

In the United States, there are several key pieces of legislation that affect the marketing and labeling of functional foods:

- *Nutritional Labeling and Education Act (NLEA), 1990*[27]: Foods must have a uniform nutrition label. A "health claim" is allowed on products if significant scientific agreement exists on the relation between a particular food (component) and disease risk. Manufacturers may petition the FDA to create a new health claim.
- *Dietary Supplement Health and Education Act (DSHEA), 1994*[28]: Dietary supplements were defined as products that contain one or more dietary ingredients used to supplement the diet. Because dietary supplements are exempted from FDA approval, a "structure/function" claim may be used by manufacturers if they market a functional food as a dietary supplement (rather than a conventional food) as long as they notify the FDA that they are being used; preapproval is not required. Any structure/function claim used under DSHEA must also be labeled as follows:

"This statement has not been evaluated by the Food and Drug Administration. This product is not intended to diagnose, treat, mitigate, cure, or prevent any disease."

- *Food and Drug Administration Modernization Act (FDAMA), 1997*[29]: This act amended the FFDCA. Manufacturers may notify the FDA to use a "health claim" that is based on position statements from "authoritative" federal public health organizations (e.g., National Institutes of Health) or the National Academy of Sciences; preapproval is not required.

The current regulations in the United States therefore allow many different types of claims that can be made on a food product, which require greater or lesser degrees of regulation by the FDA. In accordance with the above laws, there are three different types of claims that can be made for conventional foods and dietary supplements (which, through DSHEA, can appear to be a conventional food although it is legally defined as a dietary supplement), each of which is discussed below.

The first type of claim is a *Health Claim,* which describes the relationship between a food, food component, or dietary supplement ingredient and a reduction in disease or amelioration of a health condition. The legislation discussed above allows for three types of health claims:

1. NLEA-authorized health claims, including those regulated through DSHEA (health claims that meet significant scientific agreement).
2. Health claims based on authoritative statements (FDAMA claims).
3. Qualified health claims.

(The latter category of health claims, qualified health claims, indicates that research is emerging but there is not significant scientific agreement such that qualifying language must indicate that support for the claim is limited.[30])

The second type of claim is a *Nutrient Content Claim,* which characterizes the level of a nutrient in a food through the NLEA. For example, the level of a nutrient can be described as *free, high, low, more, reduced,* and *lite* to characterize it as different from similar products. The use of the word *healthy* suggests that foods have appropriate levels of total fat, saturated fat, cholesterol, and sodium as defined by the FDA. In addition, nutrient content claims can also be used regarding nutrients that do not have established daily values or recommendations, such as omega-3 fatty acids.[30]

The third type of claim currently allowed by the FDA is a *Structure/Function Claim,* which may appear on foods and dietary supplements as well as drugs. Structure/function claims are assumed to be true statements that describe the role of a nutrient or dietary ingredient in affecting normal biological structure or function.[30] Four different types of structure/function claims may be made under DSHEA[26]:

1. A claim related to prevention of classic nutrient deficiency diseases (that must disclose the prevalence of the disease in the United States).
2. A claim describing the basic role of a nutrient (or ingredient) in affecting the structure or function in human health.
3. A claim characterizing the biological mechanism by which a nutrient (or ingredient) acts to maintain structure or function in human health.
4. A claim describing the general well-being due to nutrient (or ingredient) consumption.

As summarized by Ross,[26] although structure/function claims were originally relegated to products defined as drugs, recent legislation and amendments now allow similar structure/function claims on foods if the claims derive from basic nutritional mechanisms; structure/function claims that are beyond basic nutritive value can be made only if the product is sold as a drug or dietary supplement. As a result of these recent changes in legislation, many foods now contain health claims of some kind, and the differences between a food and a drug have become obfuscated. The use of structure/function claims through DSHEA is therefore a source of considerable controversy.

Table 6–5 Current Health Claims Allowed by the FDA Under NLEA[1]

Health claims that meet Significant Scientific Agreement (SSA)
Calcium and osteoporosis
Dietary fat and cancer
Dietary saturated fat and cancer and cholesterol and risk of coronary heart disease
Dietary noncarcinogenic carbohydrate sweeteners and dental caries[2]
Fiber-containing grain products, fruits, vegetables and cancer
Folic acid and neural tube defects
Fruits and vegetables and cancer
Sodium and hypertension
Soluble fiber from certain foods and risk of coronary heart disease
Fruit, vegetables, grain products that contain fiber—particularly soluble fiber—and the risk of coronary heart disease
Soy protein and risk of coronary heart disease
Stanols/sterols and risk of coronary heart disease

FDA Modernization Act of 1997 (FDAMA) Claims
Choline
Potassium and risk of high blood pressure and stroke
Whole-grain foods and risk of heart disease and certain cancers

Qualified health claims
Selenium and cancer
Antioxidant vitamins and cancer
Nuts and heart disease
Walnuts and heart disease
Omega-3 fatty acids and coronary heart disease
B vitamins and vascular disease
Phosphatidylserine and cognitive dysfunction and dementia
0.8 mg folic acid and neural tube birth defects[3]

[1] Summarized from Reference (30).
[2] Includes sugar alcohols and D-tagatose.
[3] Note that whereas 0.4 mg of folic acid and the prevention of neural tube defects is a health claim based on SSA, the amount of 0.8 mg as a more effective dose is a qualified health claim.

In summary, through the three major pieces of legislation—NLEA, DSHEA, and FDAMA—and the three general types of claims (of which there are three different types of health claims) there are five distinct categories of claims which can be currently made. There are many nutrient content and structure/function claims that can be made in light of all that is known about the roles of nutrients in the human body and subsequent nutrient recommendations, although the list of health claims is much smaller. The health claims currently accepted by the FDA[30] appear in Table 6–5.

It should be noted that the regulation of functional foods differs around the world.[31–33] In an effort to help develop universal regulations, Codex Alimentarius, the foremost international regulatory body of the Food and Agricultural Organization and World Health Organization created in 1963, developed two specific types of health claims in 1999, as summarized by Roberfroid[7]:

- *Type A claims:* Specific beneficial effects of foods (constituents) on physiological or psychological functions or biological activities. Claims can relate to positive contributions to health, the improvement of biological functioning, or modifying or preserving health but do not include general nutrient function claims.
- *Type B claims:* Risk of disease reduction claims that can occur when foods (constituents) are consumed as part of a daily food pattern.

In summary, many foods are recognized as functional by the consumer due to the presence of health claims, nutrient content claims, and structure/function claims on the product. It is likely that the regulatory environment will continue to evolve in both the United States and abroad as the definitions and understanding of functional foods evolves.

CONSUMER ISSUES

There are several consumer issues that arise when thinking about functional foods. First, consumers must be educated about the potential use of functional foods to enhance their health, which requires a concerted communication effort. Second, education about the potential benefits of functional foods for their health does not ensure that they are selected. Therefore, understanding the factors surrounding consumer acceptance of functional foods is also important.

Consumer Communication

Like nutrition in general, educating the consumer about functional foods is imperative if these foods are able to fulfill their role in having a beneficial effect on human health. There are several mechanisms through which consumers in general and individuals can be educated.

Nutrition labels and health claims in particular are the primary source by which many consumers are educated.[7] The food industry, therefore, does play a role in providing nutrition information by labeling food products. How-

ever, the sheer quantity of claims on products arguably exacerbates extant consumer confusion about the healthfulness of foods in general. Furthermore, competition in the marketplace seen in advertising and the role of the media in conveying what are often nutrition sound bites create a din of often conflicting nutrition messages. Therefore, more direct and interactive communication may be required to help consumers sort through the bulk of information they receive. Health professionals, primarily dietitians, and nutrition and health educators all play an important role in helping educate and empower consumers to make healthy food choices. Educational programs and individual counseling are two ways of helping consumers to understand how functional foods may improve their health.

Because of the importance of both education and communication in nutritional behavior, a study was performed to assess the impact of education on intent to consume functional foods.[34] The specific objectives of the study were to assess consumer intent to consume nine functional foods (tea, broccoli, fish, garlic, purple grapes/grape juice, oats, soy, tomatoes/tomato products, and yogurt) based on a participation in a functional food education program. Among participants, who were men and women aged 18–85 years living in the state of Illinois, tomatoes and tomato products were consumed more than any other functional food. Less than 10% of younger subjects (aged 18–35 years) consumed recommended amounts of any of the nine functional foods studied, whereas a greater percentage of subjects > 65 years met or exceeded the daily recommendations for tea (24%), broccoli (27%), yogurt (31%), fish (32%), soy (33%), garlic (46%), and tomatoes/tomato products (63%). Following the educational program, more women (72%) than men (59%) indicated an intent to increase their intake of all nine functional foods. The author concluded that educating consumers about functional foods can increase their intent to consume them, reflecting that consumers are interested in choosing foods for health.[34]

Although education and communication about functional foods are important elements that will contribute to consumer understanding and acceptance, neither of these conditions is adequate to ensure consumption. Therefore, whether functional foods will play a meaningful role in an individual's diet will depend to what degree these foods can meet other consumer preferences in a food product.[35]

Consumer Acceptance

There are many psychological, sociological, and economic factors affecting how food choices are made, the most important of which are taste, cost, and convenience. Nutrition and health concerns may also play a role in food choice, to a smaller degree, among certain consumers.

Although some consumers may consider nutrition when making food choices, their perception of what foods are healthful or nutritious may vary. Bech-Larsen and colleagues[36] point out that perception of healthfulness of foods may be influenced by the type of food and food processing, origin, production date, conservation method, packaging, and use of additives, among others. The authors therefore studied the extent to which consumers' perception of food healthfulness depended on different types of health claims, functional enrichments, base-products, and processing methods, and whether there were differences among consumers in Denmark, Finland, or the United States. General attitudes toward functional foods were strongest among Finns and weakest among Danes. Also, the presence of health claims on products had a positive influence on all consumers' perception of the healthfulness of functional foods. Finns and Danes were more likely to perceive organic foods as healthier than conventional foods, although Americans were not. According to the authors, the main result of the analysis was that there were significant interactions between the functional enrichment of a product and the base-product. That is, the perception of food healthfulness is modified by whether the original (base-) product modified was healthy to begin with. For example, consumers depreciate the enrichment of juice and yogurt since these foods are already perceived as healthy, whereas they appreciate the enrichment of a spread (e.g., margarine enriched with oligosaccharides or omega-3 fatty acids), since those foods are perceived as unhealthy.[36]

Another study explored the opinions of Dutch consumers on several functional foods (yogurt, cholesterol-lowering margarines, fortified lemonade or sweets, or foods with extra calcium) and their associations with demographic and lifestyle variables.[37] Half (52%) of subjects believed that the development of functional foods was generally positive. Only 3% of subjects consumed yogurt, margarine, or sweets daily compared to 6% who consumed calcium foods; 49% never consumed yogurt, 42% never consumed the margarine, 34% never consumed fortified sweets, and 58% never consumed calcium-enriched foods. More subjects rated foods with extra calcium (39%) or yogurt (31%) as an "easy way to stay healthy," compared with the margarine (17%) and fortified sweets (17%). Women were more likely to be consumers of yogurt and men were more likely to be consumers of cholesterol-lowering margarine and fortified lemonade or candy. Smoking was also associated with use of the margarine and subjects who perceived their health as poor were more likely to consume calcium-rich foods.

In summary, communication is the first step in educating consumers about the potential role of functional foods to improve their health. However, whether consumers will ultimately accept these foods into their diet depends upon the degree to which these foods meet their other food preferences, as well as their general perceptions and attitudes toward these foods. More research is needed to both better understand factors that will increase consumer acceptance of functional foods, and will enable them to incorporate these foods into their diet.

SCIENTIFIC CONSIDERATIONS

There are several important areas of scientific research that require further study in order to support the safe and efficacious use of functional foods for health.

First, demonstrating a clear relation between functional foods and health relies on the development of biological markers that can be measured.[9,71] Biological markers need to be identified and validated for their predictive value of potential benefits to a target function or the risk of a particular disease.[8] Specifically, biomarkers need to be related to three factors: dietary exposure, biological effect or outcome, and endpoint of improved health or reduced disease.

Second, questions of toxicity and safety[2,38] of some functional food components remain since many of these components are recent discoveries and upper intake levels have not been established. Therefore, instructing consumers to consume these foods without guidelines as to the amounts in which they should be consumed may pose some, as yet unquantified, risk. Both short- and long-term research is required to establish at what levels of intake a benefit occurs and whether or not increased consumption also poses a risk. It is also important to remember that risk could be incurred not only due to potential toxicity of the particular functional food component itself, but also due to the other components in the food. For example, candies fortified with antioxidants or snack foods with echinacea are considered functional foods by the ADA[11], yet increased consumption of these foods may also deliver increased calories, sugars, and saturated fat. (Note that not all scientists would consider such products to be functional foods because of these reasons.) An increasingly complicated food supply with products such as these suggest a "risk management" approach may be required to help consumers sort through these issues to decide which foods are in fact healthiest for them.

Third, interactions among nutrients and the effect of food processing on functional foods may impact their intended health effect.[2] Nutrients and nonnutrients work together interactively and, therefore, intended effects may vary as a function of other food consumed at the same time that occurs within the total dietary pattern. In addition, food processing methods may impact bioavailability of nutrients and, therefore, effectiveness, of functional foods.

Finally, the roles of individual susceptibility and genetic variation in responses to a given functional food are also important[7] and will likely play an increasingly larger role in the nutrition and food sciences. The study of nutrient–gene interactions may in the future allow for specifically tailored dietary interventions for an individual's genetic constitution and each individual or group of individuals with similar polymorphisms, for example, may benefit from specially designed functional foods.

SUMMARY AND CONCLUSIONS

The growth of the self-care movement, high health care costs due to chronic disease and aging, technological advances, changes in food regulations, growth in the market for health and wellness products, and scientific research and discoveries linking food and its components to health[2,10,11,39] have all created an environment that is conducive to the creation of marketing of functional foods. The major points discussed in this overview of functional foods can be summarized as follows:

- Functional foods are not clearly defined and controversy remains over what foods and food components should be considered functional. Epidemiological and animal research, clinical trials, and animal models are all necessary to establish whether a food (component) is functional.
- There are thousands of bioactive food components derived from both plants and animals that play a role in human health and disease and many components play multiple roles in several physiological systems.
- The current regulatory environment allows many health claims to appear on products. Health professionals, and most importantly dietitians, are needed to help consumers understand the potential role of functional foods in health. Whether or not consumers will incorporate functional foods into their diet will depend on the degree to which functional foods meet other food preferences.
- Scientific research will help to establish the efficacy of functional foods by developing

biomarkers, assessing safety and risk, and understanding nutrient interactions and the role of individual susceptibility in disease.

In conclusion, many more functional foods and bioactive components will be discovered as nutrition science evolves and these foods will play an increasingly larger role in the global food market and human health. Although the term "functional foods" may become obsolete[38], the concept that some foods are healthier than others will always remain. Functional foods have a great potential to help improve the diet and health of consumers.

Note: This material is based upon work supported by the U.S. Department of Agriculture, under agreement No. 58-1950-4-401. Any opinions, findings, conclusions, or recommendations expressed in this publication are those of the author(s) and do not necessarily reflect the view of the U.S. Department of Agriculture.

REFERENCES

1. Weststrate JA, van Poppel G, Verschuren PM. Functional foods, trends and future. *Br J Nutr.* 2002;88 (Suppl 2):S233–S235.

2. Milner JA. Functional foods: The US perspective. *Am J Clin Nutr.* 2000;71:1654S–9S; discussion 1674S–5S.

3. International Food Information Council Foundation. *Functional foods.* 2004. URL: http://www.ific.org/ nutrition/functional/index.cfm. Accessed: 15 February 2004.

4. Clydesdale FM. ILSA North American Food Component Reports. *Crit Rev Food Sci Nutr.* 1999;39:203–316.

5. Committee on Opportunities in the Nutrition and Food Sciences, Food and Nutrition Board, Institute of Medicine. Washington, DC: National Academy Press, 1994.

6. Zeisel SH. Regulation of "nutraceuticals." *Science.* 1999;285:1853–1855.

7. Roberfroid MB. Global view on functional foods: European perspectives. *Br J Nutr.* 2002;88 (Suppl 2):S133–S138.

8. Roberfroid MB. Concepts and strategy of functional food science: The European perspective. *Am J Clin Nutr.* 2000;71:1660S–1664S; discussion 1674S–1675S.

9. Milner JA. Functional foods and health: A US perspective. *Br J Nutr.* 2002;88 (Suppl 2):S151–S158.

10. Hasler CM. Functional foods: Benefits, concerns and challenges—A position paper from the American Council on Science and Health. *J Nutr.* 2002;132:3772–3781.

11. Position of the American Dietetic Association: Functional foods. *J Am Diet Assoc.* 1999;99:1278–1285.

12. Rafter JJ. Scientific basis of biomarkers and benefits of functional foods for reduction of disease risk: Cancer. *Br J Nutr.* 2002;88 (Suppl 2):S219–S224.

13. Position of the American Dietetic Association: Phytochemicals and functional foods. *J Am Diet Assoc.* 1995;95:493–496.

14. German B, Schiffrin EJ, Reniero R, Mollet B, Pfeifer A, Neeser JR. The development of functional foods: Lessons from the gut. *Trends Biotechnol.* 1999;17:492–499.

15. Duggan C, Gannon J, Walker WA. Protective nutrients and functional foods for the gastrointestinal tract. *Am J Clin Nutr.* 2002;75:789–808.

16. Calder PC, Kew S. The immune system: A target for functional foods? *Br J Nutr.* 2002;88 (Suppl 2):S165–S177.

17. Diplock AT, Charleux JL, Crozier-Willi G, et al. Functional food science and defence against reactive oxidative species. *Br J Nutr.* 1998;80 (Suppl 1):S77–S112.

18. Schneeman BO. Gastrointestinal physiology and functions. *Br J Nutr.* 2002;88 (Suppl 2):S159–S163.

19. Roberfroid MB. Concepts in functional foods: The case of insulin and oligofructose. *J Nutr.* 1999;129: 1398S–401S.

20. Brouns F, Nieuwenhoven M, Jeukendrup A, Marken Lichtenbelt W. Functional foods and food supplements for athletes: From myths to benefit claims substantiation through the study of selected biomarkers. *Br J Nutr.* 2002;88 (Suppl 2):S177–S186.

21. Dye L, Blundell J. Functional foods: Psychological and behavioural functions. *Br J Nutr.* 2002;88 (Suppl 2):S187–S211.

22. Weaver CM, Liebman M. Biomarkers of bone health appropriate for evaluating functional foods designed to reduce risk of osteoporosis. *Br J Nutr.* 2002;88 (Suppl 2):S225–S232.

23. Hill JO, Peters JC. Biomarkers and functional foods for obesity and diabetes. *Br J Nutr.* 2002;88 (Suppl 2):S213–S218.

24. Federal Food, Drug, and Cosmetic Act. 1938.

25. *Nutrilab, Inc. v Schweiker.* (7th Circuit 1983), 1983.

26. Ross S. Functional foods: The Food and Drug Administration perspective. *Am J Clin Nutr.* 2000;71: 1735S–1738S; discussion 1739S–1742S.

27. Nutritional Labeling and Education Act. 1990.

28. Dietary Supplement Health and Education Act . 1994.

29. Food and Drug Administration Modernization Act. 1997.

30. U.S. Food and Drug Administration, Center for Food Safety and Applied Nutrition. *Claims that can be made*

for conventional food and dietary supplements. 2003. URL: http://www.cfsan.fda.gov/~dms/hclaims.html. Accessed: 15 February 2004.

31. Arai S. Global view on functional foods: Asian perspectives. *Br J Nutr.* 2002;88 (Suppl 2):S139–S143.

32. Lucas J. EU-funded research on functional foods. *Br J Nutr.* 2002;88 (Suppl 2):S131–S132.

33. Lajolo FM. Functional foods: Latin American perspectives. *Br J Nutr* 2002;88 (Suppl 2):S145–S150.

34. Pelletier S, Kundrat S, Hasler CM. Effects of an educational program on intent to consume functional foods. *J Am Diet Assoc.* 2002;102:1297–1300.

35. Newby PK. The future of food: How science, technology, and consumerism shape what we eat. In: Ulm JW, ed. *Vision: Essays on Our Collective Future.* Cambridge, MA: The Dipylon Press, 2003:3–24.

36. Bech-Larsen T, Grunert KG. The perceived healthiness of functional foods. A conjoint study of Danish, Finnish and American consumers' perception of functional foods. *Appetite.* 2003;40:9–14.

37. de Jong N, Ocke MC, Branderhorst HA, Friele R. Demographic and lifestyle characteristics of functional food consumers and dietary supplement users. *Br J Nutr.* 2003;89:273–281.

38. Milner JA. Functional foods and health promotion. *J Nutr.* 1999;129:1395S–1397S.

39. Hasler CM. The changing face of functional foods. *J Am Coll Nutr* 2000;19:499S–506S.

An Alternative Option to Weight Loss: Low/Controlled Carbohydrate Regimen

Abby S. Bloch, PhD RD, FADA

AN ALTERNATIVE APPROACH TO WEIGHT LOSS

The epidemic of obesity and diabetes is now a leading clinical issue in the United States, and is rapidly becoming global. In March 2004 Julie L. Gerberding, director of the federal Centers for Disease Control and Prevention, announced: "Obesity is catching up to tobacco as the leading cause of death in America. If this trend continues, it will soon overtake tobacco. Based on current trends, obesity will become No. 1 by 2005, with the toll surpassing 500,000 deaths a year, rivaling the annual deaths from cancer." In a statement released early in 2004, Health and Human Services Secretary Tommy G. Thompson wrote "Americans need to understand that overweight and obesity are literally killing us. To know that poor eating habits and inactivity are on the verge of surpassing tobacco use as the leading cause of preventable death in America should motivate all Americans to take action to protect their health. We need to tackle America's weight issues as aggressively as we are addressing smoking and tobacco."

Although the consumption of fat has steadily decreased over the past decade as the United States became a fat-phobic society, body weight continued to rise. Clearly, health professionals need to consider options or alternatives to the recommendation currently being offered: low fat, low calorie, portion-controlled diets, meal replacements, and other calorie-restrictive methods—since these approaches clearly are not succeeding. Is it not time to consider thinking out of the box for another approach to this serious health problem?

In a very provocative article in *Science* entitled "The Soft Science of Dietary Fat," Dr. Walter Willett is quoted:

> Mainstream nutritional science has demonized dietary fat, yet 50 years and hundreds of millions of dollars of research have failed to prove that eating a low fat diet will help you live longer. . . . NIH has spent over $100m on the three Harvard-based studies yet not one government agency has changed its primary guidelines to fit these particular data.

Dr. Willett and his colleagues have also studied the relationship between glycemic load and carbohydrate intake and the risk of heart disease and concluded:

> Our findings suggest that a high intake of rapidly digested and absorbed carbohydrate increases the risk of coronary heart disease independent of conventional coronary disease risk factors. These data add to the concern that the current low fat, high carbohydrate diet recommended in the United States may not be optimal for the prevention of coronary heart disease and could actually increase the risk in individuals with high degrees of insulin resistance and glucose tolerance.

Concerns about the increased risk factors for heart disease, kidney disease, loss of muscle mass, and other negative effects of consuming a controlled carbohydrate intake are not supported by scientific evidence. In fact, a body of emerging research exists that show the benefits of lowering carbohydrate intake and increasing the intake of healthy proteins/fats. This approach was espoused by Dr. Robert C. Atkins for over 30 years and is just beginning to gain recognition and consideration as a viable alternative by health professionals. Interestingly, the human body has an essential nutrient requirement for both protein (amino acids) and fats but no essential requirement for carbohydrate.

Alternative Dietary Approach to the Standard Low Fat Diet

Many clinicians remain skeptical that a controlled carbohydrate intake will decrease patients' potential risk of heart disease. Despite such skepticism, scientific studies now validate limiting sugars and refined carbohydrates to reducing the risk of developing heart disease by:

- lowering triglyceride levels,
- elevating HDL levels
- improving the subfractions of LDL to the more bouyant, larger pattern A vs. the smaller, denser pattern B subfraction.

Clearly the benefits of a controlled carbohydrate diet could be meaningful for the millions of individuals who are overweight or obese and who are, therefore, at increased risk of developing heart disease or diabetes.

With the mounting evidence from existing and ongoing research, common sense and an obvious public health crisis mandates a new look at the current nutritional recommendations of low fat, low calorie diets limiting saturated fats and emphasizing carbohydrates.

Current Practices

- When an individual responds to the low fat, calorie controlled approach and metabolic and physiological improvement is seen, then this successful approach should be continued for that individual.
  1. However, despite this universal approach, heart disease continues to take more lives annually (950,000) than other diseases.
  2. The American population has reached an all-time high overweight/obesity level of 65%.
  3. Diabetes, which affects 17 million Americans, has increased 49% in the last decade and is expected to increase similarly in this decade.

Clearly, reevaluating the dietary advice given and strategies used in overweight and obese individuals who are at risk for these chronic diseases is in order. An individualized diet best suited to the individual should be implemented. *One diet will not fit all patients.* Identifying specific needs and conditions is key to successful application of the best approach and management of each patient. Controlled carbohydrates should be considered a viable option or alternative to other strategies for weight loss and weight maintenance.

Metabolic Rationale for Lowering Dietary Carbohydrate Levels

- By redistributing carbohydrates, proteins, and fats to a lower carbohydrate and higher protein/fat ratio, the body burns stored fat and suppresses lipolysis.

- Excess calories, especially from high carbohydrate consumption in combination with fat, predisposes individuals to fat accumulation, especially truncally.
- Low carbohydrate levels "kick start" the fat-burning metabolic process and limit insulin secretion.

Progression of Carbohydrates on Controlled Carbohydrate Regimens

- In the first several weeks, the individual reduces carbohydrate intake to 20 g, predominantly in the form of vegetables.
- The remaining foods consist of healthy proteins, healthy fats, and lots of water and fluids along with exercise and some supplements to assure optimal nutrition.

What most practitioners fail to appreciate is that:

- this phase is of short duration
- it allows the person to begin to lose weight, especially in the truncal area
- it sensitizes the individual to excess carbohydrate consumption typically eaten

Benefits of this stepwise progression:

- Individuals lose their cravings for sweets, which in turn suppresses binge eating and snacking resulting in a steady weight loss.
- After several weeks the individual slowly and gradually introduces additional vegetables, nuts, seeds, beans, whole grains, and low glycemic fruits to the food selection.
- By gradually introducing these foods in small incremental amounts, the individual learns the appropriate amounts of carbohydrate-containing foods to select.
- Individuals arrive at their own personal threshold of carbohydrate consumption to prevent weight gain.
- By the maintenance phase, individuals should be eating a very healthy, nutritionally complete diet, which includes all food categories.

SCIENTIFIC RATIONALE FOR CONTROLLED CARBOHYDRATE MANAGEMENT

The combination of high triglycerides and low HDL levels have a common cause: hyperinsulinemia. These findings need to be addressed and then applied in individuals with hyperinsulinism, insulin resistance, prediabetes, and metabolic syndrome. All of these clinical conditions are affected by dietary constituents, specifically carbohydrates, which elevate serum glucose levels with concomitant elevation of serum insulin.

Metabolic syndrome or hyperinsulinemia manifests as:

- high triglycerides
- low HDL levels
- truncal obesity

Testing for this condition includes:

- glucose and insulin levels fasting and 2 hours postprandial reading after a carbohydrate challenge.
- when possible, a 5-hour glucose tolerance test with insulin levels every 2 hours.
- a complete lipid profile which includes:
  1. lipoprotein-A subfractions
  2. C-reactive protein
  3. homocysteine and fibrinogen
  4. ultra-fast CT scan
  5. other appropriate studies based on the patient's clinical

Studies supporting the relationship between insulin, TG, and coronary heart disease (CHD) have been done.

- One example is the finding by the Harvard Nurses Health Study where glycemic load was measured against the risk of CHD in 75,000 women. The authors conclude that "a high intake of rapidly digested and absorbed carbohydrate increases the risk of CHD independent of conventional coronary disease risk factors. These data add to the concern that the current low-fat, high carbohydrate diet recommended in the United States may not be optimal for the prevention of CHD and could actually increase the risk in individuals with degrees of insulin resistance and glucose intolerance."

- What, then, is happening to the millions of individuals who are following the low-fat, high carbohydrate diet recommended by most health professionals today?

One of the most dramatic findings of the controlled carbohydrate regimen is its beneficial effect on triglycerides. There are many studies showing the impact of triglycerides on cardiovascular disease as an extremely predictive risk factor.

Carbohydrates contribute to the elevation of:

- serum glucose
- insulin secretion
- fat mobilization

The typical American will have some degree of insulin resistance, and in this setting a high intake of highly refined carbohydrates can result in serious health problems, such as diabetes and heart disease.

In patients identified as appropriate candidates, recommending a controlled carbohydrate diet would seem to be a prudent clinical alternative to the current recommendations.

Recent studies consistently show that lipid profiles improve on a controlled carbohydrate diet.

Prior dietary studies were in the context of high levels of carbohydrate. When carbohydrates are controlled for, lipid levels improve.

Several recent dietary studies on adults showed that controlled carbohydrate diets resulted in greater weight loss, better compliance, and improved overall lipid profiles.

Another recent study showed improved body composition as well as hormonal balance.

MISCONCEPTIONS ABOUT CONTROLLED CARBOHYDRATE REGIMENS

1. Controlled carbohydrate regimens are only effective for weight loss because calories are restricted.

   Fact: While some may eat fewer calories on a controlled carbohydrate intake, it is not because the program is restrictive or unduly limits food intake. Individuals may be eating fewer calories because they are generally less hungry or have more stable blood glucose levels. It is of interest that those on ad libitum intake of controlled carbohydrates generally consume a lower caloric intake than they would normally do on a low-fat regimen. In light of the difficulty to encourage overweight individuals to control their portion sizes, this approach seems to achieve that goal without the individual having to struggle with portion control. Another interesting finding of recent research is that those on a higher caloric intake consuming controlled carbohydrates lose more weight than those on a lower calorie, low fat intake.

2. The weight lost on controlled carbohydrate regimens is mostly water, not fat.

   Fact: It is typical of any weight loss plan, including the initial phase of a controlled carbohydrate program, that during the first few days or even the first week weight loss will be primarily water (diuresis). After diuresis, however, on a controlled carbohydrate plan with adequate dietary protein/fat, the body switches from burning carbohydrate to burning stored fat, allowing an individual to use body fat along with dietary fat for energy, resulting in weight loss. Moreover, studies have shown that the weight lost is mainly fat, not lean body mass.

3. Ketosis is dangerous and causes a variety of medical problems.

   Fact: Whenever the body utilizes fat for a fuel source, the byproducts are ketones.
   a. Ketosis is very well controlled in normal individuals.
   b. The body very efficiently defends against abnormal pH levels similar to its control of temperature fluctuations, or regulation of serum glucose levels. Blood ketone levels are maintained in a safe range over extended periods of time in individuals with normal metabolic function.

c. The brain's ability to effectively utilize ketones for energy has been known for many decades.

d. Unfortunately, ketosis is often confused with *ketoacidosis,* a condition found in diabetics whose blood sugar is out of control, alcoholics, and individuals in a state of starvation.

4. Diets that promote a liberal intake of high-fat meats and dairy products raise cholesterol levels, ultimately leading to heart disease.

Fact: A growing body of scientific literature demonstrates that a controlled carbohydrate eating plan, if followed correctly, promotes heart health and improves clinical parameters. In older studies, the carbohydrate intake was high as well as the fat intake, confounding the findings that fat was the high risk constituent of the diet. In more than a dozen studies now published, cardiovascular risk factors improved on the controlled carbohydrate arm of each study. It has also been shown that a higher carbohydrate diet increases levels of triglycerides in the blood and lowers HDL levels, both of which have been associated with higher risks of myocardial infarction, ischemic heart disease, and coronary heart disease events. In addition, various researchers have demonstrated that high triglycerides and low HDL, not cholesterol alone, may be the most important factors in heart disease and stroke.

5. Because they exclude fruits, vegetables, and grains, controlled carbohydrate regimens are deficient in nutrients.

Fact: These programs do not exclude fruits, vegetables, and grains. The initial phase of the program, which people often mistake for the entire program, is the strictest phase, permitting 20 g of carbohydrates each day. However, those 20 g come in the form of three cups of green leafy salad and other vegetables each day, and thus include highly nutrient-dense, high-fiber vegetables such as broccoli, asparagus, eggplant, and spinach.

When a sample menu was analyzed the menu met or exceeded RDI requirements of most vitamins, minerals, and trace elements. Once the initial phase is completed, individuals increase their carbohydrate count in steps or a ladder format. This includes more nutrient-dense green leafy vegetables, nuts/seeds, and low-glycemic fruits such as strawberries, other berries, and melons. On maintenance, most people reintroduce legumes and whole grains into their controlled carbohydrate eating program.

6. Controlled carbohydrate regimens are deficient in bone-building calcium.

Fact: These regimens offer a variety of foods rich in calcium, including cheese and vegetables such as broccoli and spinach. Moreover, in a study published in the *American Journal of Nutrition,* researchers studied the short-term and long-term effects of a high-meat diet on calcium metabolism. The study found no significant changes of calcium balance. There was also no significant change of the intestinal absorption of calcium during the high-meat intake. Another recent study showed that in contrast to the widely held belief that increased protein intake results in calcium wasting, meat supplements, when exchanged isocalorically for carbohydrates, may have a favorable impact on the skeleton in healthy older men and women.

7. Controlled carbohydrate regimens cause renal stones and failure

Fact: No renal damage has been seen in individuals who have normal renal function with controlled carbohydrate intake. Many individuals do not follow the guidelines and recommendations of the program urging adequate fluid intake, at least three cups of vegetables, and a general multivitamin/mineral supplement to assure optimal intake. If individuals have compromised renal function, they should work with the managing physician and monitor their renal activity. The food choices should be tailored to the individual's specific needs. If weight loss and lower blood pressure are important for clinical management, the program can provide an effective tool to achieve these goals with appropriate supervision.

Conclusion

There are many variations on the controlled-carbohydrate theme. The effectiveness of restricting carbohydrates has been known for over a hundred years. Dr. Atkins began advocating for this dietary change in 1972. Current research, and rapid scientific advancement in molecular biology, genetics, elucidation of metabolic pathways, and nutrition, is helping to corroborate the metabolic rationale and efficacy for this approach. We are not solving the obesity problem with our current methods and recommendations. A new paradigm is needed. Individual needs and clinical parameters, such as metabolic syndrome or a lipoprotein subclass pattern that genetically predisposes an individual to increased risk with a low-fat regimen, are becoming widely accepted. What exciting possibilities lie ahead of us with more options, alternatives, and greater potential to improve the quality of life and the health of at-risk individuals!

REFERENCES

Abbasi F, Schulte H, Funke H, et al. High carbohydrate diets, triglyceride rich lipoproteins, and coronary heart disease risk. *Am J Cariol.* 2000;85:45–48.

Assmann G, Schulte H, Funke H, et al. The emergence of triglycerides as a significant independent risk factor in CAD. *Eur Heart J.* 1998;19(Supple. M):8–14.

Austin M, Hokanson JE, Edwards KL. Hypertriglyceridemia as a cardiovascular risk factor. *Am J Cardiol.* 1998;81:7B–12B.

Brehm BJ, Seeley RJ, Daniels SR, et al. A randomized trial comparing a very low carbohydrate diet and a calorie-restricted low fat diet on body weight and cardiovascular risk factors in healthy women. *J Clin Endocrin Metab.* 88(4):2003;1617–1623.

Dawson-Hughes B, Harris SS, Rasmussen H, et al. Effect of dietary protein supplements on calcium excretion in healthy older men and women. *J Clin Endocrinol Metab.* 2004;89:1169–1173.

Dreon DM, Fernstrom HA, Williams PT, et al: A very-low-fat diet is not associated with improved lipoprotein profiles in men with a predominance of large, low-density lipoproteins. *Am J Clin Nutr.* 1999;69:411–418.

Foster GD, Wyatt HR, Hill JO, et al. A randomized trial of a low-carbohydrate diet for obesity. *N Engl J Med.* 2003;348(21):2082–2090.

Gaziano JM, Hennekens CH, O'Donnell CJ, et al. Fasting triglycerides, high-density lipoprotein, and risk of myocardial infarction. *Circulation.* 1997;96:2520–2525.

Greene P, Willett W, Devecis J, et al. Pilot 12-week feeding weight-loss comparison: Low-fat vs low-carbohydrate (ketogenic) diets. Abstract presented at The North American Association for the Study of Obesity Annual Meeting 2003. *Obesity Research.* 2003;11S:950R.

Hays JH, Gorman RT, Shakir KM. Results of use of metformin and replacement of starch with saturated fat in diets of patients with type 2 diabetes. *Endocr Pract.* 2002;8(3):177–183.

He K, Merchant A, Rimm EB, et al. Dietary fat intake and risk of stroke in male US healthcare professionals: 14 year prospective cohort study. *BMJ.* 2003;4;327(7418): 777–782.

Heaney RP. Excess dietary protein may not adversely affect bone. *J Nutr.* 1998;128(6):1054–1057.

Jeppesen J, Hein HO, Suadicani P, et al. Triglyceride concentration and ischemic heart disease: An eight-year follow-up in the Copenhagen male study. *Circulation.* 1998;97:1029–1036.

Jiang R, Manson JE, Stampfer MJ, et al. Nut and peanut butter consumption and risk of type 2 diabetes in women. *JAMA.* 2002;27;288(20):2554–2560.

Kerstetter, JE, O'Brien KO, Insogna, KL. Low protein intake: The impact on calcium and bone homeostasis in humans. *J Nutr.* 2003;133(3):855S–861S.

Liu S, Willett WC, Stampfer MJ, et al. A prospective study of dietary glycemic load, carbohydrate intake, and risk of coronary heart disease in US women. *Am J Clin Nutr.* 2000;71:1455–1461.

Manninen V, Tenkanen L, Koskinen P, et al. Joint effects of serum triglyceride and LDL cholesterol and HDL cholestrol concentrations on coronary heart disease risk in the Helsinki heart study: Implications for treatment. *Circulation.* 1992;85:37–47.

Miller M, Seidler A, Moalemi A, et al. Normal triglyceride levels and coronary artery disease events. The Baltimore coronary observational long-term study. *J Am Coll Cardio.* 1998;31(6):1252–1257.

O'Brien KD, Brehm BJ, Seeley RJ. Greater reduction in inflammatory markers with a low carbohydrate diet than with a calorically matched low fat diet. Presented at American Heart Association's Scientific Sessions 2002 on Tuesday, November 19, 2002. Abstract ID: 117597, 2002.

Phinney SD, Bistrian BR, Wolfe RR, et al. The human metabolic response to chronic ketosis without caloric restriction: Physical and biochemical adaptation. *Metabolism.* 1983;32(8):757–768.

Pieke B, von Eckardstein A, Gülbahce E, et al. Treatment of hypertriglyceridemia by two diets rich either in unsaturated fatty acids or in carbohydrates: Effects on lipoprotein subclasses, lipolytic enzymes, lipid transfer proteins, insulin and leptin. *Int J Obes,* 2000;24(10): 1286–1296.

Samaha FF, Iqbal N, Seshadri P, et al. A low-carbohydrate as compared with a low-fat diet in severe obesity. *N Engl J Med.* 2003;348(21):2074–2081.

Schaeffner ES, Kurth T, Curhan GC, et al. Cholesterol and the risk of renal dysfunction in apparently healthy men. *Am Soc Nephrol.* 2003;4(8):2084–2091.

Sharman MJ, Kraemer WJ, Love DM, et al. A ketogenic diet favorably affects serum biomarkers for cardiovascular disease in normal-weight men. *J Nutr.* 2002;132(7): 1879–1885.

Skov AR, Toubro S, Bülow J, et al. Changes in renal function during weight loss induced by high vs. low-protein, low-fat diets in overweight subjects. *Int J Obes.* 1999;23:1170–1177.

Sondike SB, Copperman N, Jacobson MS. Effects of a low-carbohydrate diet on weight loss and cardiovascular risk factor in overweight adolescents. *J Pediatr.* 2003;142(3): 253–258.

Sondike SB, Copperman NM, Jacobson MS. Low carbohydrate dieting increases weight loss but not cardiovascular risk in obese adolescents: A randomized controlled trial. *J Adolesc Health.* 2000;26:91.

Stadler DD, Burden V, Connor W, et al. Impact of 42-day Atkins diet and energy-matched low-fat diet on weight and anthropometric indices. *FASEB Journal.* 2004;17: 4–5. Abstract of the 12th Annual FASEB Meeting on Experimental Biology: Translating the Genome; Abstract ID: 453.3, San Diego, CA, April 11–15, 2003.

Stavenow L, Kjellstrom T. Influence of serum triglyceride levels on the risk for myocardial infarction in 12,500 middle aged males: Interaction with serum cholesterol. *Atherosclerosis.* 1999;147:243–247.

Tanne D, Koren-Morag N, Graff E, et al. Blood lipids and first-ever ischemic stroke/transient ischemic attack in the Bezafibrate Infarction Prevention (BIP) Registry: High triglycerides constitute an independent risk factor. *Circulation.* 2001;104(24):2892–2897.

Taubes G. The soft science of dietary fat. *Science.* 2001;291:2536–2545.

US Department of Health and Human Services. *The Surgeon General's Call to Action to Prevent and Decrease Overweight and Obesity.* Rockville, MD: U.S. Department of Health and Human Services, Public Health Service, Office of the Surgeon General; [2001]. Available from: US GPO, Washington, DC.

Volek JS, Gómez AL, Kraemer WJ. Fasting lipoprotein and postprandial triacylglycerol responses to a low-carbohydrate diet supplemented with n-3 fatty acids. *J Am Coll Nutr.* 2000;19(3):383–391.

Volek JS, Sharman MJ, and Gomez AL, et al. An isoenergetic very low carbohydrate diet improves serum HDL cholesterol and triacylglycerol concentrations, the total cholesterol to HDL cholesterol ratio and postprandial lipemic responses compared with a low fat diet in normal weight, normolipidemic women. *J Nutr.* 2003;133(9): 2756–2761.

Volek JS, Sharman MJ, Love DM, et al. Body composition and hormonal responses to a carbohydrate restricted diet. *Metabolism.* 2002;51(7):864–870.

Volek VS, Westman EC. Very-low-carbohydrate weight-loss diets revisited. *Cleve Clin J Med.* 2002;69(11):849–862.

Westman EC, Yancy WS, Edman JS, et al. Effect of 6-month adherence to a very low carbohydrate diet program. *Am J Med.* 2002;13(1):30–36.

Willett WC, Stampfer MJ. Rebuilding the food pyramid. *Sci Am.* Jan;2003;288(1):64–71.

Willi SM, Oexmann MJ, Wright NM, et al. The effects of a high-protein, low-fat, ketogenic diet on adolescents with morbid obesity: Body composition, blood chemistries, and sleep abnormalities. *Pediatrics.* 1998;101(1):61–67.

Williams PT, Dreon DM, Krauss RM. Effects of dietary fat on high-density-lipoprotein subclasses are influenced by both apolipoprotein E isoforms and low-density-lipoprotein subclass patterns. *Am J Clin Nutr.* 1995;61:1234–1240.

Yancy WS, Bakst R, Bryson W, et al. *Effects of a Very-Low-Carbohydrate Diet Program Compared with a Low-Fat, Low-Cholesterol, Reduced Calorie Diet.* North American Association for the Study of Obesity Annual Meeting, Quebec City, Canada. October 7, 2001.

The Zone Diet: A Low-Glycemic Load Diet

Barry Sears, PhD

The Zone Diet was developed to provide a long-term control of insulin for the treatment of type 2 diabetes and cardiovascular disease.[1] The basic premise of the Zone Diet is to maintain insulin within a therapeutic zone that is neither too high, nor too low, by balancing the protein-to-carbohydrate ratio at every meal, with most of the carbohydrates coming from low-glycemic load carbohydrates.

GLYCEMIC INDEX

More than 20 years ago, some scientists began asking the question: Does a simple carbohydrate (like a sugar cube) actually enter the bloodstream slower than a complex carbohydrate (like a potato)? For years it had seemed so obvious that no one ever tried such an experiment. The result started an upheaval in nutritional thinking.[2–4]

All complex carbohydrates are simply simple sugars linked together by very weak chemical bonds that are easily broken. There are two primary simple sugars of which virtually all carbohydrates are composed: glucose and fructose. All complex carbohydrates must be broken into simple sugars for absorption by the body. While glucose can easily enter the bloodstream to stimulate insulin secretion, fructose has to be slowly converted in the liver to glucose before it can enter the bloodstream as glucose. This means that grains and starches, which are composed of pure glucose linked together by weak bonds, will have a greater impact on blood glucose levels than fruits (which are about 70% fructose) or nonstarchy vegetables (composed of about 30% fructose).[5] Since a sugar cube is composed of one half glucose and one half fructose, one can begin to understand why a potato or piece of bread would increase blood glucose levels at a faster rate than the equivalent amount of carbohydrate in the form of a sugar cube. This gave rise to the concept of the glycemic index of carbohydrates. In essence, not all carbohydrates are the same when it comes to increasing blood glucose levels.

Glycemic Load

Understanding the glycemic load of the diet is more complicated than simply looking at the rate of entry of any particular carbohydrate into the bloodstream (i.e., looking at the glycemic index). The glycemic load is a more comprehensive concept because it takes into account not only the rate of entry of a carbohydrate into the bloodstream (the glycemic index), but also the actual amount of insulin-stimulating carbohydrate that a patient is eating at a particular meal.[6] The higher the glycemic load of a meal, the more insulin the patient produces. Epidemiological research has shown that the higher the glycemic load of the total diet, the more likely a patient is to become obese, develop diabetes and heart disease, and increase inflammation.[7–9]

Understanding the glycemic load also begins to take all of the mystery out of both popular and medical diets. Yet despite the abundance of this dietary advice, there are only four types of diets and they can be described on the basis of their glycemic load.

Dietary Glycemic Load	Popular Diet Name
Very low	Atkins
Low	Zone
High	USDA Food Pyramid, American Heart Association, etc.
Very high	Typical American

The concept of the glycemic load is the universal translator that can describe any diet. Using the concept of the glycemic load, the terms such as high-protein, high-carbohydrate, low-fat, or low-carbohydrate diets become meaningless. They are simply terms that have done a poor job of describing and quantifying the glycemic load of a diet. Thus finding a lifelong diet is really finding the right glycemic load for the patient's biochemistry. Any higher glycemic load than a patient can handle genetically will start increasing the levels of insulin that can lead to hyperinsulinemia. Once you find that upper level of glycemic load for the patient, the beginnings of a lifetime dietary plan for maintaining insulin in a therapeutic zone can take place.

Defining the Glycemic Load

The glycemic load of a diet can be very different than the actual amount of carbohydrates consumed. The glycemic load can be defined mathematically as the glycemic index (GI) of a given amount of carbohydrate multiplied by the amount of that carbohydrate (g) in a meal, divided by 100 as shown below:[6]

Glycemic Load (g)

$$= \frac{\text{GI of the carbohydrate} \times \text{grams of carbohydrate per serving}}{100}$$

A glycemic load in terms of grams is more physiologically relevant because it strongly correlates with the amount of insulin that will be secreted at a meal.

The glycemic index of the two basic building blocks of all carbohydrates—glucose and fructose—is significantly different (by more than a factor of four). This means that the glycemic load of servings of different carbohydrates can vary even though the weights of the carbohydrates consumed are exactly the same. This is why diets rich in grains and starches can be considered the foundation of high glycemic-load diets, whereas a diet with exactly the same number of grams of carbohydrate coming from fruits and vegetables can be considered a low glycemic-load diet.[10] This can be seen from the following table:

Type of Carbohydrate	Glycemic Load (g) of a Typical Serving
Nonstarchy vegetables	1–5
Fruits	5–10
Grains and starches	10–30
Typical junk foods	20–30

As can be seen in the table, consuming more fruits and vegetables and fewer grains and starches is a very simple approach to maintaining a low glycemic load for a given diet. Therefore, it is not surprising that when people eat more fruits and vegetables and fewer grains and starches, they have lower rates of heart disease and overall chronic disease.[11]

Although the data for every type of carbohydrate is incomplete,[4] enough information exists so that we can further define the four different types of popular or medical diets based on their glycemic load.

Dietary Glycemic Load	Total Glycemic Load (g)	Popular Diet Name
Very low	Less than 20	Atkins
Low	50–100	Zone
High	Greater than 200	USDA Food Pyramid, American Heart Association, etc.
Very high	Greater than 300	Typical diet of an American

It is clear from the table that the dietary recommendations of the USDA Food Pyramid and even the American Heart Association have approximately three to four times the impact on insulin secretion than does the Zone Diet. This may be why epidemiological studies indicate that modification of the USDA Food Pyramid to a lower glycemic load demonstrates a significant reduction in cardiovascular disease and overall mortality.

PROTEIN-TO-CARBOHYDRATE BALANCE

The Zone Diet is more than simply a low glycemic-load diet because it also requires an appropriate balance of protein to carbohydrate to further maintain insulin in an appropriate therapeutic zone. This is because protein stimulates the counter-regulatory hormone glucagon that replenishes blood glucose levels from stored glycogen in the liver. At a low ratio of protein to carbohydrate (such as less than 0.5, as found in a high-carbohydrate, low-fat diet), insulin secretion will be dominant and blood glucose levels will drop. At a high ratio of protein to carbohydrate (such as greater than 1.0, as found in a low-carbohydrate, high-protein diet), glucagon secretion will be dominant and liver glycogen levels will be depleted, potentially leading to ketosis. The Zone Diet tries to maintain the protein-to-carbohydrate ratio between 0.5 and 1.0 at every meal. This allows an appropriate balance of insulin and glucagon and therefore maintains blood glucose levels for 4 to 6 hours. Another definition of this protein-to-carbohydrate ratio is just enough carbohydrate to prevent ketosis, but not enough to induce excess insulin secretion.[1]

INTERVENTION STUDIES

A great number of isocaloric studies have compared the Zone Diet to the dietary recommendations of the USDA Food Pyramid, the American Heart Association, and the American Diabetes Association.[12–20] In each study it has been found that the Zone Diet offers superior insulin control, greater satiety, less hunger, greater improvement in blood lipid levels, greater improvement in blood sugar control, and greater fat loss.

SUMMARY

The Zone Diet is a diet based on hormonal balance. As such it can be considered a moderate-carbohydrate (but with a low-glycemic load), moderate-protein, and moderate-fat diet designed to maintain insulin in a therapeutic zone. A quick summary of the dietary criteria of the Zone Diet follows.

Zone Diet Objectives

- To maintain insulin in a therapeutic zone that is neither too high nor too low in order to lose excess body fat and maintain long-term stable weight management.
- To reduce elevated cholesterol and/or triglyceride levels.
- To reduce inflammation induced by chronically elevated insulin levels.

Indications for Use of the Zone Diet

- Individuals seeking weight loss and weight maintenance.
- Individuals with type 2 diabetes and cardiovascular disease.
- Individuals at risk for type 2 diabetes and cardiovascular disease.

Nutritional Adequacy of the Zone Diet

- Diet is nutritionally adequate.
- Caloric intake should not be less than 1200 calories/day.

Summary of Guidelines for the Zone Diet

- Significantly reduce intake of high glycemic-load carbohydrates (primarily grains and starches) and simultaneously increase the intake of low glycemic-load carbohydrates (primarily vegetables and fruits). Total vegetable and fruit intake is approximately 10–15 servings per day.
- Use adequate amounts of low-fat protein sources. Suggested protein amounts per meal are approximately 3 oz. of low-fat protein for females and approximately 4 oz. of low-fat protein for males. Daily intake of protein is 1.5–2.0 g of protein per kg of ideal body weight.
- Maintain fat intake at 30% of total calories with majority of fat coming from monounsaturated fat sources.
- Have three meals and two snacks, each with the same macronutrient balance, per day.

REFERENCES

1. Sears B. *The Zone.* Regan Books. New York, NY (1995)
2. Jenkins DJ, Wolever TM, Taylor RH, Barker H, Fielden H, Baldwin JM, Bowling AC, Newman HC, Jenkins AL, and Goff DV. Glycemic index of foods: a physiological basis for carbohydrate exchange. *Am J Clin Nutr* 34:362–366 (1981)
3. Wolever TM, Jenkins DJ, Jenkins AL, and Josse RG. The glycemic index: methodology and clinical implications. *Am J Clin Nutr* 1991 54:846–854 (1991)
4. Foster-Powell K, Holt SH, and Brand-Miller JC. International table of glycemic index and glycemic load values: 2002. *Am J Clin Nutr* 76:5–56 (2002)
5. Liu S, Willett WC, Stampfer MJ, Hu FB, Franz M, Sampson L, Hennekens CH, and Manson JE. A prospective study of dietary glycemic load, carbohydrate intake, and risk of coronary heart disease in US women. *Am J Clin Nutr* 71:1455–1461 (2000)
6. Willett W, Manson J, and Liu S. Glycemic index, glycemic load, and risk of type 2 diabetes. *Am J Clin Nutr* 76:274S–280S (2002)
7. Liu S and Willett WC. Dietary glycemic load and atherothrombotic risk. *Curr Atheroscler Rep* 4:454–461 (2002)
8. Liu S, Manson JE, Buring JE, Stampfer MJ, Willett WC, and Ridker PM. Relation between a diet with a high glycemic load and plasma concentrations of high-sensitivity C-reactive protein in middle-aged women. *Am J Clin Nutr* 75:492–498 (2002)
9. Liu S, Manson JE, Stampfer MJ, Holmes MD, Hu FB, Hankinson SE, and Willett WC. Dietary glycemic load assessed by food-frequency questionnaire in relation to plasma high-density-lipoprotein cholesterol and fasting plasma triacylglycerols in postmenopausal women. *Am J Clin Nutr* 73:560–566 (2001)
10. Bell SJ and Sears B. Low-glycemic-load diets: impact on obesity and chronic diseases. *Crit Rev Food Sci Nutr* 43:357–377 (2003)
11. McCullough ML, Feskanich D, Stampfer MJ, Giovannucci EL, Rimm EB, Hu FB, Spiegelman D, Hunter DJ, Colditz GA, and Willett WC. Diet quality and major chronic disease risk in men and women: moving toward improved dietary guidance. *Am J Clin Nutr* 76:1261–1271 (2002)
12. Ludwig DS, Majzoub JA, Al-Zahrani A, Dallal GE, Blanco I, and Roberts SB. High glycemic index foods, overeating, and obesity. *Pediatrics* 103:E26 (1999)
13. Wolfe BM and Piche LA. Replacement of carbohydrate by protein in aconventional-fat diet reduces cholesterol and triglyceride concentrations in healthy normolipidemic subjects. *Clin Invest Med* 22:140–148 (1999)
14. Skov AR, Toubro S, Ronn B, Holm L, and Astrup A. Randomized trial on protein vs carbohydrate in ad libitum fat reduced diet for the treatment of obesity. *Int J Obes Relat Metab Disord* 23:528–536 (1999)
15. Agus MS, Swain JF, Larson CL, Eckert EA, and Ludwig DS. Dietary composition and physiologic adaptations to energy restriction. *Am J Clin Nutr* 71:901–907 (2000)
16. Dumesnil JG, Turgeon J, Tremblay A, Poirier P, Gilbert M, Gagnon L, St-Pierre S, Garneau C, Lemieux I, Pascot A, Bergeron J, and Despres JP. Effect of a low-glycaemic index–low-fat–high protein diet on the atherogenic metabolic risk profile of abdominally obese men. *Br J Nutr* 86:557–568 (2001)
17. Johnston CS, Day CS, and Swan PD. Postprandial thermogenesis is increased 100% on a high-protein, low-fat diet versus a high-carbohydrate, low-fat diet in healthy, young women. *J Am Coll Nutr* 21:55–61 (2002)
18. Gannon MC, Nuttall FQ, Saeed A, Jordan K, and Hoover H. An increase in dietary protein improves the blood glucose response in persons with type 2 diabetes. *Am J Clin Nutr* 78:734–741 (2003)
19. Layman DK, Shiue H, Sather C, Erickson DJ, and Baum J. Increased dietary protein modifies glucose and insulin homeostasis in adult women during weight loss. *J Nutr* 133:405–410 (2003)
20. Layman DK, Boileau RA, Erickson DJ, Painter JE, Shiue H, Sather C, and Christou DD. A reduced ratio of dietary carbohydrate to protein improves body composition and blood lipid profiles during weight loss in adult women. *J Nutr* 133:411–417 (2003)

Complementary and Alternative Medicine (CAM)

Sarah Laidlaw, MS, RD, MPA

DESCRIPTION

According to the National Center for Complementary and Alternative Medicine (NCCAM), CAM is defined as "a group of diverse medical and health care systems, practices, and products that are not presently considered to be part of conventional medicine." Other definitions have described CAM as being "diagnosis, treatment, and/or prevention which complements mainstream medicine by contributing to a common whole, satisfying a demand not met by orthodoxy, or diversifying the conceptual framework of medicine."

While the terms complementary and alternative are used together and appear to suggest that they are one and the same, there are some distinct differences. However, the term Integrative Medicine may be used interchangeably with CAM.

- Complementary medicine is used together with conventional medicine. An example of a complementary therapy is using yoga to help reduce the discomforts of multiple sclerosis.
- Alternative medicine is used in place of conventional medicine. An example of an alternative therapy is using a special diet to treat cancer instead of undergoing surgery, radiation, or chemotherapy that has been recommended by a conventional doctor.
- Integrative medicine, as defined by NCCAM, combines mainstream medical therapies and CAM therapies for which there is some high-quality scientific evidence of safety and effectiveness. A simplified example is the manipulation of the amount of carbohydrate in the diet while adjusting insulin to help manage blood sugar levels in diabetes.

Complementary therapies usually involve major lifestyle changes, but may be worth considering for new treatment modalities or for approaches to how one looks at health and disease

(see Table 6–6). Unfortunately, however, some therapies may be advertised as a quick fix by unscrupulous websites or practitioners, or perceived as a miracle or quick fix by those who are desperate to find a cure or solution to a major health problem. Understanding the spectrum of CAM practices and how to identify reliable—from misleading—information is essential, for those who work with patients seeking such treatments in a field that seems to grow exponentially each day.

CLASSIFICATIONS

Alternative Medical Systems

Ayurveda

- The traditional medicine of India.
- Optimal health consists of physical, mental, and spiritual harmony.
- Harmony depends on the person's constitution or "dosha."
- Doshas are defined by five elements—earth, water, fire, air, and ether—and characteristics including predominant season, taste/flavors, emotion, body part, and characteristic.
- The four pillars of Ayurvedic health maintenance are:
  1. cleansing and detoxification
  2. palliation
  3. rejuvenation
  4. mental and spiritual hygiene.
- Diet is an important consideration but is individualized, based upon a person's dosha.
- Ayurvedic treatments may include dietary modification, herbs, massage, yoga, meditation, and breathing exercises.

Holistic

- Involves the whole person, including evaluating physical, nutritional, environmental, emotional, social, spiritual, and lifestyle values.

Table 6–6 Disease Treatment Using CAM

Condition	Therapy	Support/Evidence	Contraindications/ Adverse Reactions
Cancer	**Acupuncture**	+ for nausea	Pain, bleeding, bruising
	Alternative diets	− Gerson diet	Expense, weight loss,
		− Macrobiotic diet	restrictive
	Herbal therapies	− Essiac tea	Allergic reaction
			Affect blood sugar
			Irritate GI tract
		+ Milk thistle	Allergic reaction, laxative effect
		+ Ginger	Caution in gallbladder disease
		− nausea	
	Supplements	− DMSO	Liver and kidney damage
		− Hydrazine sulfate	Interfere with blood sugar control, worsen kidney/liver disorders
			Cyanide poisoning
		− Laetril	None known
		− MGN-3	Hypercalcemia
	Hypnotherapy	− Shark cartilage	Recovering repressed
		+ palliative care	memories, false memory syndrome
	Relaxation/imagery	+ Palliative care	
	Spiritual healing/	+ Palliative care	None
	therapeutic touch	+ Palliative care	None
AIDS/HIV	**Acupuncture**	− Neuropathies	Bruising, bleeding
	Herbal therapies	± Boxwood	Diarrhea, cramps, dermatitis
		− St. John's wort	Phototoxicity
	Homeopathy	+ Individualized homeopathic treatments	Possible allergic reactions
	Massage	+ Palliative care	None
	Relaxation/imagery	+ Perceived health	None
	Spiritual/therapeutic touch	+ Palliative care	None
	Supplements	± Carnitine	None
		+ Glutamine	Sensitivity to MSG may trigger allergic reaction, not in hepatic encephalopathy, mania, seizure disorders
		± Blue-green algae/ spirulina	None
			Toxicity
		± Selenium	

continues

Table 6–6 continued

Condition	Therapy	Support/Evidence	Contraindications/ Adverse Reactions
Brain/Nervous System			
• **Alzheimer's Disease/ Dementia**	**Aromatherapy**	+ Lavender, lemon balm	Allergic reaction
	Herbal therapies	+ Ginkgo biloba	Not in bleeding disorders/with anticoagulants
		− Ginseng	Not in bleeding disorders/with anticoagulants or in heart disease
	Massage	± Hand massage as opposed to therapeutic touch	None
	Music therapy	± Soothing music	None
	Supplements	± Acetyl-l-carnitine	None
		± Vitamin E (alpha tocopherol)	Not in bleeding disorders/with anticoagulants
		+ Phosphatidyl-serine	None
• **Depression**	**Aromatherapy**	± Reducing medication use	Allergic reaction
	Acupuncture	± Symptoms	Bruising, bleeding
	Exercise/dance therapy	+ Cardiovascular fitness training	Injury if done incorrectly
	Herbal therapies	± St. John's wort	Phototoxicity, not with OCDs
	Music therapy	± Soothing music	None
	Relaxation/imagery	± Trained therapist (preferred) or books and audiotapes	None
	Yoga	± Kundalini yoga	Aggravation of psychosis possible
• **Insomnia**	**Aromatherapy**	± Lavender	Allergic reaction
		± Bitter orange	Allergic reaction
	Biofeedback	± Tailored biofeedback	None
	Exercise	+ Cardiovascular fitness training	Injury if done incorrectly
	Herbal therapies	± Kava	Liver toxicity
		+ Valerian	Not in pregnancy
	Supplements	± Melatonin	Not in pregnancy, CVD, neurological disorders, autoimmune disease, liver disease, or with immuno-suppressants/corticosteroids

continues

Table 6–6 continued

Condition	Therapy	Support/Evidence	Contraindications/ Adverse Reactions
• Migraine Headache	Acupuncture/ acupressure	+ Pain	Bleeding, bruising; caution with metal allergy
	Diet	± Avoiding MSG, chocolate, and cheese, red wine	None
	Herbal therapies	± Feverfew	Not in pregnancy or with anticoagulants
		± Ginger (eases nausea)	Not in diabetes, bleeding conditions, CVD treated with drugs with anticoagulants
		+ White willow	Not in pregnancy or with anticoagulants
• Multiple Sclerosis	Acupuncture	± Pain, bladder spasticity, bowel and bladder difficulties, walking and sleeping disorders	Bruising, bleeding, caution with fatigue, blood thinning medications, metal allergy
	Aromatherapy	± Anxiety/depression	Allergic reaction
	Biofeedback	± Anxiety, insomnia, pain, urinary/fecal incontinence, muscle stiffness	Caution with electrodermal therapy with heart disease, pacemakers
	Chiropractic	± Low back pain + Other uses	Not in osteoporosis, inflammatory spinal disease, bleeding disorders, anticoagulant use
	Diet	± Swank or low-fat diet	Extreme approach
	Exercise	+ Cardiovascular fitness training	Injury if used incorrectly
	Feldenkrais method	+ Efficient and comfortable body movement for stress, anxiety	None
	Herbal therapies	+ Cranberry for urinary tract	Not with anticoagulants Liver toxicity
		+ Kava for anxiety	Phototoxicity, not with OCDs
		+ St. John's wort	Not with sedatives
	Homeopathy	+ Valerian	Not in pregnancy
		± Anecdotal	Potential toxicity of some substances
		± Viral infections	
	Electromagnetic therapy/magnets	± Bladder function, pain, cognitive problems, walking	Not in pregnancy, or with pacemakers

continues

Table 6–6 continued

Condition	Therapy	Support/Evidence	Contraindications/ Adverse Reactions
	Relaxation/imagery	± Trained therapist (preferred) or books and audiotapes	Caution in psychiatric conditions, severe depression, anxiety
• Parkinson's Disease	Supplements	± Linoleic acid	None
		− Gamma-linoleic acid	Cost for effective dose, diarrhea, nausea
		± Omega-3 fatty acids	May worsen disease, generally no risk
	Yoga	± Hatha yoga for flexibility, pain	Safe when done correctly
	Acupuncture	± Symptoms, reduced medication use	Bleeding, bruising
	Herbal therapies	± Green tea	Contains caffeine, not with diabetes, CVD, ulcers
		± *Mucuna pruriens* (legume)	Contains levodopa, not in pregnancy
		± Fava beans	Contains levodopa, not with MAOIs or favism
	Massage	± Anecdotal reducing muscle rigidity	None
	Supplements	± Coenzyme Q-10	Nausea, insomnia, dizziness
Cardiovascular Disease/High Cholesterol	Diet	+ Oat bran	None
		+ Low fat/sat fat/ cholesterol diet	None
		+ Soy protein	Allergic reaction, not with estrogen-sensitive cancers, decreased absorption of iron
	Exercise	+ 30 minutes most days of the week of cardiovascular fitness training	Injury if done incorrectly
	Herbal therapies	+ Psyllium	Constipation
		+ Fenugreek	Lowers blood sugar
		± Garlic	Not with bleeding disorders, anticoagulants, lowers blood sugar
		+ Guggul	Monitor use in thyroid disease and diabetes
	Supplements	+ Coenzyme Q-10	None
		+ Niacin	Flushing
		+ Phytosterols	May decrease effects of immunosuppressants

continues

Table 6–6 continued

Condition	Therapy	Support/Evidence	Contraindications/ Adverse Reactions
		± Red yeast rice	Multiple interactions with herbs, dietary supplements, and drugs; caution with liver disease
Connective Tissue/ Musculoskeletal			
• **Arthritis**	**Acupuncture**	± Pain control	Bruising, bleeding
	Diet	± Fasting/ vegetarian diet	Malnutrition risk
	Exercise	+	If done incorrectly
	Herbal therapies	± Ashwagandha	Interactions with sedative drugs and herbs, immuno-suppressants, thyroid medication
		+ Devil's claw	Not with GI disease, diabetes, heart disease
		± Ginger	Not in diabetes, bleeding conditions, CVD treated with drugs with anticoagulants
		+ Frankincense	Topically, mild irritation
		+ Turmeric	Not in gallbladder disease or with anticoagulants
		+ White willow	Not in pregnancy or with anticoagulants
	Homeopathy	± Anecdotal	Allergic reactions
	Relaxation/imagery	± Trained therapist (preferred) or books and audiotapes	None
	Supplements	+ Chondroitin sulfate	Not with anticoagulants
		+ Gamma linoleic-acid (GLA)	
		+ Glucosamine	Not in liver disease or with anticoagulants
		± MSM	GI upset, increased blood sugar
		+ Omega-3 fatty acids	Caution with anticoagulant therapy
• **Chronic fatigue**	**Exercise**	+ Graded exercise	If done incorrectly
	Herbal therapies	± Evening primrose	Not with seizure or bleeding disorders
		± Ginseng	Not in bleeding disorders or with hypertension

continues

Table 6–6 continued

Condition	Therapy	Support/Evidence	Contraindications/ Adverse Reactions
	Homeopathy	± Anecdotal	Allergic reactions
	Osteopathy	+ Osteopathic body manipulation	Cost; may not be covered by insurance
	Supplements	± Amino acids	None
		+ L-carnitine	None
		± NADH	Nervousness, loss of appetite
		± Selenium	Toxicity
• Fibromyalgia	Acupuncture/ acupressure	+ Pain control	Bleeding, bruising
	Biofeedback	± Pain control	None
	Exercise	+ Cardiovascular fitness training	If done incorrectly
	Herbal therapies	+ Capsaicin	Topically, rash; internally not with GI disease, sedatives, anticoagulants
	Massage	+ Hand massage	None
	Supplements	+ SAM-e	Avoid in Parkinson's disease
Diabetes	Diet	+ Carbohydrate counting	None
	Exercise	+ Cardiovascular fitness training for blood sugar and weight control	If done incorrectly
	Herbal therapies	There are numerous dietary supplements that supposedly benefit diabetes and conditions associated with diabetes. Each one should be considered on an individual basis	Herbal therapies often affect blood sugar and other medications: consider individually
		These include:	
		+ Cinnamon	Blood sugar lowering effects
		+ Fenugreek	
		+ *Gymnema sylvestre*	
		± *Panax ginseng*	

continues

Table 6–6 continued

Condition	Therapy	Support/Evidence	Contraindications/ Adverse Reactions
	Supplements	Several supplements are thought to benefit persons with diabetes. These supplements should be considered individually as they may or may not have benefits or may cause adverse reactions:	Dietary supplements may play a role in normalizing or improving blood sugar in persons who are deficient in a particular nutrient. These should be considered individually
		± Chromium	Lowering blood sugar
		± Niacin	Flushing and hyperglycemia
		± Vandium	Increases insulin sensitivity, lowers blood sugar
Gastrointestinal			
• **Irritable bowel syndrome**	**Acupuncture**	± Reducing diarrhea	Bleeding, bruising
	Biofeedback	− Symptom reduction	None
	Exercise	± Cardiovascular fitness training	If done incorrectly
	Herbal therapies	± Peppermint	Allergic reactions, not with gallstones, hiatal hernia
		± Psyllium	Allergy; bloating, gas, drink adequate water
	Hypnotherapy	+ Trained therapist	Caution with false memory syndrome
	Relaxation/imagery	+ Trained therapist (preferred) or books and audiotapes	None
• **Constipation**	**Supplements**	+ Probiotics	Possible gas, bloating
	Biofeedback	± Self-taught or in class/therapist setting	None
	Herbal therapies	+ *Cascara sagrada*	Bloating, cramps, decreased nutrient absorption
		+ Flax	Allergy; bloating, gas, drink adequate water
		± Psyllium	Allergy; bloating, gas, drink adequate water
		+ Senna	Not with GI disease, other stimulant laxatives, may reduce absorption of other drugs

continues

Table 6–6 continued

Condition	Therapy	Support/Evidence	Contraindications/ Adverse Reactions
Reproductive Urinary Tract			
• **Benign prostatic hyperplasia**	**Herbal therapies**	± Nettle	Not in heart or kidney disease, diabetes, with sedative, herbs, anticoagulants
		+ Pumpkin seed	None
		± Pygeum	None
		+ Saw palmetto	Not with hormone therapy, bleeding disorders, immune stimulants
• **Menopause**	**Acupuncture**	± Hot flashes, mood	Bleeding, bruising
	Exercise	+ Cardiovascular fitness training	If done incorrectly
	Herbal therapies	± Black cohosh	Not with tamoxifen, GI upset, or estrogen-sensitive cancers
		± Chasteberry (vitex)	Not with oral contraceptives, antipsychotic drugs, and HRT
		± Dong quai	Photosensitivity, pregnancy, anticoagulants; decrease when menstruation begins
		+ Ginseng	Not with bleeding disorders, anticoagulants
		+ Kava	Liver toxicity
		± Red clover	None
		+ St. John's wort	Photosensitivity, not with OCDs
		+ Soy protein	Not with estrogen sensitive cancers, decreased iron absorption
	Osteopathic manipulation	± Trained practitioner	Contraindicated in osteoporosis, cancer, infections, and bleeding disorders
	Relaxation/imagery	± Trained therapist (preferred) or books and audiotapes	None
• **Premenstrual syndrome**	**Biofeedback**	± Self taught or in class/therapist setting	None
	Chiropractic therapy	± Trained practitioner	Contraindicated in osteoporosis, cancer, infections, and bleeding disorders
	Herbal therapies	± Chasteberry (vitex)	Not with oral contraceptives, antipsychotic drugs, and HRT
		± Dong quai	Photosensitivity, pregnancy, anticoagulants; decrease when menstruation begins

continues

Table 6–6 continued

Condition	Therapy	Support/Evidence	Contraindications/ Adverse Reactions
		± Evening primrose	GI upset, headache, not with anticoagulants
		+ St. John's wort	Photosensitivity, not with OCDs
	Relaxation/imagery	+ Trained therapist (preferred) or books and audiotapes	None
	Supplements	± Calcium	None
		± Vitamin B$_6$	Neuropathy
		± Vitamin E	Not with anticoagulants
• **Urinary tract infections**	**Herbal therapies**	+ Cranberry	Not with anticoagulants
		− Goldenseal	Not in pregnancy, lactation or CVD
		± Uva ursi	Not in pregnancy, lactation or kidney disease; use no more than 7 days
Respiratory Tract			
• **Asthma**	**Acupuncture**	± Improved breathing	Bleeding, bruising
	Biofeedback		
	Diet	± Avoiding food allergens	None
	Herbal therapies	± Coffee	Not in pregnancy, CVD, stimulant drugs
		± Licorice	Not in pregnancy, with CVD, high blood pressure
		± Rosemary as inhalant	Do not ingest essential oil
	Homeopathy	± Dilute preparations of allergens	Allergic reaction
	Hypnotherapy	± Self-hypnotherapy when taught by trained therapist for acute attacks and relaxation	Risk of undertreatment of acute attacks
	Massage	± Hand massage	None
	Meditation	± Self-taught or in class/therapist setting	May exacerbate psychosis
	Relaxation/imagery	± Trained therapist (preferred) or books and audiotapes	None
	Yoga	± Hatha yoga	Injury if done incorrectly

continues

Table 6–6 continued

Condition	Therapy	Support/Evidence	Contraindications/ Adverse Reactions
• **Common cold/flu**	**Aromatherapy**	± Inhalation of essential oils	Do not ingest essential oils
	Herbal therapies	± Echinacea	Not with autoimmune disorders; do not take for more than 14 days
		± Ginger for nausea	Not in gallbladder disease
		± Goldenseal, mostly anecdotal	Not in heart or digestive diseases, bleeding disorders, sedative herbs, drugs
		± Slippery elm	Not in pregnancy, lactation; may decrease absorption of other drugs
		± White willow	Not with anticoagulants, in bleeding disorders
	Homeopathy supplements	± Anecdotal	Allergic reactions
		± Vitamin C	GI distress over 1000 mg/day
		+ Zinc	Chronic use depresses immune system, interferes with copper absorption
	Acupuncture	± Improved breathing	Bruising, bleeding
• **Hay fever**	**Diet**	± Avoiding common allergens	None; avoid foods that may be common or known allergens
	Herbal therapies	± Capsaicin Internally used or used as a compress	Caution in pregnancy, lactation; may cause mild burning sensation
		+ Nettle leaf	Not with sedatives, herbs/ foods with vitamin K; not in heart, kidney disease, high or low blood pressure, pregnancy, lactation
	Homeopathy	+ Dilute preparations of allergens	Allergic reaction

- It includes numerous modalities of diagnosis and treatment, including drugs and surgery if no safe alternative exists.
- Holistic medicine focuses on education and responsibility for personal efforts to achieve health and well-being.

Homeopathy

- Derived from the Greek *homeo,* meaning same, and *pathos,* meaning suffering, homeopathy treats like with like.
- Small, highly diluted quantities of a medicinal substance are given to cure symptoms; when the same substances are given at higher or more concentrated doses they actually cause the symptoms.

Traditional Mexican Healing

- Much more than just the familiar spices in food at Mexican restaurants; however, the herbs and spices used may contribute some nutritional and healing value.
- Is more empiric than other cultural traditional healing practices or medical systems.
- Directions for use have been passed down from generation to generation, primarily by traditions and by word of mouth through family members.
- Little clinical evidence that practices or particular herbal medicines offer extraordinary health benefits; effects may be more from expectations or the placebo effect.

Naturopathy

- Draws on a combination of practices that include Ayurvedic, traditional Chinese, and Native American medicine; health is a composite of physical, mental, and spiritual well-being.
- Practitioners of naturopathy believe that the body has the innate ability to heal itself.
- Symptoms of a disease are merely signs that the body is trying to heal itself.
- The cause of disease is what is treated; disease prevention is emphasized.

- Practices may include dietary modifications, massage, acupuncture, minor surgery, and lifestyle change.

Native American Healing

- Has been practiced in North America for at least 10,000 years.
- Native American medicine is based on a spiritual view of life that stresses development of the inner life which is seen reflected in the outer world.
- Among all tribes, there are widely held beliefs about healthy living, the consequence of disease-producing behavior, and the spiritual principles that restore balance.
- Diagnosis and healing practices vary from tribe to tribe and healer to healer, as do theories of the names and causes of particular diseases.
- Many aspects of Native American healing and its traditions are not written, but passed down by word of mouth from elders, from the spirits in vision quests, and through initiation.
- There is no typical Native American healing ceremony.
- Prayer, chanting, music, smudging (burning aromatic woods), herbs, fasting, laying-on of hands, massage, counseling, imagery, harmonizing with nature, dreaming, sweat lodges, taking hallucinogens such as peyote, developing inner silence, going on a shamanic journey, and ceremony may be used in Native American healing.
- Family and community are very important in the ceremony and healing process, which may occur quickly or over time.

Traditional Chinese Medicine (TCM)

- Traditional Chinese medicine originated from Taoism some 4000 years ago.
- TCM is viewed as one of several paths to a good life—defined as the individual's harmonious interaction with the community, physical, and spiritual environment.

- Traditionally, TCM is essential to promote health and to prevent health problems.
- There are two central and essential elements of TCM:
  1. "Vital energy," "life force," or *Qi*—that which distinguishes life from death, animate from inanimate.
  2. *Yin* and *yang* referring to the Taoist concept of opposites, traditionally used to describe the functions of organs and organ systems, illnesses and conditions, and treatments.
- TCM incorporates diet, exercise (T'ai Chi and Qi Gong), the use of herbs, acupuncture, and massage into its health care system.

PRECAUTIONS FOR ALTERNATIVE MEDICAL SYSTEMS

- A major concern with the use of any CAM therapy is the forgoing of conventional medicine or therapies, resulting in delayed diagnosis and/or treatment of serious health conditions.
- Practices such as prayer, exercise, healthy dietary modifications, massage, and imagery may prove beneficial when used as a complementary therapy to conventional medicine.
- Within each therapy, precautions may vary depending on the treatment; patients should seek the advice or guidance of individuals trained, and where required, licensed, in a particular therapy.
- Supplements employed by CAM therapies should be used with caution.
  1. Some supplements may contain metals such as lead or mercury, which may be associated with toxicity or may interfere or interact with other supplements or prescription drugs.
  2. Some herbal medicines may stimulate the immune system and be contraindicated for diseases such as AIDS, multiple sclerosis, and lupus.
  3. Some preparations may cause allergic or other adverse reactions, even in very dilute forms.

4. The long-term effects of some supplement treatments have not been established.

Mind–Body Interventions

Art, Music, or Dance Therapy

Art Therapy

- Based on the belief that the creative process involved in the making of art is healing and life enhancing.
- Awareness of self; coping with symptoms, stress, and traumatic experiences; enhancing cognitive abilities; and enjoying the life-affirming pleasures of artistic creativity, are believed to be increased for those in art therapy programs.

Dance Therapy

- Dance/Movement therapy is the psychotherapeutic use of movement as a process which integrates the emotional, cognitive, social, and physical functions of the individual.
- Is based on the premise that the body and mind are interrelated, and that mental and emotional problems are often held in the body in the form of muscle tension and constrained movement patterns.
- Dance/Movement therapy provides the benefits of exercise: improved health, well-being, coordination, and muscle tone.
- Dance/Movement therapists work with individuals who have social, emotional, cognitive, and/or physical problems.
- Helps people feel more joyful and confident, and allows them to explore such issues as anger, frustration, and loss that may be too difficult to explore verbally.

Music Therapy

- The use of music to induce relaxation, promote healing, enhance mental functioning, and create an overall sense of well-being.
- Music therapy can be used alone or in conjunction with other therapies or healing treatments.
- Scientific studies have demonstrated that music can affect physiological functions, includ-

ing respiration, heart rate, and blood pressure. Music has also been shown to lower amounts of the hormone cortisol, which becomes elevated under stress, and to increase the release of endorphins, the body's natural "feel-good" hormones.

Behavioral Therapy

- Is often used in conjunction with other therapies.
- Behavioral therapy includes various forms of psychotherapy, behavior therapy, cognitive therapy, skills training, counseling, and other rehabilitative therapies.
- It helps people identify behaviors that trigger poor lifestyle choices—inactivity, unhealthy or inappropriate food choices, alcohol abuse, and many other unhealthy practices.
- It helps people establish new behaviors by directing attention to both the "wrong" and "right" assumptions they make about themselves, their actions, other people, and situations.

Biofeedback

- Monitoring, amplifying, and feeding back information on physiological responses such as breathing, heart rate, and body temperature regulation in an effort to control the body's responses.
- Any physiological response that can be monitored may be suitable for biofeedback.
- Initially a device to monitor response is used with the aim of treatment to establish a patient's mastery over the response independently of such device.

Hypnosis or Hypnotherapy

- A trancelike state that facilitates relaxation of the conscious mind resulting in enhanced suggestibility to treat medical and psychological conditions and effect behavioral changes.
- Self-hypnosis, meditation, imagery, and relaxation are related techniques.

- Has been and is used in combination with other therapies for treatment of obesity, smoking cessation, insomnia, pain, and hypertension, to name a few.

Imagery or Guided Imagery

- Guided imagery is focused relaxation that helps create harmony between the mind and body by coaching one to create calm, peaceful images in the mind.
- It is not an alternative for other treatments but can be used with other therapies treating anxiety, loss of control, panic, obesity, hypertension, and other medical conditions.
- It can decrease pain and the need for pain medication, decrease side effects and complications of medical procedures, reduce recovery time, and shorten hospital stays.
- It enhances sleep.
- It helps to strengthen the immune system and enhance the ability to heal.
- It increases self-confidence and self-control.

Meditation

- Clinical effects of meditation impact a broad spectrum of physical and psychological symptoms and syndromes, including reduced anxiety, pain, and depression, enhanced mood and self-esteem, and decreased stress.
- Meditation may be recommended as part of CAM treatment for a large and growing number of medical conditions including high blood pressure and pain management.
- Meditation can positively influence the experience of chronic illness and can serve as an illness-prevention strategy.
- Meditation involves becoming more aware and more sensitive to what is within a person.
- It focuses on quieting a busy mind by directing concentration to one healing object, such as a flower, a candle, a sound or word, or the breath, but can be objectless.
- Meditation has been shown to contribute to an individual's psychological and physiological well-being.

Prayer or Spiritual Healing

- Spiritual healing has existed since Biblical times.
- Patients with serious medical illnesses commonly use spiritual methods to cope with their illnesses.
- Recognizing patients' beliefs in the face of suffering is thought to be an important factor in health care practice.
- Spirituality appears to be associated with a range of positive outcomes in the form of an enhanced sense of well-being, improved feelings of resiliency, and decreased physical symptoms including pain and fatigue, and psychological symptoms such as anxiety.
- Spiritual healing is a term that includes all types of energy healing systems and often incorporates a healer who channels energy from a source to the patient to promote or facilitate self-healing.
- Prayer is a form of spiritual healing that has recently gained widespread popularity.

Yoga

- Yoga is a practice that was developed within Indian culture and religion, but does not require spiritual beliefs or practices.
- It is widely practiced throughout the world.
- It is a practice of gentle stretching, breath control exercises, and meditations.
- It is thought that yoga increases the body's store of vital energy and facilitates the energy's flow through improved posture.
- Yoga reportedly increases physical endurance, strength, muscle suppleness, and feelings of well-being.
- Breathing techniques help to counter reactions to stress such as rapid breathing and muscular spasm.
- It is used alone or in combination with other CAM therapies to help ameliorate symptoms in conditions such as cardiovascular disease, multiple sclerosis, asthma, epilepsy, and joint stiffness in osteoarthritis.
- It is preferable to learn yoga with a practitioner although it may be self-taught.

PRECAUTIONS FOR MIND–BODY INTERVENTIONS

- As with any therapies the indirect risk to using mind–body interventions is that access to conventional diagnosis and/or treatment may be delayed.
- There appears to be little risk involved with art or music therapy; with dance therapy there may be a risk involved if movements are not done correctly.
- It is recommended that therapies that trigger changes in mental state should be used under medical supervision due to the potential for psychosis or personality disorder. Such therapies may include behavioral, meditation, imagery, and potentially, yoga.
- When practiced by a trained professional hypnosis is considered safe, however there is the risk of exacerbation of psychological problems or false memory syndrome in some persons.
- There appear to be no adverse effects with prayer or spiritual healing; however they may be contraindicated in diagnosed psychiatric illnesses.
- There are no contraindications for the use of yoga, except that certain postures are not recommended during pregnancy and that some persons with a history of psychiatric illness may risk exacerbation of their illness when practicing yoga.

Biologically Based Systems

Aromatherapy

- A wide range of practices involving the use of plant essences of flowers, herbs, and trees to promote health and well-being and for therapeutic purposes.
- Oils can be administered through the skin, by inhalation, or by ingesting very dilute concentrations of specific oils.
- Plant essential oils, alone or in combination with other therapies, may be beneficial in treating a number of health conditions.
- The use of aromatherapy began thousands of years ago in ancient Egypt, China, and India.

- Aromatherapy massage has mild and transient anxiolytic activity.
- Aromatherapy may be beneficial in conditions such as dementia, anxiety, in palliative care, and insomnia.

Bach Flower Remedies

- A therapeutic practice that uses specially prepared plant infusions to balance emotions, and subsequently, physical complaints.
- Thirty-eight flower remedies, divided into seven therapeutic groups, are thought to be beneficial in treating illness by targeting underlying emotional imbalances.

Chelation Therapy

- Chelation therapy is an intravenous therapy recognized for treatment of heavy metal (such as lead and calcium) poisoning.
- Ethylenediamine tetraacetic acid (EDTA), when injected into the blood, will bind with the metals and remove them from the body in the urine.
- High doses of vitamins are also often given with chelation therapy.
- Chelation therapy is used to treat coronary heart disease and advocates claim that there is evidence to support the claim that it can prevent and cure heart disease, stroke, senility, other vascular diseases, multiple sclerosis, and Parkinson's disease.

Dietary Supplements

- A dietary supplement is, as defined by the Dietary Supplement Health and Education Act (DSHEA) of 1994, "any product (other than tobacco) intended to supplement the diet that contains one or more of the following ingredients: a vitamin, mineral, herb or other botanical; an amino acid; a concentrate; a metabolite, constituent, extract, or combination of any of these ingredients."
- Under DSHEA, dietary supplements are considered foods, not drugs; thus they are not regulated.

- Many dietary supplements come to market with a long history of use; a case in point is herbal therapies used for thousands of years in traditional Chinese medicine.
- Dietary supplements can carry a claim or "statement of nutritional support" that is allowed by FDA when they are or contain vitamins and minerals with established Recommended Dietary Allowances (RDAs).
- When a supplement label carries a claim, it must have the following disclaimer on the label: "This statement has not been evaluated by the FDA. This product is not intended to diagnose, treat, cure, or prevent any disease."

Gerson Therapy

- Gerson therapy requires a significant commitment on the part of the patient.
- The late Max Gerson, MD, developed cancer therapies involving a diet of fresh fruit and vegetable juices, and juice extract from fresh calves' liver.
- It also promotes the use of coffee enemas for detoxifying the body.

Hoxey Therapy

- Based on various herbs, this treatment consists of a tonic and some caustic external pastes for burning away skin cancers.
- Harry Hoxey, a naturopath, developed the treatment from a formula his great-grandfather concocted after watching a horse with cancer graze on various herbs.

Herbal Therapy

- Herbal therapies include the medical use of preparations that contain exclusively botanical materials—plant parts such as flowers, leaves, stems, and roots.
- It has been practiced for thousands of years in several traditional medical healing practices or therapies.
- Many current prescription drugs are made from herbs or botanical materials. Digoxin, a powerful heart drug made from *Digitalis purpurea,* is an example of one.

- Herbal therapies treat a wide range of conditions from anxiety to weight control.
- Herbs are not regulated, although they are considered drugs and are most often used for self-treatment of medical conditions.
- Since herbs are considered drugs, caution should be exercised when using them together or in combination with prescription drugs.

Natural, Nonvitamin/Mineral/Nonherbal Supplements

- Although considered in the realm of dietary supplements, there are some nonherbal and nonvitamin/mineral supplements that are used for a variety of conditions and disease prevention.
- Among these supplements are dehydro-epiandrosterone (DHEA), creatine, carnitine, acidophilus, Coenzyme-Q 10, glucosamine, chondrotin, and MSM, to name just a few.

Therapeutic Diets

- Therapeutic diets are considered to fall within the CAM arena since they may complement a medical therapy.
- Therapeutic diets must be individualized; one diet does not fit all.
- Some diets may pose as therapeutic, to treat a particular disease or condition, but in fact may be contraindicated; a raw food diet to treat cancer is an example of such a diet.

PRECAUTIONS FOR BIOLOGICALLY BASED SYSTEMS

- Although aromatherapy has been used for centuries, only a few high-quality, randomized, controlled trials have examined it.
- Studies suggest that aromatherapy massage has mild and transient anxiolytic activity in patients with cancer. The effects are likely to be small; they may benefit cancer patients by enhancing feelings of well-being.
- There are few risks associated with aromatherapy. Some oils are potentially carcinogenic but the exposure rate for patients, when used appropriately, is likely to be too low to constitute a real danger.
- Some oils may produce a skin rash; because of toxic effects of some oils, essential oils should not be taken internally.
- The hypothesis that Bach flower remedies are associated with effects beyond a placebo response is not supported by data from rigorous clinical trials.
- Bach flower remedies are dispensed in homoeopathic dosages, appear to be safe, and do not appear to interfere with any other medication.
- Chelation therapy for conditions such as intermittent claudication and ishemic heart disease has not been found to be superior to placebo treatment.
- Chelation therapy should not be used in patients with renal disease, who are pregnant, or who have bleeding abnormalities.
- Just because a dietary supplement is available for sale legally, it does not prove that it is safe or effective.
- Some vitamins and minerals have been shown to have protective effects against certain diseases including cancer and heart disease. However, massive doses of vitamins and minerals (megadoses) have not been proven to cure disease and may in fact interfere with prescription medication and with one another.
- The Gerson therapies have not been shown to be an effective means of cancer treatment, according to the National Cancer Institute.
- There is no reliable evidence of the clinical efficacy of coffee enemas used in Gerson therapies.
- Coffee enemas are associated with adverse reactions (e.g., electrolyte imbalances), some of which are severe.
- The effectiveness of Hoxey therapies have not been proven effective in clinical research studies.
- There is good evidence for some herbal preparations. However, each herbal therapy or supplement should be evaluated on its own merit. Sweeping statements regarding the efficacy and safety of all herbs cannot be made.

- Precautions exist for each herb or herbal preparation and the potential for interactions with other herbs, drugs and foods, as well as disease conditions may exist.
- A fundamental problem with herbal preparations has been whether different products, extracts, or even the same brand are comparable and equivalent and are without adulteration; with improving dietary supplement regulations, this concern is beginning to abate.
- As with other dietary supplements (vitamins, minerals, and herbs) nonvitamin/mineral/nonherbal supplements may prove to be preventive or curative of some conditions, but must be individualized.
- As with herbs and vitamin/mineral supplements, these supplements have the potential to interact with other supplements, prescription drugs, and/or be contraindicated in certain conditions. Care must be taken to know which supplements may pose a risk with other supplements, drugs, or conditions.
- Therapeutic diets are beneficial in some conditions such as heart disease and diabetes.
- Therapeutic diets must be tailored to the individual. Some radical diets may prove to be inadequate in nutrients and or calories; in conditions where weight loss is a concern, such as in cancer and some pulmonary diseases, restrictive diets may be counterproductive.
- Macrobiotic, vegan, and vegetarian diets, to name a few, are often touted as beneficial and may have some possible disease preventive properties. They have not been proven to stop or reverse cancer, but may offer some hope in heart disease when used under medical supervision.

Manipulative and Body-Based Therapies

Acupuncture or Acupressure

- Acupuncture involves stimulation of defined points on the skin, usually by inserting small needles.
- Acupressure is the manual stimulation of acupuncture points.

- Acupuncture is used with herbal therapies and other modalities as part of TCM.
- In Western medicine, acupuncture is used as a single treatment.
- The concept behind acupuncture is that a person's Chi, or vital energy, is disturbed, and in order to prevent or correct this disturbance appropriate points on the body surface are stimulated.
- Acupuncture has been used for treating nausea, smoking cessation, weight management, headaches, osteoarthritis, and pain control.

Chiropractic

- Based on the belief that the nervous system determines the health of an individual, and that most diseases are caused by spinal malalignment and respond to manipulation of the spine.
- Recently chiropractors have become accepted health care providers.
- Chiropractic treatments are now being evaluated objectively based on the principles of evidence-based medicine.
- Chiropractic treatments are used to treat musculoskeletal problems, especially spinal pain syndromes.
- Some practitioners maintain that spinal manipulation can treat other conditions including asthma, heart disease, headaches, and irritable bowel syndrome, to name a few.

Massage

- The manipulation of muscle and connective tissue to enhance function of the tissues and promote relaxation and well-being.
- Massage improves circulation of blood and lymph, resulting in increased oxygen supply to tissues. It also relieves tension, stimulates nerves, and stretches and loosens muscles and connective tissue to keep them elastic.
- Massage purportedly helps the body rid itself of waste products.
- Massage is used to help relieve muscular tension, back pain, constipation, depression, stress, and other conditions.

- Massage is frequently used for the treatment of minor sports injuries and repetitive stress injuries, and to enhance physical conditioning.

Osteopathic

- A form of conventional medicine that, in part, emphasizes that diseases arise in the musculoskeletal system and that structure and function are closely related.
- It is thought that the primary role of the osteopathic physician is to facilitate the body's inherent ability to heal itself.
- There is an underlying belief that all of the body's systems work together, and disturbances in one system may affect function elsewhere in the body.
- Osteopathic manipulation—a full-body system of hands-on techniques to alleviate pain, restore function, and promote health and well-being—may be used by some physicians.
- In the United States, osteopathic physicians (DOs) use allopathic therapeutic therapies along with osteopathic manipulative techniques, and are considered mainstream health care professionals.

Feldenkrais

- A type of body work which focuses on efficient and comfortable body movements.
- A method of "breaking" the pattern of dysfunctional improper body movements.
- It is claimed that it can decrease stress, relieve pain, and improve balance and coordination.

PRECAUTIONS FOR MANIPULATIVE AND BODY-BASED THERAPIES

- As with other CAM therapies, there is a concern regarding delay of access to conventional medical treatment for potentially serious or life-threatening illnesses.
- Acupuncture may be useful for nausea/vomiting, for mild relaxation, and for pain/anxiety in persons with cancer.

- Acupuncture is contraindicated in bleeding conditions and first-trimester pregnancy (other than for treatment of nausea).
- Mild, transient effects that are common with acupuncture include drowsiness, bruising, bleeding, and pain.
- Acupuncture employing the use of electrical stimulation is contraindicated in persons with pacemakers.
- Chiropractic treatments are contraindicated in person with bleeding disorders, including those on anticoagulant therapies, those with osteoporosis, and those with malignant or inflammatory spinal disease.
- Some practitioners of chiropractic medicine overuse x-ray diagnostics and advise against the use of immunizations.
- Massage therapy is currently contraindicated in deep vein thrombosis, phlebitis, burns, skin infections, eczema, open wounds, high fever, low platelet count, bone fractures, and osteoporosis.
- Adverse reactions have rarely been reported when massage is done by trained and licensed therapists.
- The use of osteopathic manipulations appear to be contraindicated in conditions such as osteoporosis, cancer, infections, and bleeding disorders.
- Feldenkrais may exacerbate symptoms of injury, disease, degeneration, or psychological-related disorders if used inappropriately.

Energy Therapies

Biofield Therapies

Biofield therapies generally involve nontactile, noncontact interactions between practitioner and patient to attain healing. Biofield therapies employ the human body's subtle energy using a wide variety of practices, and are administered by practitioners who work with the biofield of the patient.

- *Qi gong*
  1. A component of traditional Chinese medicine that combines movement, meditation,

and regulation of breathing to enhance the flow of Qi (Chi) or vital energy in the body, improve blood circulation, and enhance immune function.

- *Reiki*
  1. A Japanese word representing Universal Life Energy. Reiki is based on the belief that when spiritual energy is channeled through a Reiki practitioner, the patient's spirit is healed, which in turn heals the physical body.
  2. Healing, it is felt, can also occur at a distance through intention.
- *Therapeutic touch*
  1. Life energy is believed to be manipulated therapeutically by the hands or touch of a practitioner.
  2. It is based on concepts similar to the religious practice of "laying on of hands," where healing energy is thought to pass from one person to another.
  3. It is a modern variation of ancient healing methods such as TCM and Ayurvedic medicine.
  4. Although the name implies touching, the practice involves the practitioner's hands being held 2 to 4 inches from the patient's body; undesirable energy is removed from the patient and beneficial energy is transferred.

Bioelectromagnetic-Based Therapies

Bioelectromagnetic-based therapies are called "energy medicine" and use external medical devices. Magnets and electricity have been used for centuries for medicinal purposes.

- *Magnet therapies*
  1. Magnets are used as bracelets, mattresses, shoe inserts, and belts.
  2. It is thought that they help to correct disease-causing electrical imbalances in the body.
  3. Magnets have been used for treatment of low back pain.

- *Pulsed therapies*
  1. Devices produce weak, pulsing electromagnetic fields.
  2. As with magnets, pulsed therapies are alleged to produce beneficial effects by correcting the body's disease-causing electrical imbalances.
  3. Pulsed therapies have been used to treat multiple sclerosis, fractured bones, arthritis, bed sores, depression, anxiety, and neurological disorders.

PRECAUTIONS FOR ENERGY THERAPIES

- Qi gong appears to have no adverse reactions, although psychosis has been observed in persons with latent condition.
- There are no known contraindications or adverse reactions associated with Reiki.
- Therapeutic touch may be contraindicated in persons who have difficulty with closeness or being touched.
- There has been very little scientific investigation of the effectiveness of magnets.
- Magnetic field therapies are contraindicated in pregnancy, persons with pacemakers, myasthenia gravis, and bleeding disorders, including the use of anticoagulant therapies.

REFERENCES

Aldridge D. Spirituality, healing and medicine. *Br J Gen Pract.* 1991;41:425–427.

Astin JA, Shapiro SL, Eisenberg DM, Forys KL. Mind-body medicine: State of the science, implications for practice. *J Am Board Fam Prac.* 2003;16:131–147.

Bent S. Aromatherapy: Ineffective treatment or effective placebo? *Effective Clinical Practice.* http://www. acponline.org/journals/ecp/julaug00/aromatherapy_ editorial.htm. Accessed 01/05/2004.

Bonadonna R. Meditation's impact on chronic illness. *Holist Nurs Pract.* 2003;17(6):309–319.

Bowling AC. *Alternative Medicine and Multiple Sclerosis.* New York, NY: Demos Publishing, Inc.; 2001.

Chrisman L. Native American medicine. *Gale Encyclopedia of Alternative Medicine.* http://www.gwu.edu/~english/

ccsc/2002%20Pages/Rodriguez.htm. Accessed January 03, 2004.

Ernst E, ed. *The Desktop Guide to Complementary and Alternative Medicine.* New York, NY: Mosby; 2001.

Ernst E. Flower remedies: A systematic review of the clinical evidence. *Wien Klin Wochenschr.* 2002;114:963–966.

Ernst E. A primer of complementary and alternative medicine commonly used by cancer patients. *Med J Australia.* http://www.mja.com.au/public/issues/174_02_150101/ernst/ernst.html. Accessed January 05, 2004.

Hoffman F, Manning M. *Herbal Medicine and Botanical Medical Fads.* New York, NY: The Haworth Press; 2002.

Holden K. Parkinson's disease and complementary therapies. *Nutr Comp Care.* 2003:6;21,27–28.

Jellin J, ed. *Natural Medicines Comprehensive Database.* Stockton, CA: Therapeutic Research Facility; 2003.

Laidlaw SH. *Herbs for Health and Healing.* Minnetonka, MN: National Health and Wellness Club; 2003.

Mehl-Madronna LE. Native American healing. http://www.healing-arts.org/mehl-madrona/mmtraditionalpaper.htm. Accessed January 03, 2004.

National Center for Complementary and Alternative Medicine. *What is Complementary and Alternative Medicine (CAM)?* http://www.nccam.nih.gov/health/whatiscam. Accessed January 03, 2004.

Shannahoff-Kahlsa DS. An introduction to Kundalini yoga meditation techniques that are specific for the treatment of psychiatric disorders. *J Altern Complement Med.* 2004. Feb;10(1):91–101.

Snyder M, Egan EC, Burns KR. Interventions for decreasing agitation behaviors in persons with dementia. *J Gerontol Nurs.* 1995. Jul;21(7):34–40.

Talbott SM. *A Guide to Understanding Dietary Supplements.* New York, NY: The Haworth Press; 2003.

Thorgrimsen L, Spector A, Wiles A, Orrell M. Aromatherapy for dementia. *Cochrane Database Syst Rev.* 2003;(3): CD003150.

The American Art Therapy Association. http://www.arttherapy.org/aboutarttherapy/about.htm. Accessed January 04, 2004.

The American Dance Therapy Association. http://www.adta.org. Accessed January 04, 2004.

http://www.camreports.hs.columbia.edu/diseases.html. Accessed January 03, 2004.

Medicomm Corporation. http://www.medicomm.net/Consumer%20Site/am/music.htm. Accessed January 04, 2003.

Merck manual online, 2nd ed. http://www.merck.com/mrkshared/mmanual_home2/sec25/ch302/ch302c.jsp. Accessed January 06, 2003.

FDA/CFSAN Dietary Supplement Overview. http://vm.cfsan.fda.gov/~dms/supplmnt.html. Accessed January 05, 2004.

Reimbursement for Medical Nutrition Therapy

Carol Frankmann, MS, RD, LD, CNSD

DESCRIPTION

Medical Nutrition Therapy (MNT) involves a comprehensive assessment of the patient's overall nutritional status, medical data and diet history, intervention to an individualized course of treatment, and reassessment and follow-up interventions. In 2001, the establishment of current procedural terminology (CPT) codes for MNT provided registered dietitians and nutrition professionals with billing codes that are specific to nutritional diagnostic, therapy, and counseling services.

CODES

MNT Codes are included in the *American Medical Association's Current Procedural Terminology CPT* book.[1] The codes are updated and published annually, and decisions regarding the addition, deletion, or modification of codes are made by the American Medical Association (AMA). Table 6–7 lists MNT CPT codes as defined by the AMA, the American Dietetic Association (ADA), and the Centers for Medicare and Medicaid Services (CMS).

With the establishment of MNT CPT codes, these codes should be used to bill for professional nutrition services. It is no longer appropriate to bill with codes "incident to" physician services.

In January 2003, CMS established two new codes for MNT. These codes are to be used when the treating physician determines that there is a change in diagnosis or medical condition of the Medicare beneficiary and additional hours of MNT services are needed beyond the hours typically covered by Medicare.[2] These additional codes are listed in Table 6–8.

These codes were established by CMS to meet an operational need for Medicare beneficiaries prior to the update of AMA CPT codes. Although they are considered to be temporary codes, they could remain in use indefinitely.[3]

Coverage

Codes are used to describe services that are billed; however, coverage of services is determined on a policy-specific basis. In addition, coverage of services changes as health care plans and/or CMS regulations are revised. Communication with the third party payor is essential to identify current MNT coverage. Health plan websites may provide coverage information,[4,5] and the CMS website provides extensive information on coverage for Medicare beneficiaries.[6]

Health plans often define coverage for MNT based on the patient's diagnosis, as well as specify the treatment setting and number of visits. The Medicare guidelines define MNT coverage for medical nutrition therapy services for their beneficiaries as follows.

- Medicare Part B provides MNT coverage for outpatient care only. MNT is not covered for an inpatient stay in a hospital or skilled nursing facility because nutrition services are bundled into facility charges and billed under Medicare Part A in these settings.
- Coverage is restricted to patients with diabetes mellitus type 1 and type 2, gestational diabetes, patients with chronic renal insufficiency (nondialysis), and patients provided posttransplant care for 36 months after discharge from the hospital for a kidney transplant. Diagnostic criteria are outlined below[7].
  1. Diabetes mellitus type 1 or 2: fasting glucose greater than or equal to 126 mg/dl.
  2. Gestational diabetes: any degree of glucose intolerance with onset or first recognition during pregnancy.
  3. Chronic renal insufficiency: a reduction in renal function not severe enough to require dialysis or transplantation (glomerular filtration rate (GFR) 13–50 ml/min/1.73 m^2).
- A maximum of 3 hours of MNT may be reimbursed in the initial calendar year and 2 follow-up hours in subsequent years.

Table 6–7 Medical Nutrition Therapy CPT Codes

Code	*Description*
97802	Medical nutrition therapy: initial assessment and intervention, individual, face-to-face with the patient, each 15 minutes
97803	Reassessment and intervention, individual, face-to-face with patient, each 15 minutes
97804	Group (2 or more individuals), each 30 minutes

Table 6–8 Additional Medical Nutrition Therapy Codes

Code	Description
G0270	Medical nutrition therapy; reassessment and subsequent intervention(s) following second referral in same year for change in diagnosis, medical condition, or treatment regimen (including additional hours needed for renal disease), individual face-to-face with the patient, each 15 minutes
G0271	Medical nutrition therapy; reassessment and subsequent intervention(s) following second referral in same year for change in diagnosis, medical condition, or treatment regimen (including additional hours needed for renal disease) group (2 or more individuals), each 30 minutes

From Medical Nutrition Therapy (MNT) Services for Beneficiaries with Diabetes or Renal Disease—Policy Change.

Additional hours are permitted when there is a referral due to a change in diagnosis or medical condition.[8]

General conditions of MNT coverage for Medicare beneficiaries are listed below.

- The treating physician must make a referral and indicate a diagnosis of diabetes or renal disease, including the International Classification of Diseases, 9th Revision, Clinical Modification (ICD-9-CM) code to the highest level of specificity.[9]
- Prior to providing the service, a signed copy of the referral and a physician order is required during each calendar year when nutrition services are needed.[7]

ADVANCED BENEFICIARY NOTICE

If the provider is unsure if MNT will be covered for a Medicare beneficiary with diabetes or nondialysis renal disease, it is necessary to inform the patient prior to the delivery of MNT. An Advanced Beneficiary Notice (ABN) is used to provide written notice that a patient is responsible for the payment if Medicare denies the claim. The provider may be *unsure* of coverage when the frequency and duration of MNT exceeds the coverage guidelines or when it may not be considered medically necessary. Providers should not give ABNs to all Medicare pa-

tients. If the provider is certain the MNT will not be covered by Medicare (i.e., it is not a covered diagnosis), an ABN is not needed.[10,11]

MNT services cannot be billed to Medicare for beneficiaries with any condition other than the covered diagnoses. If no other insurance coverage is available, the patient would pay for the MNT services provided out-of-pocket.[10] This has major implications in practice settings that primarily treat patients with conditions not covered by Medicare. Decisions about billing for MNT in those settings should be made in consultation with professionals with expertise in billing, compliance, and legal areas.

Providers

Medicare regulations define Registered Dietitians or nutrition professionals as providers of MNT. To enroll and receive a Medicare Provider Identification Number (PIN), practitioners should contact their local/state Medicare carrier and receive enrollment forms. Carrier information is available from CMS.[12] Dietitians employed by physician clinics or other outpatient facilities must also complete a reassignment form to allow the employer to submit claims and collect payment for MNT services provided by the RD. The enrolled practitioner will be subject to all of the rules, regulations, and quality issues of Medicare providers. Documentation, billing procedures, and standardized protocols will need to be followed and closely monitored for probable audits.

OPTING OUT

The decision to "opt out" of Medicare is a serious one. The following factors should be considered.

- Dietitians who are not Medicare providers can provide MNT to Medicare beneficiaries with covered diagnoses only if the patient pays for the service out-of-pocket. The practitioner is required to
  1. Provide Medicare beneficiaries with specific documentation that he/she has chosen to "opt out" of Medicare and that the patient is responsible for full payment.
  2. Inform the patient that the MNT service is available from Medicare providers, hence the patient would pay only the co-pay.
- The practitioner who decides to "opt out" of Medicare must sign a formal affidavit and mail this detailed statement to each Medicare carrier. The document is effective for 2 years and remains in effect even if the practitioner's place of employment changes.[11]

Dietitians are advised to consult with the Compliance Officer in their facility or with a health care attorney for appropriate counsel and assistance in reviewing regulations and determining the impact that Medicare private contracts have on their professional practice and business decisions. Providers are advised to carry malpractice insurance.[11]

Documentation

CMS has not yet established documentation standards that are specific to MNT for Medicare beneficiaries. However, the following elements are pertinent to requirements by CMS and should be included, along with nutritional assessment and intervention documentation:

- Receipt of referral
- Diagnosis
- Date of visit and start/stop times.

Billing

Billing issues are complex and need to be addressed in consultation with professionals that have expertise in billing regulations and knowledge of the practice setting. The following basic principles should help clarify the Medicare Part B billing requirements.

- Registered dietitians and nutrition professionals must either bill Medicare utilizing their own PIN or reassign their reimbursement.
- Medicare should only be billed for MNT that is appropriately provided to beneficiaries with covered diabetes or renal diagnoses.
- Medical nutrition therapy should not be billed as an "incident to" physician services for Medicare beneficiaries.[7]
- Registered dietitians who are Medicare providers and part of a multidisciplinary team that provides Diabetes Self-Management Training (DSMT) services, may bill on behalf of a DSMT program. However, only one person or entity from the program bills Medicare for the whole program, and payment is made as if rendered to a physician. The DSMT benefit is completely separate from the MNT benefit. Both DSMT and MNT cannot be billed on the same date of service.[8]

The CMS-1500 (HCFA-1500) is used for billing for professional services. It is the accepted billing form with Medicare, Medicaid, and many insurers. The Unique Physician Identification Number (UPIN) of the referring physician must be on the claim form submitted by the provider.[7] It is important that practitioners establish systems to track billing transactions for the MNT services that they provide.

Compliance

The Compliance Officer is responsible for coordinating activities that safeguard against fraud and abuse, improve the quality of health care, and reduce the costs of care. Every physician practice, billing company, and health care organization should designate a Compliance Officer. To ensure compliance with regulations, audits may be conducted within the organization, as well as by Medicare and other payors.

FEES

Medicare payment rates for the MNT CPT codes are made under the physician fee schedule by geographical area. The rates are established by CMS and are a calculation of RVUs (relative value units), a conversion factor, and a geographical location factor. As a Medicare provider, the dietitian agrees to accept the payment rate established by Medicare and agrees to collect the co-pay from the beneficiary. Any further billing of the patient would be illegal.[7]

Reimbursement

Reimbursement by Medicare is the lesser of the actual charge or 85% of the physician fee schedule amount. Coinsurance is 20% of the lesser of these two amounts.[2] A sample Medicare beneficiary payment is shown in Table 6–9.

Payment of codes 97802 (initial) and 97803 (follow-up) are the same value; it is assumed that the difference between these two types of visits is the time spent performing the service. Group 97804 (group) is paid at a lower rate.

Providers for managed care organizations often negotiate a discounted fee-for-service rate. In managed care markets with capitated payment systems, practitioners can negotiate to receive fee-for-service or a percentage of the capitation from a physician practice for providing MNT to patients.

DENIED CLAIMS

Claims can be denied for a range of reasons, including incorrect or insufficient information. When investigating or resubmitting a denied claim, submit a letter and supporting documentation to substantiate that the MNT was medically necessary. In addition, ask the insurer what additional information or clarification is desired.

Medicare Prescription Drug, Improvement, and Modernization Act of 2003

The Medicare Modernization Act of 2003 expanded MNT in two major areas. For the first time, an initial preventive physical examination will be available to new beneficiaries within the first 6 months of Medicare eligibility. MNT is included in the screening and other preventive services covered by this benefit. In addition, the bill provides for the establishment of voluntary Chronic Care Improvement (CCI) programs to be phased in over 3 to 5 years, beginning January 1, 2006. Chronic diseases are defined as "congestive heart failure, diabetes, chronic obstructive pulmonary disease, or other diseases or conditions as selected by the Secretary of

---

Table 6–9 Medicare Payment Method

Medicare Payment	Amount (Hypothetical)
Actual bill for MNT*	$130
Physician fee schedule amount	$ 90
MNT approved amount (85% of assigned physician fee)	$ 76.50
Medicare beneficiary payment (20% of approved amount)	$ 15.30

*Note: Beneficiary has met Part B Deductible.

Health and Human Services." Each chronic care management plan will include appropriate self-care education through approaches such as disease management or MNT and education for primary caregivers and family members. A CCI will provide programs under contract with Medicare, so the dietitian that provides MNT will do so as an employee of (or under contract with) the CCI. Reimbursement rates may be individually negotiated and not governed by CMS.[13]

ADA continues to actively advocate for expansion of the coverage for nutrition services. The establishment of CPT codes for MNT was a major milestone, achieved after a decade of work. Medicare reforms legislation offers additional opportunities. To maximize these opportunities, it is essential for dietitians to actively support ADA's initiatives in this arena, as well as to stay abreast of reimbursement issues.

REFERENCES

1. *American Medical Association Current Procedural Terminology CPT 2004.* Chicago, IL: AMA Press, 2003.

2. *Medical Nutrition Therapy (MNT) Services for Beneficiaries with Diabetes or Renal Disease—Policy Change.* Program Memorandum Intermediaries/Carriers, Department of Health and Human Services, Centers for Medicare and Medicaid Services (CMS); November 1, 2002. Transmittal AB-02-115, Change Request 2404, CMS Pub 60A.

3. Procedures for coding and payment determinations for clinical laboratory tests and durable medical equipment. Centers for Medicare and Medicaid Services website. Available at http://www.cms.hhs.gov/medicare/hcpcs/codpayproc.asp. Accessed December 17, 2004.

4. Clinical Policy Bulletins: Nutritional Counseling. Aetna website. Available at http://www.aetna,com/cpb/data/CPBA0049.html. Accessed December 17, 2004.

5. TUFTS Health Plan Nutritional Counseling Guidelines. TUFTS Health Plan website. Available at http://www.tuftshealthplan.com/providers/provider.php?sec=billing_guidelines&content=b_nutr-counseling&rightnav=billing. Accessed December 17, 2004.

6. Centers for Medicare and Medicaid Services website. Available at http://www.cms.hhs.gov/. Accessed June 1, 2004.

7. *Additional clarification for Medical Nutrition Therapy (MNT) Services.* Program Memorandum Intermediaries/Carriers, Department of Health and Human Services, Centers for Medicare and Medicaid Services (CMS); May 1, 2002. Transmittal AB-02-059, Change Request 2142, CMS Pub 60AB.

8. *Clarification Regarding Non-physician Practitioners Billing on Behalf of a Diabetes Outpatient Self-Management Training Services (DSMT) Program and the Common Working File Edits for DSMT and Medical Nutrition Therapy (MNT).* Program Memorandum Intermediaries/Carriers, Department of Health and Human Services, Centers for Medicare and Medicaid Services (CMS); October 25, 2002. Transmittal AB-02-151, Change Request 2372, CMS Pub 60AB.

9. *ICD-9-CM, International Classification of Diseases, 9th Revision, Clinical Modification.* Vol 1-3. 6th ed. Los Angeles, CA: Practice Management Information Corporation; 2003.

10. Infante M, Michael P. Medicare Part B coverage and billing for medical nutrition therapy. *J Am Diet Assoc.* 2002:102(1):32.

11. Infante MC, Michael P, Pritchett E. Opting out of Medicare: A serious business decision. *J Am Diet Assoc.* 2002;102(8);1061–1062.

12. Medicare Fee-for-Service Provider/Supplier Enrollment. Centers for Medicare and Medicaid Services website. Available at: http://www.cms.hhs.gov/providers/enrollment/default.asp? Accessed December 15, 2004.

13. Smith R. Medicare reform: What it means to the future of dietetics. *J Am Diet Assoc.* 2004;104:734–735.

CHAPTER 7

Meal Planning

Chris Biesemeier, MS, RD, LD

STANDARD DIETS

Regular Diet

Objectives

- To meet nutritional needs for optimal health
- To provide a basis for modified diets

Indication for Use

- Individuals who do not need dietary modification

Nutritional Adequacy

- Diet is nutritionally adequate.
- Diet meets Dietary Reference Intakes (DRIs).

Summary of Guidelines

- Refer to the U.S. Department of Agriculture (USDA) *Dietary Guidelines for Americans* for a description of an overall approach to healthful eating.
- Use the Food Guide Pyramid to determine the kinds and amounts of foods to eat each day and the Nutrition Facts Label to select foods.
- Use the Interactive Healthy Eating Index to assess nutritional adequacy of intake (http://www.cnpp.usda.gov/ihei.html).

High-Protein/High-Calorie Diet

Objective

- To provide protein- and calorie-rich foods for individuals with increased requirements

Indications for Use

- Individuals with increased requirements due to illness or injury
- Individuals who are malnourished and desire repletion of energy stores and lean body mass

Nutritional Adequacy

- Diet is nutritionally adequate.
- Diet meets DRIs.

Summary of Guidelines

- Use the suggested servings in the "moderate" and "higher" categories of the Food Guide Pyramid to make food selections.
- Consider between-meal snacks and use of nutritional supplements.
- Vitamin and mineral supplementation may be indicated.

Vegetarian Diet

Objective

- To consume a healthful, plant-centered diet

Nutritional Adequacy

- Nutritional adequacy varies according to the type of vegetarian diet, variety of foods consumed, and individual food choices. Most vegetarian diets can be nutritionally adequate.
- Special attention is needed to ensure adequate intake of calories, iron, calcium, zinc, vitamin D, vitamin B_{12}, and the omega-3 fatty acids, especially in vegetarian diets with limited food variety.
- Omission of milk products makes it difficult to meet the calcium needs of children, teenagers, and pregnant or lactating women, without supplementation.

Summary of Guidelines

- Determine the type of vegetarian diet being followed and individualize nutrient recommendations accordingly.
- Pay special attention to adequacy of protein, vitamin B_{12}, vitamin D, calcium, zinc, iron, and omega-3 fatty acids.
- Combine complementary plant proteins over the course of the day to meet protein needs.
- Assess fat intake, especially when dairy foods are consumed. Consumption of high-fat versions of dairy products may result in high intake of saturated fat.
- Supplementation may be required during pregnancy, lactation, infancy, and adolescence and after loss of a large amount of blood.
- Women in their childbearing years may need to take an iron supplement.

Pregnancy and Lactation Diet

Objective

- To meet the nutritional needs of mother and baby during pregnancy and lactation in order to support optimal growth and development

Nutritional Adequacy

- Diet is nutritionally adequate.
- Diet meets DRIs.

Summary of Guidelines

- Use the Food Guide Pyramid as a tool in making healthful food choices.
- Increase calories above nonpregnant needs by an average of 300 kcal/day during the second and third trimesters of pregnancy and 500 kcal/day for lactation.
- Energy needs may be increased for adolescents during pregnancy, depending on age and activity level and for adolescents who are lactating. Energy needs may be increased for women who are breastfeeding more than one infant, pregnant while breastfeeding, or underweight.
- Include 60 g/day protein for adults and adolescents during pregnancy. Include 65 g/day for the first 6 months of lactation and 62 g/day during the second 6 months. Protein needs may be increased if breastfeeding more than one infant.
- Emphasize consumption of dairy products and an iron-rich diet to meet calcium and iron needs. Supplemental calcium may be needed for complete vegetarians and for women under the age of 25 years who are not consuming dairy products. Supplemental iron (30 mg of elemental iron; 60–120 mg for iron-deficiency anemia) is needed daily during pregnancy and may be recommended for a short interval postdelivery. Iron needs are not increased above normal during lactation.
- Supplementation with folic acid is recommended preconception (0.4 mg/day), during pregnancy (0.6 mg/day), and during lactation (0.5 mg/day). Women who have already had a birth with a neural tube defect will have increased needs during current pregnancy, with levels of supplementation per physician prescription.
- Meet requirements for other vitamins and minerals by selecting a variety of foods.

- Discourage alcohol during pregnancy, even moderate amounts.
- The evidence on the effect of caffeine during pregnancy is mixed, with some studies reporting a small increase in risk of spontaneous abortion and low birth weight in women who consume > 150 mg/day, the approximate amount in 1–2 cups of coffee. However, other research has reported no correlation with adverse outcomes at levels of consumption up to 300 mg/day. Consumption of moderate amounts of caffeine during lactation is acceptable. However intake > 650 mg/day has been associated with caffeine stimulation of the infant.
- Use of moderate amounts of sugar substitutes during pregnancy and lactation is considered acceptable.
- High fluid intake (8–12 cups daily) is needed for lactation.

Diet for Infants and Children

Objective

- To meet nutritional needs, especially during periods of accelerated growth, in a form that is compatible with developmental ability

Indications for Use

- Infants and children who are developing in a normal manner and do not need dietary modifications

Nutritional Adequacy

- Diet is nutritionally adequate. DRIs are only estimates of needs, making it important to monitor the growth and development of each infant.
- Breastfed infants and infants fed less than 500 ml of formula per day should be given a vitamin D supplement (200 IU/day), due to potentially inadequate exposure to sunlight.
- DRIs for 7- to 12-month-old infants can be met with a combination of breast milk or formula and complementary foods.

- Inclusion of "empty calorie foods" by older infants and toddlers reduces achievement of DRIs and should be limited.
- For toddlers, special attention is needed to meet DRIs for iron, essential fatty acids, and vitamin E. It may be difficult to achieve adequate intake (AI) of fiber.

Summary of Guidelines

- Promote breastfeeding to meet infants' nutritional needs and to provide other advantages. Exclusively breastfed infants are exposed to a variety of flavors, depending on maternal diet, suggesting the importance of early diet variety.
- Encourage breastfeeding of infants with a strong family history of food allergy (those whose parents or siblings have or had significant food allergies) for as long as possible. Encourage these nursing mothers to limit their intake of particularly allergenic foods. Delay introduction of complementary foods in infants at risk for food allergy until after 6 months of age. Complementary foods are defined by the American Academy of Pediatrics (AAP) as "any energy-containing foods that displace breastfeeding and reduce the intake of breast milk."
- If breastfeeding is not selected, use an iron-fortified formula. Use an iron-fortified formula if breastfed infants need supplementation.
- Use careful handling techniques during collection and storage to ensure that expressed breast milk is clean and does not get contaminated. Follow manufacturers' directions for use and storage of infant formulas.
- For most infants, breast milk and/or iron-fortified formula provide all required nutrients for about the first 6 months after birth.
- By approximately 6 months, term breastfed infants require an additional source of iron to meet needs. Good iron sources include meats, especially red meats, and iron-fortified cereals. One ounce of iron-fortified cereal provides the daily iron requirement. Feed with a vitamin C source, such as baby fruits, to enhance iron absorption from the cereal.

- After 6 months of age, term breastfed infants also require complementary foods to meet DRIs for energy, manganese, fluoride, vitamin D, vitamin B₆, niacin, zinc, vitamin E, magnesium, biotin, phosphorus, and thiamin.
- Introduce a variety of flavors and foods during the first 2 years to promote acceptance of a wider variety of flavors and foods in later childhood and the likelihood of greater willingness to try new foods. Up to 10–15 exposures may be needed before a particular food is accepted.
- Introduce new foods one at a time and watch for adverse reactions. A reasonable schedule for introducing foods is one new food every 2 to 4 days. Give combination foods after tolerance to the individual components has been established.
- Introduce foods in a general progression that promotes achievement of nutrient needs. Evidence about the order of introduction of foods is limited.
- Readiness for and acceptance of different food textures appears to depend on child's developmental stage and prior experience with particular textures. In most infants, developmental skills needed to begin complementary foods are present between 4 and 6 months of age.
- Exposure to a variety of textures appears to promote acceptance. Gradually expose infants to solid textures during the sensitive period for learning to chew (from the time complementary foods are introduced through 10 months of age) to reduce likelihood of rejection of certain textures, refusal to chew, or vomiting.
- Delay introduction of cow's milk until after 1 year of age and provide only whole milk. If milk is limited to 2 cups per day, use an additional tablespoon of oil in food preparation or added to prepared foods to provide needed amounts of linoleic and alpha-linolenic acids. Soybean oil will provide adequate amounts of both essential fatty acids. If soybean oil cannot be used, a mixture of 50% canola and 50% safflower or corn oils will provide needed amounts.
- In infants with a strong family history of food allergy, delay introduction of the major food allergens (e.g., eggs, cow's milk, wheat, and soy) until well after 1 year of age and the introduction of foods associated with "lifelong" sensitization (e.g., peanuts, tree nuts, fish, and shellfish) even longer.
- There is no evidence that the precautions for infants with a strong family history of food allergy are of any benefit to infants who are not at risk for allergy.
- Avoid wheat, rye, barley, and oats in infants with a family history of celiac disease. Oats do not contain gluten but may be contaminated with wheat gluten during processing.
- Delay introduction of gluten-containing and gluten-free cereals before 4 months in infants with a strong family history of type 1 diabetes (parents and first-degree relatives) to decrease the risk of developing islet immunity.
- Encourage parents to develop a healthy feeding relationship with their infant/child. Promote a role for parents in setting the eating environment and providing appropriate healthy foods. Encourage parents to respond appropriately to infant cues of hunger and satiety and to allow children to decide whether to eat and how much.
- Encourage parents to demonstrate feeding skills rather than relying on verbal prompts alone.
- Encourage fiber-rich foods.
- Encourage an appropriate level of activity in order to allow a level of food intake that meets nutrient needs but does not promote excessive weight gain.
- Promote physical activity by encouraging parents to limit excessive use of infant restraints, balance sedentary pastimes with active ones, and make a conscious effort to include movement and physical activity in play.
- DRI for physical activity in older children is 60 minutes of accumulated activity most if not all days.

- Discourage television viewing by children under the age of 2, in accordance with the AAP position, because of potential negative effects on development and physical activity. Limit TV viewing in children over the age of 2 to fewer than 2 hours per day.
- Encourage parents to provide a good example in their own food choices and physical activity patterns.

Diet for Older Adults

Objective

- To provide a variety of nutrient-dense foods that will meet the nutritional needs of older adults, incorporate individual food habits and lifestyle, and address physical limitations and health status.

Nutritional Adequacy

- Diet is nutritionally adequate.
- Diet meets DRIs.

Summary of Guidelines

- Requirements for specific nutrients are generally the same as for younger adults. However, DRIs for calcium, vitamin D, and vitamin B_6 are increased in individuals over the age of 50.
- Ten to thirty percent of older adults do not have the ability to absorb adequate amounts of vitamin B_{12} from food and will need to meet the DRI from synthetic sources of B_{12}-fortified foods, supplements, or injections.
- Emphasize nutrient-dense foods to ensure nutritional adequacy.
- Reduce caloric intake as needed to accommodate reductions in lean body mass and physical activity.
- Modify food consistency as needed for chewing and swallowing problems.
- Encourage insoluble fiber, additional fluids, and intake of fruits, vegetables, and whole-grain breads and cereals as needed for constipation.
- Evaluate psychosocial factors that may affect eating and food availability.

MODIFIED-CONSISTENCY DIETS

Soft Diet

Objective

- To provide foods that are soft in texture, easily digested, moderately low in roughage, and mildly seasoned.

Indications for Use

- May be used as a transition diet for individuals who cannot tolerate the texture and seasoning of food on a regular diet.
- Traditionally has been used for patients who are experiencing gas or distention, though the benefit derived may arise more from perception than from actual physiological effect. Postoperative symptoms of nausea, vomiting, gas, and distention arise from anesthesia, gut immobility, and the general effect of bed rest, not from specific foods or a particular diet. Many patients will be able to tolerate resumption of their regular diet by the second postoperative meal.

Nutritional Adequacy

- Diet is nutritionally adequate.
- Diet meets DRIs.

Summary of Guidelines

- Include food selections based on individual tolerance. Limit highly-seasoned foods based on preference. Modify texture and methods of food preparation according to tolerance.
- Smaller, more frequent meals may be helpful in relieving gas and distention.
- For persistent nausea and vomiting, provide small quantities of dry foods and progress to small meals of palatable foods.

Diet for Peptic Ulcer Disease

Objective

- To reduce intake of known gastric irritants and foods that stimulate gastric acid secretion

Indications for Use

- Patients with chronic peptic ulcer disease, as an adjunct to treatment with medications, such as antacids and antibiotics
- Evidence does not support the use of the traditional bland diet to reduce gastric acid secretion.

Nutritional Adequacy

- Diet is nutritionally adequate.
- Diet meets DRIs.

Summary of Guidelines

- Encourage consumption of a regular, well-balanced diet.
- Remove foods from the diet only after repeated intolerance has been demonstrated.
- Avoid frequent meals and evening snacks, in order to reduce gastric acid secretion.
- Avoid alcohol and all caffeine-containing beverages.
- Limit foods and seasonings that stimulate gastric acid secretion, such as black pepper, garlic, cloves, and chili powder.

Dysphagia Diet

Objective

- To provide foods that can be tolerated by individuals with chewing and swallowing disorders, meet nutrient requirements, and avoid complications from food intolerance, such as choking, aspiration pneumonia, and undernutrition

Indications for Use

- Individuals with chewing and swallowing disorders, including bulbar palsy, myasthenia gravis, amyotrophic lateral sclerosis, polymyositis, complications from radiation therapy, cerebrovascular accident, head injuries, brain tumors, cerebral palsy, Parkinson's disease, multiple sclerosis, Huntington's chorea, stricture of the esophagus, inflamma-

tion of the pharynx, and history of aspiration pneumonia

Nutritional Adequacy

- Diet is nutritionally adequate.
- Diet meets DRIs.

Summary of Guidelines

- Individualize the diet and foods provided according to ability to chew and swallow. Foods that hold some shape are the easiest to swallow. Avoid thin liquids, which are difficult to swallow, until tolerance is determined.
- Provide thickened foods and liquids according to the directions of the speech pathologist. Use thickeners such as baby rice cereal, mashed potatoes, or bananas to thicken liquids to appropriate consistency.
- Ability to tolerate liquids is assessed separately from tolerance to solids. Use the National Dysphagia Diet in order to promote consistency in terminology and content of levels of dysphagia diets.
- Liquids are described as thin (allows all fluids including water, ice, milk, coffee, tea, and carbonated beverages), nectar-like (can be sipped from a cup or through a straw and will slowly fall off a spoon that is tipped), honey-like (can be eaten with a spoon but do not hold their shape on a spoon), and spoon-thick (very thick and must be eaten with a spoon).
- Diet stages include: National Dysphagia Diet 1 (NDD-1)-"Dysphagia Pureed" (thick, smooth, homogeneous, semi-liquid textures with no lumps; foods are pudding-like); National Dysphagia Diet 2 (NDD-2)-"Dysphagia Mechanically Altered" (moist, soft-textured foods that are easily formed into a bolus, such as tender ground or finely diced meats, soft-cooked vegetables, soft ripe or canned fruits, and slightly moistened dry cereals with no texture); and National Dysphagia Diet 3 (NDD-3)-"Dysphagia Advanced" (foods of nearly regular textures with the exception of very hard, sticky, or crunchy foods).

- Taste sensation may be decreased. Enhance flavorings as needed unless tissue irritation is present. Use broths and gravies to moisten foods.
- Avoid foods with mixed textures such as stews and gelatin with fruit.
- Provide nutrition supplements as needed to meet nutrient requirements.
- Consider six small meals instead of three large meals. Ensure that staff is available to assist with feedings between scheduled meals.

Clear Liquid Diet

Objectives

- To provide fluids and electrolytes in order to prevent dehydration
- To reduce amount of residue present in the intestinal tract and to stimulate minimal digestive activity

Indications for Use

- May be used as a transition from NPO order to a regular diet
- May be used prior to bowel surgery and gastrointestinal (GI) diagnostic procedures

Nutritional Adequacy

- Inadequate in all nutrients without the use of low-residue nutrition supplements. Should be used for short intervals only.

Summary of Guidelines

- Provide liberal amounts of coffee, tea, clear fruit juices and drinks, broth, and gelatin.
- Other foods included on the diet are Popsicles, plain hard candy, gumdrops, and fruit ices.
- Patients with diabetes mellitus should receive the same foods provided to patients who do not have diabetes, including sweetened carbonated beverages and gelatin. An initial suggested amount of carbohydrate is 200 g/day, provided in small feedings spaced throughout the day. Frequent blood glucose monitoring is recommended, with adjustments in medications and diet based on results.

GASTROINTESTINAL DISORDER DIETS

Anti-Reflux Diet

Objectives

- To provide foods that reduce cardiac sphincter pressure and gastric acidity
- To avoid irritation of an inflamed esophagus

Indications for Use

- Individuals who have gastroesophageal reflux disease (GERD), esophagitis, and hiatal hernia

Nutritional Adequacy

- Diet is nutritionally adequate.
- Individual food selections and avoidance of groups of food may limit nutritional adequacy.

Summary of Guidelines

- Avoid high-fat foods such as fried foods, gravies, pastries, and high-fat meats.
- Limit use of added fats such as margarine, butter, cream, oil, and salad dressing.
- Avoid coffee and foods and beverages containing chocolate, cocoa, caffeine, peppermint oil, and spearmint oil.
- Avoid tomatoes, tomato juice, citrus juices, and alcohol.
- Choose foods according to individual tolerance.
- Achieve and maintain a healthy weight.
- Avoid large meals. Eat small, frequent meals.
- Avoid bending over after eating and lying down within 45 to 60 minutes of eating.
- Avoid eating within 2 hours of bedtime.

Fiber-Restricted Diet

Objectives

- To limit the amount of fiber consumed in order to decrease stool volume and frequency
- To prevent distention of the bowel and further aggravation of inflamed tissue

Indications for Use

- Individuals experiencing complications of radiation therapy
- Individuals experiencing acute exacerbations of diverticulosis, Crohn's disease, ulcerative colitis, and other inflammatory bowel disease
- Used for longer periods of time when inflammatory changes have resulted in stenosis of the lumen of the intestine or esophagus to prevent blockage
- Used as a pre- and postoperative regimen for lower bowel surgery

Nutritional Adequacy

- Diet is nutritionally adequate.
- Nutritional adequacy may be limited by individual food selections and avoidance of groups of food.

Summary of Guidelines

- Include beverages and juices without pulp; refined breads and cereals; potatoes without skin; refined pasta; most meats; cheese; canned, cooked, and selected fresh fruits; selected canned and cooked vegetables; selected raw vegetables; plain cakes and cookies; sugar; hard candies; jelly; margarine; plain sauces; gravies; and salad dressings. Selection of foods will depend on individual tolerance.
- Avoid whole-grain flour, bran, oatmeal, granola, seeds, nuts, coconut, fruit and vegetable pulp, dried fruits, berries, dried beans, peas, lentils, legumes, and popcorn.
- Number and size of food portions on diet are limited. Consult a diet manual for detailed listing of foods.
- Diet may cause a delay in intestinal transit.
- Terms *fiber* and *residue* are not synonymous. *Residue* refers to the total amount of material in the colon and includes undigested fiber and food, intestinal secretions, bacteria, and sloughed cells. Residue can be reduced by limiting milk on Fiber-Restricted Diet to 2 cups a day and avoiding prune juice.

High-Fiber Diet

Objectives

- To increase the amount of fiber consumed to 20–35 g/day (10–13 g/100 kcal).
- To reduce intracolonic pressure and promote regular elimination.
- To normalize serum lipids.

Indications for Use

- Used in treatment of atonic constipation, diverticulosis, hemorrhoids, and irritable bowel syndrome
- Used in treatment of elevated LDL-cholesterol level (soluble fiber)

Nutritional Adequacy

- Diet is nutritionally adequate.
- There is no DRI for fiber.

Summary of Guidelines

- Include whole-grain, bran, and granola-type breads and cereals; oatmeal; fruits and vegetables, especially raw and with skin; and legumes, nuts, and seeds. Consult a diet manual for fiber content of foods and recommended servings.
- Increase fiber intake gradually to avoid abdominal gas and cramping.
- Drink 8 or more glasses of fluid daily.
- Diet includes sources of both insoluble and soluble fiber. Insoluble fiber does not dissolve in water and is found in wheat bran, whole grains, and vegetables. Soluble fiber has a high water-holding capacity and turns to a gel during digestion. It is found in oat bran, barley, kidney beans, other dried beans, and some fruits and vegetables.

CALORIE-CONTROLLED DIETS

Postgastrectomy Diet

Objectives

- To prevent rapid passage of food from the stomach into the intestine and the creation of a hyperosmolar load in the small intestine
- To maintain optimal nutrition status

Indications for Use

- Individuals who have had a partial gastrectomy or another operation that interferes with the function of the pylorus or the ability of the stomach to serve as a reservoir

Nutritional Adequacy

- Nutritional adequacy will depend on the extent of the individual's surgery, food tolerances, and food selections. Undernutrition and poor intake are common due to the problems that accompany eating and digestion.
- Vitamin and mineral supplementation is recommended.
- Injections of vitamin B_{12} may be required due to a lack of intrinsic factor.

Summary of Guidelines

- Avoid sugars and concentrated sweets.
- Choose high-protein, moderate-fat foods. Suggested level of protein intake is 20% of calories. Suggested level of fat is 30%–40% of calories.
- Use the American Diabetes Association and the American Dietetic Association's "Exchange Lists for Meal Planning" for carbohydrate control. Carbohydrate counting may be a helpful approach to regulating carbohydrate intake.
- Divide food into small, frequent meals.
- Avoid liquids with meals. Drink low-carbohydrate liquids up to 30–60 minutes before a meal and 30–60 minutes after meals.
- Choose foods and fluids of moderate temperature. Avoid temperature extremes.
- Avoid alcohol.
- Determine lactose intolerance by gradual introduction of milk and dairy products into the diet.

Diet for Reactive Hyperglycemia

Objective

- To prevent a marked rise in blood glucose after meals, thereby avoiding the stimulation of excessive insulin secretion

Indications for Use

- Individuals with diagnosed reactive hypoglycemia

Nutritional Adequacy

- Diet is nutritionally adequate.

Summary of Guidelines

- Calorie level of diet is based on individual requirements.
- Use the American Diabetes Association and the American Dietetic Association's "Exchange Lists for Meal Planning" for carbohydrate control. Carbohydrate counting may be a helpful approach to regulating carbohydrate intake.
- Avoid sugars and concentrated sweets.
- Divide food into small, mixed meals and include complex carbohydrates, protein, fat, and fiber at each meal.
- Limit alcohol.
- Determine tolerance of caffeine by restricting initially and establishing individual tolerance.

Diet for Diabetes Mellitus

Objectives

- To provide a variety of nutrients: carbohydrate, protein, fat, vitamins, and minerals
- To attain and maintain blood glucose levels that are as near normal as possible
- To promote the achievement of normal blood lipid levels
- To attain and maintain a healthy, reasonable weight and normal growth and development for children and adolescents
- To prevent long-term complications

Indications for Use

- Individuals with diabetes mellitus

Nutritional Adequacy

- Diet is nutritionally adequate.
- Caloric levels below 1200 kcal/day may not meet DRIs.

Summary of Guidelines

- The focus of glycemic control is on the total amount of carbohydrate consumed at each meal and snack, not the type of carbohydrate. Scientific evidence does not support the elimination of sucrose from the diet.
- Limit total calories as needed to achieve a reasonable weight. Encourage moderate-intensity exercise on most if not all days, unless contraindicated.
- Provide 60%–70% of calories from carbohydrates and monounsaturated fats. Determine total percent of carbohydrate calories based on glucose, lipid, and weight goals. For healthful eating, emphasize complex carbohydrates over simple carbohydrates.
- Determine the total percent of fat calories based on glucose, lipid, and weight goals. Provide less that 10% of calories from saturated fats and not more than 10% of calories from polyunsaturated fats.
- Provide 10%–20% of calories from protein. With nephropathy, limit protein to 0.8 g/day or approximately 10% of calories.
- Distribute food throughout the day to promote better blood glucose control. Develop an individualized nutrition prescription and choose an approach to meal planning that is suited to the individual's diabetes management goals, diabetes medications, lifestyle, and activity level.
- Available approaches to meal planning include:
  1. *Menu approaches*—individualized menus or the use of a food choice plan
  2. *Guideline approaches*—Food Guide Pyramid or Canada's Food Guide to Healthy Eating
  3. *Exchange lists*—Exchange Lists for Meal Planning and Canada's Good Health Eating Guide Food Choice Values
  4. *Carbohydrate counting*—estimating carbohydrate intake using Exchange Lists for Meal Planning, Canada's Good Health Eating Guide Food Choice Values, food labels, or a carbohydrate counter book.

- While the use of low-glycemic foods may help to control postprandial glucose levels, there is insufficient evidence to warrant use of low-glycemic index diets as a primary approach in food/meal planning.
- The role of fiber in glycemic control may not be significant. This is primarily due to the large amount of fiber needed to produce the desired effect and the inability of many people with diabetes mellitus to consume this amount of fiber.
- Soluble fiber may help lower blood lipid levels.
- Choose high-fiber foods to achieve a goal of 20–35 g/day of fiber, the same recommendation as for the general population.
- Limit cholesterol to less than 300 mg/day and sodium to less than 2400 mg/day for mild to moderate hypertension and less than 2000 mg/day for nephropathy, hypertension, and edema.
- Alcohol may be used occasionally in moderate amounts with well-controlled blood glucose levels according to established guidelines and precautions, including consumption with food. Intake should be limited to one drink per day for adult women and two drinks per day for adult men.
- Use the American Dietetic Association's *Evidence-Based MNT Guides for Practice for Type 1 and Type 2 Diabetes Mellitus* as protocols for assessment and counseling.

Diet for Pre-Diabetes

Objective

- To delay or prevent the development of type 2 diabetes mellitus in persons at risk of the disease

Indications for Use

- Individuals with elevated blood glucose levels (100–125 mg/dl)
- Individuals at risk for type 2 diabetes mellitus due to presence of one or more risk factors (excess weight, family history, ethnicity, gestational diabetes, elevated blood pressure, elevated cholesterol, and inactivity)

Nutritional Adequacy

- Diet is nutritionally adequate.

Summary of Guidelines

- Lose 5%–7% of current weight by limiting calorie and fat intake.
- Increase physical activity over time to 30 minutes on 5 or more days each week.

Diet for Gestational Diabetes Mellitus

Objective

- To promote normal blood glucose levels in the absence of ketones, an appropriate pattern of weight gain, and optimal nutrition for a healthy pregnancy

Indications for Use

- Pregnant women with the diagnosis of gestational diabetes mellitus

Nutritional Adequacy

- Diet is nutritionally adequate.

Summary of Guidelines

- Determine calorie level of diet based on desired pattern of weight gain. Women who are overweight before pregnancy need a lower caloric level; women who are underweight before pregnancy need a higher caloric level.
- Determine percent of carbohydrate calories based on individual eating habits, blood glucose goals, and data from self-blood glucose monitoring. Consistency of meals and amounts eaten is important. Decide use of sucrose based on its effect on blood glucose levels.
- Distribute carbohydrate throughout the day in three small to moderate meals and two to four snacks, including a bedtime snack.
- Limitation of carbohydrate at breakfast may be beneficial in some women, due to increased morning release of cortisol and resulting insulin resistance.
- Provide 60 g/day protein.

- Determine percent of fat calories based on goals, limiting saturated fat to less than 10% of calories.
- Develop an individualized meal plan, and choose a meal planning approach that is suited to the woman's management goals, medications, lifestyle, and emotional needs.
- Choose high-fiber sources to achieve a goal of 20–35 g/day.
- Counsel on postpartum weight management strategies aimed at reducing weight or preventing weight gain and increasing physical activity, in order to lower risk of developing gestational diabetes in subsequent pregnancies and type 2 diabetes later in life.
- Use the American Dietetic Association's *Evidence-Based MNT Guide for Practice for Gestational Diabetes* as a protocol for assessment and counseling.

Weight Management Diet

Objective

- To limit calories and increase physical activity in order to prevent weight gain or reduce body weight

Indications for Use

- Individuals who are overweight or obese who desire to lose weight
- Individuals who are experiencing undesirable weight gain
- Individuals who are trying to maintain weight loss

Nutritional Adequacy

- Diet can be nutritionally adequate with use of the Food Guide Pyramid for food choices.
- Use of a vitamin-mineral supplement may be necessary in individuals with low to very low caloric intake and those with limitated variety of food choices.

Summary of Guidelines

- Emphasize the importance of calorie reduction (500 to 1000 kcal/day deficit) to achieve weight loss. Calorie deficit appears to be more important that diet composition in achieving weight loss.

- Individualize the approach to weight loss. Emphasize improved eating habits, nutritious food choices, regular physical activity, and reduced time spent in sedentary activities (such as watching TV, talking on the phone, and working on the computer). Children and adolescents are encouraged to watch less than 2 hours of TV each day.
- Set a reasonable weight goal (5%–10% reduction from baseline weight in 6 to 12 months) based on personal and family history and the evidence on weight loss, rather than on a value from a height/weight table or a calculated ideal body weight.
- For some individuals, maintenance of weight without further gain is a suitable goal.
- Choose a variety of foods, using the Food Guide Pyramid to make food choices. Encourage 5-A-Day (5 or more servings of fruits and vegetables) and 3-A-Day (3 or more servings of dairy foods). Limit fat to control caloric intake.
- Avoid restricting a food or a group of foods. Encourage eating in response to internal hunger and satiety cues.
- Encourage self-monitoring of intake, weight, and physical activity. Self-monitoring records enhance awareness of needed lifestyle changes and progress made in achieving goals. Encourage keeping of food records at "problem eating times" if recording total intake is not feasible.
- Stress role of physical activity in weight management, especially weight loss maintenance. Encourage 60 minutes of moderate-intensity physical activity (such as walking at 3–4 mph) on most if not all days. Inactive individuals will need to start at lower levels of activity and work toward this goal over time. Use screening tools to identify individuals who need physician approval prior to beginning activity (such as PARQ).
- Data from the National Weight Control Registry indicate that weight loss can be maintained with lifelong changes in food and activity habits, including using a low-fat meal plan, engaging in 60 min/day of physical activity such as walking, self-monitoring, eating breakfast, and limiting fast-food meals to fewer than once a week.
- Encourage development of a realistic attitude about weight loss and appearance. Promote self-acceptance and positive self-esteem. Focus on reducing risk factors for chronic disease.
- Weight management in children and adolescents requires family-based intervention that emphasizes parenting skills, such as appropriate nurturing and limit-setting, a sensible approach to eating such as the Stop Light Diet, regular physical activity, and reduced sedentary activity.
- Make referral to other health care professionals when signs of eating disorders are identified in both adult and pediatric patients.

Diet for Metabolic Syndrome

Objective

- To reduce the risk factors for metabolic syndrome and likelihood of developing type 2 diabetes mellitus and coronary heart disease

Indications for Use

- Individuals with diagnosis of metabolic syndrome or risk factors for metabolic syndrome (abdominal obesity, elevated triglycerides, low HDL-cholesterol, elevated blood pressure, and elevated fasting glucose)

Nutritional Adequacy

- Diet can be nutritionally adequate with use of Food Guide Pyramid to make food choices.
- Use of a vitamin-mineral supplement may be necessary in individuals with low to very low caloric intake and those with limited variety of food choices.

Summary of Guidelines

- Implement interventions aimed at reducing weight and increasing physical activity as first-line treatment that will have a positive impact on all risk factors. Use strategies for control of LDL-cholesterol as needed.

- Implement other strategies aimed at control of lipid (elevated triglycerides and low HDL-cholesterol) and non-lipid risk factors (elevated blood pressure and elevated blood glucose).
- Interventions for specific dyslipidemias should be used when indicated by lab values and diagnosis. Consult a diet manual for guidelines.

PROTEIN-, FLUID-, AND ELECTROLYTE-CONTROLLED DIETS

Renal Diet

Objectives

- To achieve and maintain optimal nutrition status
- To lessen the work of the kidney by decreasing the amount of waste products produced from protein metabolism
- To replace protein lost in dialysis
- To prevent or correct fluid and electrolyte imbalances
- To prevent or correct imbalances in phosphorus and calcium

Indications for Use

- Individuals with renal failure or renal insufficiency

Nutritional Adequacy

- A diet that is restricted in protein, sodium, potassium, phosphorus, and fluid does not contain adequate amounts of calcium, iron, and water-soluble vitamins.

Summary of Guidelines

- Provide 30–45 kcal/kg/day for adult renal failure. Provide 30–35 kcal/kg/day for end-stage renal failure and dialysis if age 60 and above and 35 kcal/kg/day if under 60 years of age.

- Provide adequate caloric intake in order to prevent weight loss and to promote positive nitrogen balance. Caloric requirements for individuals on peritoneal dialysis (PD) should take into account carbohydrate absorption from the dialysate, estimated via the peritoneal equilibration test (PET) method. Consult reference for PET formula.
- Limit protein during acute failure, before dialysis, or when dialysis is not indicated to 0.6 to 1.0 g/kg (not less than 40 g/day), according to assessed needs.
- Increase protein during dialysis to compensate for losses. Provide 1.2–1.3 g/kg for hemodialysis (HD) and patients undergoing PD.
- Provide at least 50% of protein allowance in the form of high-biological value proteins.
- Limit sodium according to symptoms of hypertension, fluid retention, edema, and congestive heart failure. Usual limitation in end-stage renal failure (ESRD) is 2–3 g/day and 3–4 g/day in PD. In some persons, a high-sodium diet may be indicated to prevent low blood pressure and dehydration.
- The usual potassium restriction for ESRD is 2–3 g/day, although this should be individualized. The usual potassium restriction for automated peritoneal dialysis (APD) is 3–4 g/day. Restriction may not be indicated for persons under continuous ambulatory peritoneal dialysis (CAPD). Food sources of potassium include fruits, vegetables, meat, cheese, and milk.
- Phosphorus is limited in order to minimize bone demineralization, which occurs as a result of a high serum phosphorus and the resulting low serum calcium level. Calcium mobilization from the bones produces weakened bones and can lead to mineralization of soft tissues. The usual range of phosphorus restriction is 800–1200 mg/day in HD and 1200 mg/day in PD. Phosphorus sources in the diet include foods high in protein and potassium, especially dairy products.
- For HD, when appropriate, limit daily fluid intake to an amount equal to urine output plus 500–1000 ml for insensible losses. Fluid is usually not restricted in CAPD and is limited to 3000–4000 ml in APD.

- Consider use of a water-soluble vitamin supplement designed for dialysis patients (usually contain folic acid, vitamin B complex, and vitamin C) to meet needs and replace losses. Do not use a vitamin A supplement, due to elevated vitamin A levels in uremia. Due to inability to activate vitamin D, supplementation with either oral or intravenous calcitriol may be needed, in order to increase calcium absorption and suppress parathyroid hormone. The need for supplementing vitamins E and K has not been clearly defined. Consider between-meal calcium supplements to compensate for dietary inadequacy, based on individual needs. Consider zinc supplement to improve taste acuity (not more than 100 mg/day). Evaluate need for an iron supplement on an individual basis. Iron supplementation is usually required with the use of recombinant human erythropoietin (rHuEPO) and should be taken separately from phosphate binders.
- Dietary measures to control serum lipids to prevent or treat coronary heart disease have not been shown to be effective. Prevention of malnutrition takes precedence over tight control of serum lipids. Increased use of monounsaturated fats is suggested to increase calories.
- For persons with renal disease who also have diabetes mellitus, improvement in uremic symptoms takes precedence over tight blood glucose control. The carbohydrate and fat content of the renal diabetic diet will be higher, and simple sugars may be included in the meal plan. High blood glucose can cause thirst which makes fluid limitation more difficult to achieve. Small, frequent meals may help maintain more normal blood glucose levels.
- See Renal Conditions section in Chapter 3.

Diet for Liver Disease

Objectives

- To maintain or improve nutrition status
- To manage the metabolic derangements commonly associated with liver disease
- To prevent or improve the symptoms of hepatic encephalopathy
- To prevent further damage to the liver and promote regeneration of new tissue when possible

Indications for Use

- Individuals with liver disease including hepatitis, cirrhosis, and hepatic encephalopathy

Nutritional Adequacy

- Nutritional adequacy will depend on the protein level of the diet. Generally a 40-g protein diet is adequate in all nutrients except vitamin B_6, vitamin B_{12}, iron, zinc, calcium, niacin, vitamin D, and vitamin E.

Summary of Guidelines

- Determine energy needs via indirect calorimetry if possible. Estimated needs are 25–35 kcal/kg or estimated basal energy expenditure plus 20%.
- Provide 1.2–1.5 g/kg protein per day to maintain nitrogen balance. Provide a minimum of 0.8 g/kg protein per day.
- Protein restriction is not recommended to prevent encephalopathy or the progression of liver disease.
- Reserve use of branch-chain amino acids to patients in encephalopathy who do not tolerate adequate amounts of standard protein.
- Provide carbohydrate to meet energy needs. Monitoring of blood glucose levels is important, due to the impact of liver disease on glucose metabolism. Insulin is used to manage hyperglycemia.
- Fat restriction may be needed if maldigestion, malabsorption and/or steatorrhea are present. Use MCTs for malabsorption.
- Monitor fluid and electrolyte status closely. Restrict sodium to 2000 mg for ascites and consider need for fluid restriction. If ascites is severe, a more restricted sodium diet (1000–2000 mg) may be needed. Monitor potassium levels, renal status, and medications such as potassium-wasting diuretics. En-

sure adequate potassium intake as needed to prevent hypokalemia, when renal function is adequate.

- Supplementation with water and fat-soluble vitamins may be needed, since deficiencies and excess losses (fat-soluble) are common in liver disease.
- Monitor for signs of mineral deficiency. Avoid excess copper and manganese in patients with biliary obstruction. Provide iron for esophageal or GI bleeding. Avoid iron therapy in patients with hemochromatosis or hemosiderosis.
- Consult renal conditions section in Chapter 3.

Diet for Urolithiasis

Objectives

- To inhibit or prevent the reformation of renal calculi

Indications for Use

- Individuals who are predisposed to calcium oxalate and calcium phosphate stones
- Reformation of calculi composed primarily of uric acid, cysteine, and struvite is less responsive to dietary intervention.

Nutritional Adequacy

- Adequacy will depend on the extent of dietary restriction.
- Long-term calcium intake of less than 800 mg/day may be detrimental to bone mineral content.

Summary of Guidelines

- Reduce intake of sodium, calcium, oxalate, and protein in conjunction with a generous intake of fluid. Encourage consumption of 3 L of fluid or more per day.
- Limit sodium intake to 100–150 mmol/day to promote decreased calcium excretion.
- Limit calcium to 800 mg/day for absorptive hypercalciuria and to 1000 mg/day for idiopathic hypercalciuria, with simultaneous oxalate restriction

- Limit oxalate intake to 50–60 mg/day. Consider oxalate bioavailability of food sources. Limit these foods which have been shown to increase urinary oxalate content: spinach, rhubarb, beets, nuts, chocolate, tea, wheat bran, and strawberries.
- Encourage moderate protein intake (0.8–1.0 g/day) and consumption of vegetable proteins to reduce intake of animal proteins which contain higher levels of purines.
- Consult diet manual for specific diet guidelines, food choices, and portion sizes.

High-Potassium Diet

Objectives

- To restore, maintain, or prevent the depletion of body potassium due to potassium-wasting medications and physiological disorders

Indications for Use

- Individuals prescribed long-term potassium-wasting diuretics
- Hypokalemia resulting from antibiotics
- Conditions of mineralocorticoid or glucocorticoid excess such as primary or secondary aldosteronism, Cushing's syndrome, or use of steroids
- Excess losses of potassium, as might occur with vomiting, diarrhea, laxative abuse, fistulas, GI suctioning, and renal tubular necrosis

Nutritional Adequacy

- Diet is nutritionally adequate.

Summary of Guidelines

- Plan daily food choices by using a reference list of the potassium content of foods.
- Consume 2000–4000 mg/day above baseline intake level.
- For prevention of hypokalemia, with careful planning, potassium can be obtained from dietary sources without supplementation. Supplements may be needed once hypokalemia has occurred. Consult physician prior to initiating supplementation with potassium chloride.

SODIUM-CONTROLLED DIETS

Objectives

- To restore normal sodium balance
- To control hypertension
- To prevent, treat, and eliminate edema
- To prevent stimulation of thirst in individuals on a fluid-restricted regimen

Indications for Use

- The level of sodium restriction depends on disease severity, amount of edema, and prescribed medications.
- A moderate sodium restriction ($<$ 2400 mg/day) is considered prudent, especially for individuals who are sodium sensitive.
- The 3000-mg sodium diet is used for individuals with mild hypertension and mild fluid retention and for individuals who are receiving corticosteroid therapy.
- The 2000-mg sodium diet is used for individuals with congestive heart failure, hypertension, edema, renal disease, and cirrhosis with ascites and for individuals who are receiving corticosteroid therapy.
- The 1000-mg sodium diet is used for individuals with severe cases of hypertension, congestive heart failure, cirrhosis with ascites, pulmonary edema, and renal disease. Use in the home setting is not practical.
- The 500-mg-sodium diet is used on a short-term basis for hospitalized patients needing a severe sodium restriction.

Nutritional Adequacy

- The 3000-mg sodium diet and the 2000-mg sodium diet are nutritionally adequate.
- The 1000-mg sodium diet is nutritionally adequate with the use of low-sodium products.
- Nutritional adequacy of the 500-mg sodium diet is difficult to achieve, due to low palatability and the unavailability of required low-sodium products.

Summary of Guidelines

3000-mg (130 mmol) Sodium Diet

- Includes most foods from a regular diet.
- Omit or eat infrequently high-sodium foods, condiments, and beverages. High-sodium foods include convenience foods such as pizza, TV dinners, frozen meat entrees, and canned, boxed, and frozen convenience foods; processed, cured, pickled, and smoked meats such as bacon, bologna, Canadian bacon, corned beef, frankfurters, ham, sausage, and luncheon meats; salted snack foods; regular canned soups and frozen and dried soup mixes; sauerkraut, pickled vegetables, hominy, vegetable juice, and tomato juice; and salt and salt seasonings, barbecue and other meat sauces, meat tenderizers, soy sauce, olives, pickles, commercial salad dressings, and ketchup.
- May include foods that have been lightly salted in cooking.
- Omit the addition of salt to food at the table.

2000-mg (87 mmol), 1000-mg (44 mmol), and 500-mg (22 mmol) Sodium Diets

- Avoid the use of salt during cooking.
- Check the sodium content of water used in food preparation.
- Omit high-sodium foods. Limit milk to 16 oz/day. On the 500-mg sodium diet, use low-sodium bread; omit vegetables that are naturally high in sodium; and limit meat to 5 oz/day.
- Consult a diet manual for specific diet guidelines, food choices, and portion sizes.
- Include low-sodium products to replace the higher sodium versions of these items.
- Assess use of nonfood sources of sodium such as chewing tobacco, snuff, and selected toothpastes and antacids.
- Read labels carefully to determine the sodium content of foods.
- Consider the use of a sodium point system for calculating sodium intake at home as an alternate to the use of food lists that are allowed and not allowed. With this system, in which a

point equals 1 mmol (23 mg) of sodium, the individual decides the use of allotted points daily, using a reference list of the sodium point values of different foods.

DASH Eating Plan

Objectives

- To lower blood pressure
- To reduce the amount of sodium consumed

Indications

- Individuals with hypertension or pre-hypertension
- Eating plan is suitable for all adults.

Nutritional Adequacy

- Diet is nutritionally adequate.
- Diet meets DRIs.
- Eating plan is rich in protein, magnesium, potassium, calcium, and fiber.

Summary of Guidelines

- Eating plan is low in saturated fat, cholesterol, and total fat. It emphasizes fruits, vegetables, and low-fat dairy foods and includes whole-grain products, fish, poultry, and nuts.
- Eating plan is reduced in red meat, sweets, and sugar-containing beverages.
- Reducing sodium intake in addition to the DASH eating plan produces further reduction in blood pressure. The largest reductions have been achieved with both 1500 mg/day sodium and the DASH eating plan. Individuals trying to reduce sodium intake may find it easier to adopt the eating plan at the 2400 mg/day level and work toward the 1500 mg/day level over time.
- Eating plan is based on 2000 cal/day. Daily servings of allowed foods will depend on weight status and resulting need for calorie balance or reduction.
- Because the eating plan is high in fiber, encourage gradual increase in intake of fruits, vegetables, and whole-grain foods.

- Consult a diet manual for specific diet guidelines, food choices, and portion sizes.

FAT-CONTROLLED DIETS

Diets for Dyslipidemia

Objectives

- To reduce elevated LDL-cholesterol, total cholesterol, and/or triglyceride levels and increase HDL-cholesterol
- To control intake of saturated fat and cholesterol
- To promote achievement of a desirable body weight
- To achieve optimal nutrition status and reduce risk of chronic disease and related complications

Indications for Use

- Individuals with dyslipidemia, diabetes mellitus, or coronary heart disease (CHD)
- Individuals at risk for type 2 diabetes mellitus or CHD

Nutritional Adequacy

- Diet is nutritionally adequate.

Summary of Guidelines

- Dietary guidelines have been established by an expert panel of the National Cholesterol Education Program (*Detection, Evaluation, and Treatment of High Blood Cholesterol in Adults*—Adult Treatment Panel III)
- The primary focus of nutrition intervention is on strategies that reduce serum LDL-cholesterol level. First emphasize reduced intake of saturated fat to less than 7% of total calories and intake of cholesterol to < 200 mg/day. Allow total fat in the range of 25%–35% of total calories, limiting saturated fat and trans fatty acids and including monounsaturated fats up to a level of 20% of total calories and polyunsaturated fats up to a level of 10% of total calories.

- Provide protein up to 15% of total calories and carbohydrate to a maximum of 50%–60% of total calories. If triglycerides are elevated, consider a lower level of carbohydrate.
- Check LDL-cholesterol after 6 weeks and if LDL-goal has not been met, initiate other strategies such as introduction of plant sterols and stanols (2 g/day) and increased intake of soluble fiber (10–25 g/day).
- After maximum reduction in LDL-cholesterol has been achieved, shift emphasis to management of the metabolic syndrome and associated lipid risk factors (low HDL-cholesterol and elevated triglyceride levels).
- Provide calorie level based on weight goals, reducing calories to achieve weight loss when indicated. Encourage regular moderate-intensity physical activity.
- Nutrition-related factors contributing to an elevated triglyceride level include obesity and overweight, inactivity, excess alcohol intake, and high carbohydrate ($> 60\%$ of energy intake). In borderline (150–199 mg/dl) and high (200–499 mg/dl) triglycerides, aim primary therapy at reduction in elevated LDL-cholesterol if present. Emphasize weight reduction and increased physical activity as secondary goals. Drug therapy may be prescribed for high levels.
- Use a very low fat ($\leq 15\%$ of calorie intake) diet in conjunction with drug therapy for very high (≥ 500 mg/dl) triglycerides to prevent acute pancreatitis. Once triglycerides are below 500 mg/dl, return primary attention to LDL-cholesterol reduction.
- Diabetic dyslipidemia includes a combination of high triglycerides, low HDL, and small dense LDL. Aim primary treatment at reduction in LDL-cholesterol. When triglycerides are ≥ 200 mg/dl, direct secondary intervention at reducing non-HDL cholesterol.
- Consult a diet manual for specific diet guidelines, food choices, and portion sizes.

Fat-Restricted Diet

Objective

- To limit fat intake to 40–50 g/day

Indications for Use

- Individuals with diseases of the biliary tree, including the liver, gallbladder, and pancreas
- Individuals with diseases of the intestinal mucosa and lymphatic system
- Individuals with impaired digestion and absorption of fat
- Individuals with gastroesophageal reflux

Nutritional Adequacy

- Diet is nutritionally adequate.

Summary of Guidelines

- Limit fats, including margarine, butter, oils, salad dressings, and cream to 3–5 servings daily.
- Limit lean meat and meat substitutes to 6-oz. cooked portion per day.
- Restrict fat sources in the diet, including whole, 2%, and 1% milk and dairy products and foods made with these ingredients; breads made with large amounts of fat; high-fat desserts and sweets; avocados; fried foods; high-fat soups and stews; vegetables seasoned with fat, cheese, or cream sauces; and gravies.
- Monitor individual tolerance of fat closely. Adjust fat intake if symptoms of intolerance persist.
- When a very-low-fat diet (< 25 g/day) is indicated, reduce meat and meat substitutes to 4 oz/day and fats to 1 serving per day. Diet may not be nutritionally adequate depending on food choices.

FOOD ALLERGY/INTOLERANCE DIETS

Lactose-Restricted Diet

Objectives

- To restrict foods containing lactose
- To prevent the symptoms associated with lactose ingestion

Indications for Use

- Individuals with lactose intolerance or lactase deficiency

Nutritional Adequacy

- Diet may be deficient in calcium, phosphorus, vitamins A and D, and riboflavin, depending on the extent to which milk and dairy products are eliminated from the diet. Use of small amounts of milk and dairy products if tolerated or use of lactose-restricted, soy, or rice milks may meet needs.
- Use a calcium supplement if diet is restricted in sources of calcium.
- Consider use of a vitamin D supplement if exposure to sunlight is limited.
- Consider use of a riboflavin supplement if fluid milk is not consumed.

Summary of Guidelines

- Individualize the amount of lactose in the diet on the basis of individual tolerance. Small amounts of milk (4–6 oz.) and dairy products may be tolerated by some individuals, if eaten at separate times throughout the day.
- Establish tolerance by gradually adding sources of lactose to a lactose-free diet.
- Encourage use of milk and dairy products at meals, due to slower gastric emptying and allowance of more time for endogenous lactase activity.
- Consumption of complex carbohydrates and soluble fiber with lactose-containing foods may improve lactose tolerance. In addition, cocoa and chocolate milk may improve tolerance.
- Consult a diet manual for specific diet guidelines, food choices, and portion sizes.
- Consider use of yogurt in place of milk. Yogurt contains bacterial lactase, which substitutes for the lactase that is missing in the individual's intestinal tract.
- Consider use of special commercially prepared lactose-reduced products; use of lactose-hydrolyzed milk; or ingestion of an enzyme tablet or drops just prior to meals containing lactose or added to milk and milk products before consumption.
- Read food labels carefully. Be alert to the presence of lactose when the ingredient list includes milk, milk solids, lactose, whey, or casein. Consult with a pharmacist about the lactose content of medications for severe lactose intolerance.
- The amount of lactose in products varies from one brand to another, due to differences in production. For example, lactose is an optional ingredient used in the process of creaming cottage cheese.
- Cheese spreads have more lactose than aged cheese or processed cheese, due to the addition of dry milk solids and whey powder.

Gluten-Restricted Diet

Objectives

- To eliminate gluten from the diet
- To control or eliminate the malabsorption that results from a sensitivity to gluten in individuals with celiac disease
- To promote healing of the small intestine

Indications for Use

- Individuals with celiac disease or secondary gluten-induced enteropathy
- Treatment of the skin lesions associated with dermatitis herpetoformis

Nutritional Adequacy

- Diet is nutritionally adequate, as planned, for individuals whose intestinal villi have regenerated. Nutritional adequacy will depend on individual tolerance of food and food selections made.
- Nutrient supplementation may be needed when malabsorption is present. This includes supplementation of potassium, folic acid, vitamin B_{12} and other water-soluble vitamins, vitamin D and other fat-soluble vitamins; calcium; iron; and magnesium. Supplements can be discontinued as intake and absorption improve.

Summary of Guidelines

- Diet must be followed for life.
- Eliminate foods containing wheat, rye, and barley. Oats appear to be safe for most

individuals with celiac disease, but are not recommended because of possible contamination with gluten during processing.

- Read food labels carefully. Be alert to the presence of one of the grains not allowed on the diet when the ingredient list includes cereal, cereal additive, cereal product, emulsifier, flavoring, hydrolyzed vegetable or plant protein, malt, malt flavoring, modified food starch, soy sauce, stabilizer, starch, vegetable gum, or vegetable protein.
- Plan diet to be high in protein and carbohydrate in order to correct poor nutritional status.
- Assess tolerance of lactose. Limit milk and dairy products, if necessary, until tolerance improves.
- Determine existence of steatorrhea. When present, limit fat in the diet. Reintroduce gradually, as recovery progresses.
- Consult a diet manual for specific diet guidelines, food choices, and portion sizes.

Low-Purine Diet

Objectives

- To limit foods high in purine and fat in order to reduce hyperuricemia
- To increase fluid intake in order to promote excretion of uric acid and prevent calculi
- To attain and maintain a desirable weight

Indications for Use

- Individuals with hyperuricemia, gout, or uric acid stones, as an adjunct to drug therapy

Nutritional Adequacy

- Diet is nutritionally adequate, with the exception of iron for women in their childbearing years.

Summary of Guidelines

- Limit meat, shellfish, poultry, nuts, peanut butter, and beans and peas.
- Omit anchovies, sardines, mackerel, scallops, herring, meat extracts, game, brains, and organ meats (liver and kidneys).
- Limit fat to 30% of total calories due to slowing of uric acid excretion.
- Provide moderate protein intake (10%–15% of total calories), with a large proportion of protein coming from low-fat or skim milk, low-fat cheeses, eggs, vegetables, and refined breads and cereals.
- Consume 2–3 L of fluid daily.
- Encourage gradual weight loss in obese individuals. Rapid weight loss or fasting can precipitate an attack of gout, due to reduced uric acid excretion secondary to ketone formation.
- Eliminate alcohol.

REFERENCES

ADA MNT Evidence-Based Guides for Practice. American Dietetic Association Publication. Chicago, IL: 2002.

American Academy of Pediatrics. *Pediatric Nutrition Handbook.* 5th ed. Kleinman RD, ed. Elk Grove Village, IL: American Academy of Pediatrics; 2004:103.

American Diabetes Association and American Dietetic Association. *Exchange Lists for Meal Planning.* Chicago, IL: American Dietetic Association; 2003.

American Diabetes Association. Nutrition principles and recommendations in diabetes. *Diabetes Care. Suppl. 1.* 2004;27:S36–S46.

American Dietetic Association and Dietitians of Canada. *Manual of Clinical Dietetic.* 6th ed. Chicago, IL: American Dietetic Association; 2000.

Butte N, Cobb K, Dwyer J, Graney L, Heird W, Rickard K. The Start Healthy Feeding Guidelines for Infants and Toddlers. *J Am Diet Assoc.* 2004;104:442–454.

Food and Nutrition Board: Institute of Medicine. *Dietary Reference Intakes for Calcium, Phosphorus, Magnesium, Vitamin D, and Fluoride.* Washington, DC: National Academy Press, 1997.

Food and Nutrition Board: Institute of Medicine. *Dietary Reference Intakes for Energy, Carbohydrate, Fiber, Fat, Fatty Acids, Cholesterol, Protein, and Amino Acids.* Washington, DC: National Academy Press, 2002.

Food and Nutrition Board: Institute of Medicine. *Dietary Reference Intakes for Thiamin, Riboflavin, Niacin, Vitamin B_6, Folate, Vitamin B_{12}, Pantothenic Acid, Biotin, and Choline.* Washington, DC: National Academy Press, 1998.

Food and Nutrition Board: Institute of Medicine. *Dietary Reference Intakes for Vitamin A, Vitamin K, Arsenic, Boron, Chromium, Copper, Iodine, Iron, Manganese, Molybdenum, Nickel, Silicon, Vanadium, and Zinc.* Washington, DC: National Academy Press, 2001.

Food and Nutrition Board: Institute of Medicine. *Dietary Reference Intakes for Vitamin C, Vitamin E, Selenium, and Carotenoids.* Washington, DC: National Academy Press, 2000.

Foster GD, Nonas C. *Managing Obesity: A Clinical Guide.* Chicago, IL: American Dietetic Association; 2003.

National Dysphagia Diet Task Force. *National Dysphagia Diet: Standardization for Optimal Care.* Chicago, IL: American Dietetic Association; 2002.

National Heart, Lung, and Blood Institute and North American Association for the Study of Obesity. *The Practical Guide: Identification, Evaluation and Treatment of Overweight and Obesity in Adults.* October, 2000. http://www.nhlbi.nih.gov/guidelines/obesity/prctgd_c.pdf. Accessed: July 26, 2004.

National Heart, Lung, and Blood Institute. Third Report of the National Cholesterol Education Program Expert Panel. *Detection, Evaluation, and Treatment of High Blood Cholesterol in Adults (ATPIII). Executive Summary.* May, 2001. http://www.nhlbi.nih.gov/guidelines/obesity/prctgd_c.pdf. Accessed: July 26, 2004.

National Heart, Lung, and Blood Institute. *JNC 7 Express. The Seventh Report of the Joint National Committee on Prevention, Detection, Evaluation, and Treatment of High Blood Pressure.* May, 2003. http://www.nhlbi.nih.gov/guidelines/hypertension/jncintro.htm. Accessed: July 26, 2004.

National Heart, Lung, and Blood Institute. *Facts about the Dash Eating Plan.* May, 2003. http://www.nhlbi.nih.gov/health/public/heart/hbp/dash/index.htm. Accessed: July 26, 2004.

National Institutes of Health. *Consensus Development Conference Statement, Celiac Disease (Draft).* Jun28–30, 2004. http://consensus.nih.gov/cons/118/118celiacPDF.pdf. Accessed: July 26, 2004.

Appendix 1

Algorithm for Treatment of Diarrhea

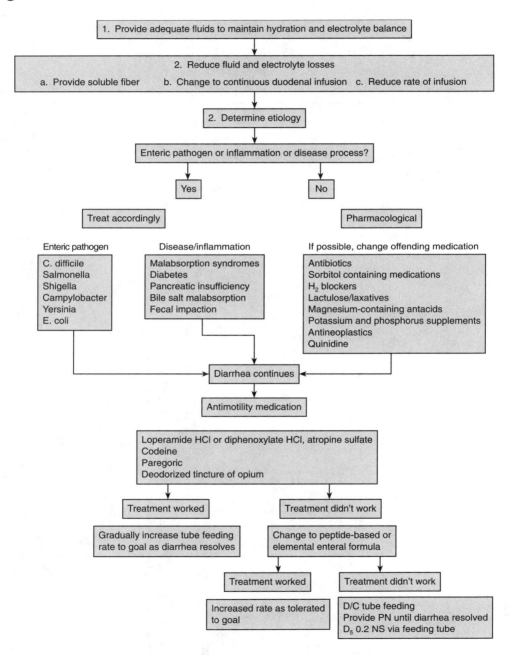

Source: Reprinted from Fuhrman MP. Diarrhea and tube feeding. *Nutr Clin Pract.* 1999;14:84 with permission from the American Society for Parenteral and Enteral Nutrition (A.S.P.E.N.)

Appendix 2

Anemia

	Hemoglobin	Hematocrit	Mean Corpuscular Volume	Serum Iron	Total Iron-Binding Capacity	Transferrin	Reticulocytes
Fe deficiency	→↓	→↓	→↓	→↓	→↓	→↓	↑↓
B₁₂, folate deficiency	→↓	→↓	←↑	←↑	→↓	→↓	↑↓
Fe plus megaloblastic	→↓	→↓	↓↑	↓	→↓	→↓	↑↓
Dehydration	←↑	←↑	→↓	→↓	→↓	→↓	↑↓
Malnutrition	→↓*	→↓*	↓←↑	↓←↑	↓←↑	↓←↑	↑↓
Malabsorption	→↓	→↓	←↑	→↓	→↓	→↓	↑↓
Liver disease	↓→*	↓→*	↓←↑	↓←↑	→↓	↓←↑	↓→
Kidney disease	↓→*	↓→*	↓←↑↓↑	→↓	→↓	→↓	↑↓
Gastrectomy	→↓	→↓	←↑→↓	→↓	↓←↑	→↓	←↑↓
Small bowel surgery	↓→	↓→	→↓	→↓	↓←↑	↓←↑	↑↓
Blood loss	→↓	→↓	→↓	→↓	→↓	→↓	↑↓
Sepsis	↓→*	→↓*	↓←↑	→↓	↓←↑	→↓	↑↓

*Mild decrease.

Source: Copyright 1993, The American Dietetic Association. Winkler MF, Lysen LK, eds. "Suggested Guidelines for Nutrition and Metabolic Management of Adult Patients Receiving Nutrition Support." Used by permission.

Appendix 3

Anthropometric Measures

- Body Mass Index (BMI) = $\dfrac{\text{Weight (kg)}}{\text{Height}^2 \ (\text{m}^2)}$

19–25	Appropriate weight (19–34 years)
21–27	Appropriate weight (> 35 years)
> 27.5	Obesity
27.5–30	Mild obesity
30–40	Moderate obesity
> 40	Severe or morbid obesity

- Stature from knee height (for ages 65–90):

  Men = (2.02 × knee height) – (0.04 × age) + 64.19
  Women = (1.83 × knee height) – (0.24 × age) + 84.88

- Determination of Ideal Body Weight by Hamwi method:

  Females: 100 lb for the first 5 ft plus 5 lb for each additional inch above 5 ft.
  Males: 106 lb for the first 5 ft plus 6 lb for each additional inch above 5 ft. + 10% for large frame;
     – 10% for small frame

- Amputee weight calculations:

  Ideal amputee weight = preamputation ideal body weight (IBW) – (IBW × % amputation)
  Segmental body weights:
     entire arm = 6.5%
     upper arm = 3.5%
     lower arm = 2.3%
     hand = 0.8%
     entire leg = 18.5%
     thigh = 11.5%
     knee, lower leg, and foot = 7.1%
     foot = 1.8%

continues

Appendix 3 continued

- Evaluation of Body Weight

    - Percentage usual body weight $= \dfrac{\text{Actual weight}}{\text{Usual weight}} \times 100$

        85%–90%   Mild malnutrition
        75%–84%   Moderate malnutrition
        < 74%   Severe malnutrition

    - Percentage IBW $= \dfrac{\text{Actual weight}}{\text{IBW}} \times 100$

        ≥ 200%   Morbid obesity
        ≥ 130%   Obesity
        110%–120% Overweight
        80%–90%   Mild malnutrition
        70%–79%   Moderate malnutrition
        < 69%   Severe malnutrition

    - Percentage weight loss $= \dfrac{\text{Usual body weight} - \text{Actual body weight}}{\text{Usual body weight}} \times 100$

Significant weight loss	*Severe weight loss*
5% over 1 mo	> 5% over 1 mo
7.5% over 3 mo	> 7.5% over 3 mo
10% over 6 mo	> 10% over 6 mo

- Measurement of total body fat (arm fat area)

    $$\text{AFA (cm}^2) = \frac{\text{MAC} \times \text{TSF}}{2} - \frac{\pi \times (\text{TSF})^2}{4}$$

    where MAC = midarm circumference.

- Measurement of skeletal protein mass:

    $$\text{MAMC (cm)} = \text{MAC (cm)} - 3.14\ \text{TSF (cm)}$$

    $$\text{AMA (cm}^2) = \frac{[\text{MAC (cm)} - 3.14\ \text{TSF (cm)}]^2}{4\pi}$$

    Bone Free AMA (cm²):

    $$\text{Women: AMA (cm}^2) = \frac{[\text{MAC (cm)} - 3.14\ \text{TSF (cm)}]^2}{4\pi} - 6.5\ \text{cm}^2$$

    $$\text{Men: AMA (cm}^2) = \frac{[\text{MAC (cm)} - 3.14\ \text{TSF (cm)}]^2}{4\pi} - 10\ \text{cm}^2$$

    where MAMC = mid–upper-arm muscle circumference and AMA = arm muscle area.

Source: Courtesy of Laura E. Matarese, Cleveland Clinic Foundation, Cleveland, Ohio.

Appendix 4

Assessment of Vitamin Nutriture

Vitamin	Requirement	Recommended Intake	Methods of Evaluation	Deficiency Symptoms	Treatment of Deficiency	Toxicity Symptoms
Water-Soluble Vitamins						
Thiamin	0.35 mg/1000 kcal	Enteral: 1–1.5 mg/d* Parenteral: 3 mg/d	Urinary excretion: Reflects intake, not stores Decreased with deficient intakes Blood: Whole blood thiamin Erythrocyte transketolase activity: Estimates deficiency of body stores Increased with deficiency	Beriberi: Mental confusion Weakness Peripheral neuropathy Heart disease Edema (wet) Muscle wasting (dry) Wernicki's encephalopathy	Thiamin hydrochloride Wernicki's: 50-mg bolus 50 mg/d until stores repleted Limited intake: 1–2 mg/d	(Rare) Irritability Headache Insomnia Interferes with riboflavin and B_6
Riboflavin	0.4–5.0 mg/100 kcal	Enteral: 1.2–1.8 mg/d* Parenteral: 3.6 mg/d	Urinary excretion: Correlates with intake, not stores Decreased with limited intakes Increased with (–)N^2 balance Blood: Erythrocyte riboflavin Glutathione reductase + flavin adenine dinucleotide reflects body stores deficiency: Increased stimulation	Angular stomatitis Chellosis Glossitis Scrotal or vulval dermatitis	5 times RDA per day	Unknown

continues

Appendix 4 continued

Vitamin	Requirement	Recommended Intake	Methods of Evaluation	Deficiency Symptoms	Treatment of Deficiency	Toxicity Symptoms
Niacin	8.8–12.3 mg niacin equivalents (NE)/d	Enteral: 12–20 mg/d Parenteral: 40 mg/d RDA: 13–19 mg/d	Urinary excretion: Reflects intake, not stores N1-methylnicotinamide 2-pyridone/N1-methylinicotinamide decreased excretion with intake Serum: Represents body stores, usually Body stores: none	Pellagra: Diarrhea Dementia Dermatitis Death Scarlet tongue Tongue fissuring	40–200 mg of nicotinic acid or nicotinamide per day	Liver damage Vascular dilation Flushing Irritation
Vitamin B_6	0.2 mg/g of protein ingested	Enteral: 1.6–2.0 mg/d* Parenteral: 4 mg/d	Urinary excretion: Reflects recent intakes Decreased with limited intakes Aminotransferase activity Stimulated: deficiency Measures body stores Plasma levels Tryptophan load test: Tryptophan to nicotinic acid—B_6 dependent Measure tryptophan metabolites Reflects body stores Methionine load test	(Rare except in presence of B_6 antagonist) Polyneuritis Nasolabial seborrhea Glossitis Microcytic anemia Oxalate stones	Pyridoxine hydrochloride 5 mg/d	None known
Pantothenic acid	4–7 mg/d	Enteral: 5–10 mg/d Parenteral: 15 mg/d No RDA	Body stores: none Serum level: Red blood cell (RBC) content responds to changes in dietary intakes Urinary excretion: Correlates with intake	(Rare) Lethargy Abdominal pain Nausea Flatulence Vomiting	10–100 mg	Diarrhea

Biotin	50 µg/1000 kcal	Enteral: 150–300 µg/d Parenteral: Normal: 60 µg/d Repletion: 300 µg/d No RDA	Body stores: none Evaluation of intake: Whole blood RBC Plasma Urinary excretion	Skin rash Alopecia Lethargy Anorexia Paresthesias	10–300 µg/d	None known
Folic acid	100 µg/d	Enteral: 200–400 µg/d Parenteral: 400 µg–10 mg/d RDA: 180–200 µg/d	Urine: Formiminoglutamic acid Histidine load Increased excretion with deficiency Not accurate Blood: Serum folate Reflects dietary change Not a single parameter to assess deficiency Used in conjunction with red cell folate Affected by hypoalbuminemia Red cell folate: Most accurate Evaluated with serum folate	(Folate stores last 3–6 mo after cessation of folate ingestion) Macrocytic anemia Stomatitis Glossitis Lethargy Diarrhea	0.5–1.0 mg/d	Not known

continues

Appendix 4 continued

Vitamin	Requirement	Recommended Intake	Methods of Evaluation	Deficiency Symptoms	Treatment of Deficiency	Toxicity Symptoms

Vitamin B_{12}	Minimal amount for hematologic response: 0.1 µg/d
	Maximum response: 0.5–1.0 µg/d
		Enteral: 3 µg/d*
		Parenteral: 5 µg/d
		RDA: 2 µg/d
			Methylmalonic acid:
			Increased excretion with B_{12} deficiency
			Not as useful as serum
			Shilling test:
			Assesses absorption of B_{12}
			Part 1 of test
			  Normal: no malabsorption, test ends
			  Abnormal: positive test, complete part 2
			Part 2 of test
			  Normal: malabsorption secondary to lack of intrinsic factor
			  Abnormal: malabsorption secondary to ileal disease, decreased absorptive capacity, bacterial overgrowth
			Does not assess body stores with transcobalamin II deficiency
			Low in folate deficiency with normal stores
				Megaloblastic anemia
				Neuropathy
				Stomatitis
				Glossitis
				Anorexia
				Diarrhea
					Deficient diet: 1 µg/d
					Inadequate absorption: 1 µg/d parenterally or 100 µg/mo
						None known

Vitamin C	10 mg/d prevents scurvy but does not provide for adequate reserves	Enteral: 60 mg/d* maintains body pool of 1500 mg Parenteral: Normal: 100 mg/d Catabolic stress: 500 mg/d	Blood: Plasma: Assesses intake, not deficiency state Whole blood: Assesses intake, not deficiency state Buffy coat: Anticoagulated centrifuged whole blood Accurate Closely related to stores Leukocyte ascorbate: Closely related to stores Radioactive-labeled vitamin C: Most accurate measurement Closely related to stores	Hemorrhaging: Skin Nose GI tract Weakness Irritability Bleeding gums	10 mg/d alleviates scurvy 60–100 mg/d replenishes stores	Interferes with tests for glucosuria May cause osmotic diarrhea and formation of oxalate stones Interferes with anticoagulation therapy Inactivates or destroys vitamin B_{12} in presence of heat

continues

Appendix 4 continued

Vitamin	Requirement	Recommended Intake	Methods of Evaluation	Deficiency Symptoms	Treatment of Deficiency	Toxicity Symptoms
Fat-Soluble Vitamins						
Vitamin A	500–600 retinol equivalents (RE)/d (1 RE = 1 μg RE)	Enteral: 800–1000 RE/d* Parenteral: 1000 RE/d	Urine: known Blood: Serum vitamin A: Reflects body stores, but only at very low levels Retinyl ester (fasting): Reflects toxicity Serum carotene: Used to assess malabsorption Variable since it reflects intake of carotenoids Does not measure stores	Visual changes: Poor dark adaptation Bitot's spots Xerosis Irreversible corneal ulceration Scarring and softening of cornea Male sterility	37,500–45,000 RE/d	Acute (200,000 RE/d): Nausea Vomiting Headaches Increased cerebrospinal pressure Vertigo Double vision Chronic (10,000 RE/d): Desquamation of skin Gingivitis Alopecia Swelling of bone Hepatomegaly Pruritis Anorexia

Vitamin	Function	Requirement	Assessment	Deficiency	Treatment	Toxicity
Vitamin D	Exact amount not established 2.5 μg of cholecalciferol/d prevents rickets, promotes growth, ensures adequate absorption of calcium 10 μg of cholecalciferol/d promotes better absorption of calcium, increases growth rate	Enteral: 5–10 μg/d* Parenteral: 5 μg/d	Urine: none Blood: Serum phosphate: Decreased with deficiency Serum calcium: Decreased with deficiency Serum 25-hydroxyvitamin D: Decreased with deficiency Alkaline phosphatase: Increased with deficiency 1,25-dihydroxyvitamin D: Correlates with function, not intake/stores X-ray of bones	Decreased body stores of calcium and phosphorus Rickets Osteomalacia	Amount varies with cause of deficiency (1250–2500 μg cholecalciferol/d)	Excess bone calcification Stiffness Soft tissue calcification Kidney stones Hypercalcemia
Vitamin K	30 μg/d	Enteral: 50–200 μg/d Parenteral: 150 μg/d RDA: 65–80 μg/d	Prothrombin time Serum prothrombin Serum vitamin K	Primary vitamin-K deficiency is uncommon Excessive bruising Purpura Bleeding	Dependent on cause of deficiency	Jaundice

continues

Appendix 4 continued

Vitamin	Requirement	Recommended Intake	Methods of Evaluation	Deficiency Symptoms	Treatment of Deficiency	Toxicity Symptoms
Vitamin E	2 mg of α-tocopherol per day	Enteral: 8–10 mg of α-tocopherol* Parenteral: 10 mg of α-tocopherol	Serum vitamin E Erythrocyte peroxide hemolysis: Nonspecific Rules out deficiency if normal Serum tocopherol esters: Chromatography High-performance liquid chromatography	Hemolysis Anemia Retinal degeneration Neuronal axonopathy Myopathy	180 mg of α-tocopherol per day	300 mg of α-tocopherol Prolonged clotting time

*Range same as RDA.
Source: Reprinted from Hopkins B. Assessment of Nutritional Status. In: Gottschlich MM, Matarese LE, Shronts EP, eds. *Nutrition Support Dietetics Core Curriculum.* 2nd ed. 1993:44–51, with permission from the American Society for Parenteral and Enteral Nutrition (A.S.P.E.N.).

Appendix 5

Average Daily Fluid Gains and Losses in Adults

Fluid Gains		*Fluid Losses*	
Sensible		Sensible	
Oral fluids	1100–1400 ml	Urine	1200–1500 ml
Solid foods	800–1000 ml	Intestinal	100–200 ml
Insensible		Insensible	
Oxidative metabolism	300 ml	Lungs	400 ml
		Skin	500–600 ml
Total	2200–2700 ml	Total	2200–2700 ml

Source: Adapted from Horn MM, Swearingen PL (eds): *Pocket Guide to Fluid, Eectrolyte and Acid-Base Balance,* 2nd ed. St. Louis, MO: Mosby; 1993:23.

Appendix 6

Body Mass Index
Weigh Your Risk with BMI

BMI	Good Weights								Increasing Risk					
HEIGHT	19	20	21	22	23	24	25	26	27	28	29	30	35	40
	WEIGHT (in pounds)													
4'10"	91	96	100	105	110	115	119	124	129	134	138	143	167	191
4'11"	94	99	104	109	114	119	124	128	133	138	143	148	173	198
5'	97	102	107	112	118	123	128	133	138	143	148	153	179	204
5'1"	100	106	111	116	122	127	132	137	143	148	153	158	185	211
5'2"	104	109	115	120	126	131	136	142	147	153	158	164	191	218
5'3"	107	113	118	124	130	135	141	146	152	158	163	169	197	225
5'4"	110	116	122	128	134	140	145	151	157	163	169	174	204	232
5'5"	114	120	126	132	138	144	150	156	162	168	174	180	210	240
5'6"	118	124	130	136	142	148	155	161	167	173	179	186	216	247
5'7"	121	127	134	140	146	153	159	166	172	178	185	191	223	255
5'8"	125	131	138	144	151	158	164	171	177	184	190	197	230	262
5'9"	128	135	142	149	155	162	169	176	182	189	196	203	236	270
5'10"	132	139	146	153	160	167	174	181	188	195	202	209	243	278
5'11"	136	143	150	157	165	172	179	186	193	200	208	215	250	286
6'	140	147	154	162	169	177	184	191	199	206	213	221	258	294
6'1"	144	151	159	166	174	182	189	197	204	212	219	227	265	302
6'2"	148	155	163	171	179	186	194	202	210	218	225	233	272	311
6'3"	152	160	168	176	184	192	200	208	216	224	232	240	279	319
6'4"	156	164	172	180	189	197	205	213	221	230	238	246	287	328

The health risk from any level of BMI is increased if you have gained more than 11 pounds since age 25 or if you have a waist circumference above 40 in (100 cm) due to central fatness.

Source: Courtesy of Pennington Biomedical Research Center, Baton Rouge, Louisiana.

Appendix 7

Calculation of Daily Water Requirements

Method 1	
Body Weight	**Water Requirement**
1st 10 kg	100 ml/kg
2nd 10 kg	50 ml/kg
Each additional kg	20 ml/kg ($\leq$ 50 yrs)
	15 ml/kg ($>$ 50 yrs)

Method 2	
Age	**Water Requirement**
Young athletic adult	40 ml/kg
Most adults	35 ml/kg
Elderly adults	30 ml/kg

Method 3
1 ml/kcal energy expenditure

Source: Reprinted from Whitmire SJ. Fluid and electrolytes. In: Gottschlich MM, ed. *The Science and Practice of Nutrition Support: A Case-Based Core Curriculum.* Dubuque, IA: Kendall/Hunt Publishing Co; 2001:56 with permission from the American Society for Parenteral and Enteral Nutrition (A.S.P.E.N.).

Appendix 8

Clinical Determinants of the Metabolic Syndrome

Risk Factor	Defining Level

Abdominal obesity	Waist circumference:
	  males > 40 in (> 102 cm)
	  females > 35 in (> 88 cm)

Triglycerides	≥ 150 mg/dl
HDL cholesterol	Males < 40 mg/dl Females < 50 mg/dl
Blood pressure	Systolic ≥ 130 mm Hg Diastolic ≥ 85 mm Hg
Fasting plasma glucose	≥ 110 mg/dl

Source: Adapted from National Cholesterol Education Program. 2001. *Third report of the expert panel on detection, evaluation, and treatment of high blood cholesterol in adults.* Bethesda, MD: US Department of Health and Human Services, Public Health Service; National Institutes of Health; National Heart, Lung, and Blood Institute.

Appendix 9

Daily Protein and Calorie Requirements for Adults*

Protein
Maintenance   0.8–1.0 g/kg
Catabolic patients   1.2–2 g/kg

Energy
Total calories   25–30 kcal/kg
Volume   20–40 ml/kg

*Assumes normal organ function.
Source: Reprinted from Mirtallo J, Canada T, Johnson D, Kumpf V, Petersen C, Sacks G, Seres D, Guenter P; Task Force for the Revision of Safe Practices for Parenteral Nutrition. Safe practices for parenteral nutrition. *JPEN J Parenter Enteral Nutr.* 2004 (Suppl); 28: S55 with permission from the American Society for Parenteral and Enteral Nutrition (A.S.P.E.N.).

Appendix 10

Daily Protein Requirements (g/kg) for Pediatric Patients*

Neonates	2.5–3.0
Infants	2.0–2.5
Children	1.5–2.0
Adolescents	0.8–2.0

*Assumes normal age-related organ function.

Daily Energy Requirements (Nonprotein kcal/kg) for Pediatric Patients

Preterm neonate	120–140
< 6 months	90–120
6–12 months	80–100
1–7 yr	75–90
7–12 yr	60–75
>12–18 yr	30–60

Source: Reprinted from Mirtallo J, Canada T, Johnson D, Kumpf V, Petersen C, Sacks G, Seres D, Guenter P; Task Force for the Revision of Safe Practices for Parenteral Nutrition. Safe practices for parenteral nutrition. *JPEN* 2004 (Suppl); 28: S55 with permission from the American Society for Parenteral and Enteral Nutrition (A.S.P.E.N.).

Appendix 11

Serum Proteins Used in Nutritional Assessment

Serum Protein	Normal Value, Mean ± SD or (Range)*	Half-Life	Function	Comments[†]
Albumin	45 (35–50)	18–20 days	Maintains plasma oncotic pressure; carrier for small molecules	In addition to protein status, other factors affect serum concentrations.
Transferrin	2.3 (2.6–4.3)	8–9 days	Binds iron in plasma and transports to bone marrow	Iron deficiency increases hepatic synthesis and plasma levels; increases during pregnancy, during estrogen therapy, and in acute hepatitis; reduced in protein-losing enteropathy and nephropathy, chronic infections, uremia, and acute catabolic states; often measured indirectly by total iron-binding capacity; equations for indirect prediction should be developed locally.
Prealbumin	0.30 (0.2–0.4)	2–3 days	Binds T_3 and, to a lesser extent, T_4; carrier for retinol-binding protein	Level is increased in patients with chronic renal failure on dialysis due to decreased renal catabolism; reduced in acute catabolic states, after surgery, in hyperthyroidism, in protein-losing enteropathy; increased in some cases of nephrotic syndrome; serum level determined by overall energy balance as well as nitrogen balance.
Retinol-binding protein (RBP)	0.372 ± 0.0073[‡]	12 hours	Transports vitamin A in plasma; binds noncovalently to prealbumin	It is catabolized in renal proximal tubular cell; with renal disease, RBP increases and half-life is prolonged; low in vitamin A deficiency, acute catabolic states, after surgery, and in hyperthyroidism.
Insulin-like growth factor-1 (IGF-1)	0.83 IU/ml (0.55–1.4)	2–6 hours	One of a family of insulin-like peptides that have anabolic actions on fat, muscle, cartilage, and cultured cells	It was referred to earlier as somatomedin-C; levels fall rapidly with fasting and quickly recover during refeeding; low values in hypothyroid patients, with estrogen administration, and possibly in obesity; may be a valid nutritional marker during acute-phase response.

continues

Appendix 11 continued

Serum Protein	Normal Value, Mean ± SD or (Range)*	Half-Life	Function	Comments[†]
Fibronectin	Plasma: 2.92 ± 0.2 Serum: 1.82 ± 0.16	4–24 hours	A glycoprotein found in many tissues; a soluble form appears in blood and behaves as an opsonic glycoprotein; may exert chemotactic activity and be involved in wound healing	Plasma fibronectin deficiency may contribute to host defense suppression with malnutrition; may be a sensitive marker during nutritional depletion and repletion; levels may be influenced by acute-phase response; more clinical studies needed; reference ranges not well studied.

*All units are g/l. Normal range varies among centers; check local values.
[†]All the listed proteins are influenced by hydration and the presence of hepatocellular dysfunction.
[‡]Normal values are age- and sex-dependent. Table value is for pooled subjects.
Source: Adapted from Heymsfield SB, Tighe A, Wang ZM. Nutritional assessment by anthropometric and biochemical methods. In: Shils ME, Olson JA, Shike M, eds. *Modern Nutrition in Health and Disease,* 8th ed. Philadelphia, PA: Lea and Febiger; 1994.

Appendix 12

Determine Your Nutritional Health Checklist

The Warning Signs of poor nutritional health are often overlooked. Use this checklist to find out if you or someone you know is at nutritional risk.

Read the statements below. Circle the number in the yes column for those that apply to you or someone you know. For each yes answer, score the number in the box. Total your nutritional score.

DETERMINE YOUR NUTRITIONAL HEALTH

	YES
I have an illness or condition that made me change the kind and/or amount of food I eat.	2
I eat fewer than 2 meals per day.	3
I eat few fruits or vegetables, or milk products.	2
I have 3 or more drinks of beer, liquor, or wine almost every day.	2
I have tooth or mouth problems that make it hard for me to eat.	2
I don't always have enough money to buy the food I need.	4
I eat alone most of the time.	1
I take 3 or more different prescribed or over-the-counter drugs a day.	1
Without wanting to, I have lost or gained 10 pounds in the last 6 months.	2
I am not always physically able to shop, cook, and/or feed myself.	2
TOTAL	

Total Your Nutritional Score. If it's –

0-2 **Good!** Recheck your nutritional score in 6 months.

3-5 **You are at moderate nutritional risk.** See what can be done to improve your eating habits and lifestyle. Your office on aging, senior nutrition program, senior citizens center or health department can help. Recheck your nutritional score in 3 months.

6 or more **You are at high nutritional risk.** Bring this checklist the next time you see your doctor, dietitian or other qualified health or social service professional. Talk with them about any problems you may have. Ask for help to improve your nutritional health.

Remember that warning signs suggest risk, but do not represent diagnosis of any condition. Turn the page to learn more about the Warning Signs of poor nutritional health.

These materials are developed and distributed by the Nutrition Screening Initiative, a project of:

AMERICAN ACADEMY
OF FAMILY PHYSICIANS

THE AMERICAN
DIETETIC ASSOCIATION

THE NATIONAL COUNCIL
ON THE AGING, INC.

continues

Appendix 12 continued

The Nutrition Checklist is based on the Warning Signs described below. Use the word <u>DETERMINE</u> to remind you of the Warning Signs.

DISEASE

Any disease, illness or chronic condition which causes you to change the way you eat, or makes it hard for you to eat, puts your nutritional health at risk. Four out of five adults have chronic diseases that are affected by diet. Confusion or memory loss that keeps getting worse is estimated to affect one out of five or more of older adults. This can make it hard to remember what, when, or if you've eaten. Feeling sad or depressed, which happens to about one in eight older adults, can cause big changes in appetite, digestion, energy level, weight, and well-being.

EATING POORLY

Eating too little and eating too much both lead to poor health. Eating the same foods day after day or not eating fruit, vegetables, and milk products daily will also cause poor nutritional health. One in five adults skip meals daily. Only 13% of adults eat the minimum amount of fruit and vegetables needed. One in four older adults drink too much alcohol. Many health problems become worse if you drink more than one or two alcoholic beverages per day.

TOOTH LOSS/MOUTH PAIN

A healthy mouth, teeth, and gums are needed to eat. Missing, loose, or rotten teeth or dentures which don't fit well, or cause mouth sores make it hard to eat.

ECONOMIC HARDSHIP

As many as 40% of older Americans have incomes of less than $6,000 per year. Having less—or choosing to spend less—than $25-$30 per week for food makes it very hard to get the foods you need to stay healthy.

REDUCED SOCIAL CONTACT

One-third of all older people live alone. Being with people daily has a positive effect on morale, well-being, and eating.

MULTIPLE MEDICINES

Many older Americans must take medicines for health problems. Almost half of older Americans take multiple medicines daily. Growing old may change the way we respond to drugs. The more medicines you take, the greater the chance for side effects such as increased or decreased appetite, change in taste, constipation, weakness, drowsiness, diarrhea, nausea, and others. Vitamins or minerals, when taken in large doses, act like drugs and can cause harm. Alert your doctor to everything you take.

INVOLUNTARY WEIGHT LOSS/GAIN

Losing or gaining a lot of weight when you are not trying to do so is an important warning sign that must not be ignored. Being overweight or underweight also increases your chance of poor health.

NEEDS ASSISTANCE IN SELF-CARE

Although most older people are able to eat, one of every five have trouble walking, shopping, buying and cooking food, especially as they get older.

ELDER YEARS ABOVE AGE 80

Most older people lead full and productive lives. But as age increases, risk of frailty and health problems increase. Checking your nutritional health regularly makes good sense.

Source: Reprinted from the Nutrition Screening Initiative, a project of the American Academy of Family Physicians, the American Dietetic Association and the National Council on Aging, Inc., and funded in part by a grant from Ross Products Division, Abbott Laboratories, Inc.

Appendix 13

Dietary Reference Intakes

Years	Thiamin (mg)*	Riboflavin (mg)*	Niacin (mg)*	Biotin (µg)†	Pantothenic acid (mg)†	Vitamin B_6 (mg)*	Folate (µg)*	Choline (mg)†	Vitamin B_{12} (µg)*	Vitamin C (mg)*	Vitamin A (µg)*	Vitamin D (µg)†	Vitamin E (mg)*	Vitamin K (µg)†
Infant														
0–0.5	0.2	0.3	2	5	1.7	0.1	65	125	0.4	40	400	5	4	2
0.5–1.0	0.3	0.4	4	6	1.8	0.3	80	150	0.5	50	500	5	5	2.5
Child														
1–3	0.5	0.5	6	8	2	0.5	150	200	0.9	15	300	5	6	30
4–8	0.6	0.6	8	12	3	0.6	200	250	1.2	25	400	5	7	55
Male														
9–13	0.9	0.9	12	20	4	1	300	375	1.8	45	600	5	11	60
14–18	1.2	1.3	16	25	5	1.3	400	550	2.4	75	900	5	15	75
19–50	1.2	1.3	16	30	5	1.3	400	550	2.4	90	900	5	15	120
51–70	1.2	1.3	16	30	5	1.7	400	550	2.4	90	900	10	15	120
>70	1.2	1.3	16	30	5	1.7	400	550	2.4	90	900	15	15	120
Female														
9–13	0.9	0.9	12	20	4	1	300	375	1.8	45	600	5	11	60
14–18	1	1	14	25	5	1.2	400	400	2.4	65	700	5	15	75
19–50	1.1	1.1	14	30	5	1.3	400	425	2.4	75	700	5	15	90
51–70	1.1	1.1	14	30	5	1.5	400	425	2.4	75	700	10	15	90
>70	1.1	1.1	14	30	5	1.5	400	425	2.4	75	700	15	15	90

Source: Reprinted with permission from Dietary Reference Intakes for Thiamin, Riboflavin, Niacin, Vitamin B_6, Folate, Vitamin B_{12}, Pantothenic Acid, Biotin and Choline © 1998 by the National Academy of Sciences, courtesy of the National Academies Press, Washington, D.C.

Appendix 14

Drug-Induced Nutrient Alterations in Enteral Patients

Drug*	Nutrient Altered	Mechanism	Notes on Nutritional Care
Antacids			
Numerous	Riboflavin	Increased pH alters absorption	Recommend a multivitamin product or B-complex vitamin with up to 200% of DRI for riboflavin if antacids used regularly (>3 days/wk)
Anticonvulsants			
Phenytoin, primidone, phenobarbital	Folate, Vitamins B_{12} and D	Accelerates vitamin D metabolism in liver; mechanism in folate absorption unclear	Monitor nutrient levels in patients on long-term therapy (>3 to 6 months) supplement as necessary
Antihypertensive			
Methyldopa	Folate, iron, vitamin B_{12}	Autoimmune	Monitor nutrient levels; supplement as necessary
Anti-infectives			
Neomycin, cycloserine, erythromycin, kanamycin	Nitrogen, fat, Ca, Na, K, Mg, vitamins A and B_{12}, folate	Structural defect; bile acid sequestration	Monitor nutrient levels; supplement as necessary
Irritable Bowel Therapy			
Sulfasalazine, tetracyclines	Folate	Mucosal block Di- and trivalent cations (effect on iron absorption not clinically significant)	Monitor for anemia (uncommon) Forms chelates Hold tube feeding for 1 and 2 hours after drug administration Take drug 1 hour before or 2 hours after meal
Anti-inflammatory			
Colchicine	Fat, carotene, vitamin B_{12}	Mitotic arrest; structural (for gout) damage	Monitor vitamins A and B_{12}; Na, K defect; enzyme and electrolyte status; supplement as necessary
Antineoplastic			
Methotrexate	Folate, vitamin B_{12}, Ca	Mucosal damage	Monitor folate and vitamin B_{12} status; supplement as necessary
Antitubercular			
p-Aminosalicylic acid	Fat, Ca, Mg, iron, folate, vitamin B_{12}	Musocal block in vitamin B_{12} uptake can cause megaloblastic anemia; mechanism of absorption unclear	Monitor nutrient levels; supplement as necessary
Contraceptive			
Estrogen-containing	Vitamin C, folate, vitamin B_6	Altered metabolism	Recommend multivitamin or B complex plus C vitamin with up to 200% of RDI; folate especially critical if pregnancy planned when drug stopped
Glucocorticoids			
Dexamethasone, prednisone	Folate		Monitor folate level and for megaloblastic anemia

Drug	Nutrient Altered	Mechanism	Notes on Nutritional Care
Glucose-lowering			
Metformin	Vitamin B_{12}		Monitor vitamin B_{12} status
Hypocholesterolemia			
Cholestyramine	Fat, fat-soluble vitamins, carotene	Binding of bile acids, salts, and nutrients	Monitor vitamin B_{12}, A, and D long-term therapy (>3 months) or recommend multivitamin that includes fat-soluble vitamins at 100% RDI; monitor iron status; supplement as necessary
Clofibrate	Vitamins A, D, E, and B_{12}	Unknown action on liver	Monitor nutrients and/or recommend multivitamin as with cholestyramine
Colestipol	Fat, fat-soluble vitamins	Binds and promotes excretion of bile acids	Monitor nutrients and/or recommend multivitamin as with cholestyramine
Laxatives			
Castor oil	Ca, K	Malabsorption of fat-soluble vitamins	Monitor Ca and K; supplement as necessary; recommend multivitamin as with cholestyramine
Mineral oil	Carotene, vitamins A, D, and K	Physical barrier; nutrients dissolve in oil and are lost	Avoid use near mealtimes
Potassium Repletion			
KCl	Vitamin B_{12}	Change in ileal pH inhibits vitamin B_{12} absorption	Monitor vitamin B_{12} status

*Only drugs that alter vitamin status are included in this table. The reader should seek alternate sources of information for the many drugs that alter electrolyte status.

Source: From ASPEN Board of Directors and the Clinical Guidelines Task Force: Guidelines for the use of parenteral and enteral nutrition in adult and pediatric patients. Section IX: Drug-nutrient interactions. *JPEN.* 2002;26 (1 suppl):42SA.

Appendix 15

Electrolyte Disorders

Electrolyte Disorder	Diagnosis/Etiology

1. Hyponatremia (must evaluate serum osmolality and extracellular fluid volume)	Check serum osmolality
	A. Pseudohyponatremia (normal osmolality)
	  1. Hypertriglyceridemia (multiply triglyceride value in g/dl by 0.002 to yield the mEq/l reduction in serum Na).
	  2. Hypoproteinemia (multiply total protein by 0.25 to yield the mEq reduction in serum Na).
	B. Hypertonic hyponatremia (> 290 mOsm)
	  1. Hyperglycemia and infusion of hypertonic solutions (glucose, mannitol) causing Na-free water to move from cells to the extracellular fluid space, diluting serum Na.
	  2. Hyperglycemia (serum Na falls 1.6 mEq/l for each 100 mg/dl rise in blood sugar above normal).
	Evaluate extracellular volume
	C. Hypotonic hyponatremia (evaluate extracellular volume)
	  1. Hypovolemic hyponatremia: loss of Na-containing fluid (gastrointestinal [GI] tract, skin, lungs, kidneys, sequestration of plasma volume) and replacement with Na-free fluid.
	  2. Hypervolemic hyponatremia: reduced effective arterial blood volume (i.e., congestive heart failure [CHF], severe hypoalbuminemia limits the excretion of ingested water) causing Na and water retention with a disproportionately greater water retention.
	  3. Isovolemic hyponatremia: due to altered mechanism, antidiuretic hormone (ADH) secretion and defective renal diluting mechanisms, syndrome of inappropriate secretion of ADH (SIADH), excessive water intake with loss of salt-containing body fluids.

2. Hypernatremia (osmolality is always elevated)	Extracellular fluid volume
	  1. Hypovolemic hypernatremia: loss of hypotonic body fluids without replacement or replacement of hypotonic body fluids with hypertonic solutions, diuresis (urea- or diuretic-induced or glycosuria).
	  2. Hypervolemic hypernatremia: infusion of large amounts of hypertonic solutions.
	  3. Isovolemic hypernatremia: inappropriate replacement of daily isotonic and hypotonic body fluid loss (ie, skin and respiratory loss) with normal saline; diabetes insipidus.

3. Hypokalemia	A. Potassium depletion: due to cation loss from skin, GI tract, renal potassium wasting (drug-induced or renal tubular acidosis [RTA]). B. Redistribution hypokalemia: secondary to movement of potassium intracellularly as in alkalosis (K^+ falls 0.6 mEq/0.1 pH unit rise), insulin administration, B_{12} therapy, and stimulation of glycolysis and the Krebs cycle by feeding.

Electrolyte Disorder	Diagnosis/Etiology
4. Hyperkalemia	A. Pseudohyperkalemia: secondary to test-tube hemolysis, ischemic blood drawing, leukocytosis, and thrombocytosis. B. Redistribution: from hyperglycemia, acidosis, tissue necrosis. C. Excessive K^+ ingestion; renal failure.
5. Hypercalcemia	A. Malignancies and hyperparathyroidism are responsible for 70%–80% of all cases. B. Acute tubular necrosis (ATN) recovery after myoglobinuria-induced disease.
6. Hypocalcemia	A. Hypoalbuminemia: (4.0 − actual serum albumin level) × 0.8 yields the amount of hypocalcemia due to protein depletion. B. Hypomagnesemia: impairs parathyroid hormone (PTH) secretion and its peripheral action on the bone. C. Vitamin D deficiency: causes decreased bone responsiveness to PTH or decreased intestinal Ca absorption. D. Hyperphosphatemia: causes decreased conversion of vitamin D to its active form, reduced bone absorption. E. Pancreatitis: mechanism unclear.
7. Hypomagnesemia	A. Renal magnesium wasting. B. Stimulation of glycolysis by feeding enhances magnesium uptake in the cell.
8. Hypermagnesemia	A. Renal failure.
9. Hypophosphatemia	A. Stimulation of glycolysis by feeding enhances phosphorus uptake in the cell. B. Phosphorus binding by albumin- or magnesium-containing antacids. C. Renal phosphate binding.
10. Hyperphosphatemia	A. Renal failure.
11. Hypobicarbonatemia	A. Overproduction of acid (i.e., lactic acid). B. Diarrheal loss of sodium bicarbonate with renal retention of sodium chloride. C. Renal failure or ATN, causing retention of acid or urinary wastage of alkali. D. Total parenteral nutrition (TPN), which causes a mild metabolic acidosis. E. Addition of 15 to the serum bicarbonate estimates the last two digits of the pH.
12. Hyperbicarbonatemia	A. Caused by a source of a new alkali and reduced bicarbonaturia. B. Contraction alkalosis as seen in diuresis (bicarbonate concentration in interstitial fluid is similar to that in blood). C. Excessive GI loss of acid (nasogastric suction and vomiting), which leaves unneutralized bicarbonate behind.

Source: Reprinted from *Handbook of Total Parenteral Nutrition,* JP Grant, ed., Administration of Parenteral Nutrition Solutions, p. 94, Copyright (1980), with permission from Elsevier.

Appendix 16

Energy Expenditure Equations

ENERGY CONVERSIONS

1 kilocalorie (Kcal) = 1000 calories = 4.184 kilojoules (KJ)

FICK EQUATION

1. CaO_2 (ml/dl) = 1.39 (Hgb) $\times$ SaO_2/100 + 0.0031 (PaO_2)
2. CVO_2 (ml/dl) = 1.39 (Hgb) $\times$ SVO_2/100 + 0.031 (PVO_2)
3. VO_2 (ml/min) = Cardiac output $\times$ 10 CaO_2 − CVO_2

BASAL ENERGY EXPENDITURE (HARRIS-BENEDICT EQUATION)

Males: BEE = 66.4730 + 13.7516 (w) + 5.0033 (s) − 6.7550 (a)
Females: BEE = 655.0955 + 9.5634 (w) + 1.8496 (s) − 4.6756 (a)
Where w is weight in kg
   s is stature (height) in cm
   a is age in years

SWINAMER

REE = BSA (941) − age (6.3) + T_{max} (104) + RR(24) + V_T(804) − 423
Where BSA is body surface area
   T_{max} is maximum body temperature (centigrade)
   RR is respiratory rate (breaths/min)
   V_T is tidal volume (L)

IRETON-JONES

REE = wt (5) − age (10) + sex (281) + trauma (292) + burns (851) + 1925
Where sex was male = 1 and female = 0
   Trauma and burns were yes = 1, no = 0

FRANKENFIELD

REE = BEE(1.5) + body temp(250) + V_e(100) + dobut (40) + MOF(300) − 11,000
Where body temp is body temperature during study (degrees centigrade)
   V_E is expired minute volume (L/min)
   dobut is dobutamine dose (mcg/kg per minute)
   MOF is presence of multiple organ failure

Implications of Respiratory Quotient (RQ)

RQ	Significance
<0.70	Oxidation of alcohol
	Oxidation of ketones
	Carbohydrate synthesis
	Measurement problem
0.70–0.75	Mostly lipid oxidation
	Possible starvation
0.85–0.95	Mixed substrate oxidation
	Calories adequate
>1.00	Lipogenesis
	Primarily carbohydrate oxidation
	Hyperventilation
	Measurement problem

WEIR FORMULA

REE = [3.941 (VO_2) + 1.106 (VCO_2)]1.44 − 2.77(UN)
REE = resting energy expenditure (kcal/day)
VO_2 = oxygen consumption (ml/min)
VCO_2 = carbon dioxide production (ml/min)
UN = urinary nitrogen (g/d)

Abbreviated Weir Formula

REE = [3.941 (VO_2) + 1.106 (VCO_2)]1.44

Source: Taken from Nutrient Requirements. In: Matarese LE, Gottschlich MM, eds. *Pocket Guide Companion to Contemporary Nutrition Support Practice; Clinical Guide.* Philadelphia, PA: Elsevier Science (USA); 2003:28–29.

Appendix 17

Examples of Typical Parenteral Nutrition Solutions

For Peripheral Administration:*

Amino acids	35 g
Dextrose	70 g
Sodium chloride	15 mEq
Potassium acetate	30 mEq
Sodium phosphate	20 mEq
Magnesium sulfate	8 mEq
Calcium gluconate	9.4 mEq
Multiple vitamins	10 ml
Trace elements	3 ml
Heparin	200 units

Administer 250 ml of 20% lipids daily to provide 878 kcal and 35 g of protein in 1250 ml of fluid.

For Central Administration:*

Amino acids	60 g
Dextrose	250 g
Sodium chloride	35 mEq
Potassium acetate	30 mEq
Sodium phosphate	20 mEq
Magnesium sulfate	8 mEq
Calcium gluconate	9.4 mEq
Multiple vitamins	10 ml
Trace elements	3 ml
Heparin	1000 units

Administer 250 ml of 20% lipids daily to provide 1590 kcal and 60 g of protein in 1250 ml of fluid.

*Nutrient content expressed per liter.

Appendix 18

Guidelines to Determine Metabolic Stress

	Stress Levels			
	0 *Starvation*	*1* *Low* *Stress*	*2* *Moderate* *Stress*	*3* *Severe* *Stress*
Urinary nitrogen loss (g/day)	<5	5–10	10–15	>15
Estimated caloric requirements	BEE	BEE × 1.3	BEE × 1.5	BEE × 2.0
Nonprotein calorie-nitrogen ratio (kcal/g N)	150:1	100:1	100:1	80:1
Amino acids (g/kg/day)	1	1.5	2	2–2.5 or more
Total nonprotein calories (kcal/kg/day)	25	25	30	35
Total calories (kcal/kg/day)	28	32	40	50

BEE = basal energy expenditure.
Source: Adapted from Cerra FB: *Pocket Manual of Surgical Nutrition.* St. Louis, MO: Mosby; 1984:8–20.

Appendix 19

Ideal Weight for Height (Male Patients)

Height (cm)	Weight (kg)	Height (cm)	Weight (kg)	Height (cm)	Weight (kg)
145	51.9	159	59.9	173	68.7
146	52.4	160	60.5	174	69.4
147	52.9	161	61.1	175	70.1
148	53.5	162	61.7	176	70.8
149	54.0	163	62.3	177	71.6
150	54.5	164	62.9	178	72.4
151	55.0	165	63.5	179	73.3
152	55.6	166	64.0	180	74.2
153	56.1	167	64.6	181	75.0
154	56.6	168	65.2	182	75.8
155	57.2	169	65.9	183	76.5
156	57.9	170	66.6	184	77.3
157	58.6	171	67.3	185	78.1
158	59.3	172	68.0	186	78.9

Ideal Weight for Height (Female Patients)

Height (cm)	Weight (kg)	Height (cm)	Weight (kg)	Height (cm)	Weight (kg)
140	44.9	150	50.4	160	56.2
141	45.4	151	51.0	161	56.9
142	45.9	152	51.5	162	57.6
143	46.4	153	52.0	163	58.3
144	47.0	154	52.5	164	58.9
145	47.5	155	53.1	165	59.5
146	48.0	156	53.7	166	60.1
147	48.6	157	54.3	167	60.7
148	49.2	158	54.9	168	61.4
149	49.8	159	55.5	169	62.1

Source: Reprinted from Blackburn GL, Bistrian GR, Haini BS, Schlamm HT, Smith MF. Nutritional and metabolic assessment of the hospitalized patient. *JPEN.* 1977;1:14 with permission from the American Society for Parenteral and Enteral Nutrition (A.S.P.E.N.).

Appendix 20

Interdisciplinary Home Enteral Nutrition Education Checklist

1. Explain rationale for enteral feedings, short-term and long-term goals.
2. Explain type of feeding tube by the entrance site and where the terminal tip is placed.
3. Describe care of access site:
   a. skin care and cleaning of site
   b. appropriate dressing
   c. monitoring for signs of infection
4. Demonstrate proper handwashing and clean technique when preparing and giving feeding.
5. Describe proper use and storage of formula and equipment.
6. Explain feeding schedule:
   a. name of formula
   b. volume of formula and amount to provide for each feeding
   c. times feeding to be given
   d. method of administration
   e. appropriate amount of flush before and after each feeding and between feedings as indicated
7. Demonstrate proper administration of formula and flush:
   a. verify tube placement
   b clamp tube prior to opening
   c. flush tube with water prior to instilling formula
   d. place appropriate amount of formula into feeding receptacle
   e. mixing of modular components/formulas as appropriate
   f. prime tubing
   g proper use of pump if appropriate
   h. set roller clamp at correct setting for drip desired if appropriate
   i. flush tube at end of feeding with correct amount of flush
8. State/demonstrate medication administration:
   a. appropriate time to give medications
   b. food–drug interactions
   c. drug–drug interactions
   d proper crushing and mixing technique for medications
   e. proper flushing technique when giving medications
9. List potential complications and interventions:
   a. occlusion of feeding tube
   b. leakage from or around stoma site
   c. displaced feeding tube
   d. signs of infection at stoma site such as redness, drainage, tenderness, fever
   e. vomiting, diarrhea, constipation, cramping, flatulence
   f. weight loss
   g weight gain of greater than 2 pounds per week
   h. excessive thirst or urination
10. Identify appropriate contact for questions or emergencies.

Source: Adapted from Romano M. Home enteral nutrition: What the hospital-based dietitian needs to know. *Support Line.* 25(5):17–19. Reprinted with permission.

Appendix 21

Metabolic Complications of Tube Feeding

Problem	Possible Causes	Prevention or Therapy
Glucose intolerance	Refeeding syndrome in malnourished patient	Monitor serum glucose daily until stable (< 200 mg/dl) at goal TF rate.
	Specific disease states or condition such as diabetes mellitus, sepsis, or trauma	Maintain last tolerated TF rate, then gradually increase as tolerated.
	Metabolic stress	Provide 30%–50% total kcal as fat; may need modular formula.
Hypertonic dehydration	Inadequate fluid intake	Monitor daily fluid intake and output; monitor body weight daily; weight change >0.2 kg/day reflects decrease or increase of extracellular fluid.
	Excessive fluid losses	Monitor serum electrolyte values, serum osmolality, urine specific gravity, and BUN and Cr levels daily. (BUN/Cr ratio is usually 10:1 in patients with normal hydration status.)
	Administration of hypertonic, high-protein formula in patient unable to express thirst	Assess fluid status; estimate fluid loss (mild loss, 3% body weight decrease; moderate loss, 6% body weight decrease; severe loss, 10% body weight decrease); replace fluid loss in addition to maintenance fluid needs enterally or parenterally.
Overhydration	Excessive fluid intake	Assess fluid status; monitor daily fluid intake and output.
	Rapid refeeding in malnourished patient	Monitor serum electrolyte values daily.
	Increased extracellular mass catabolism causing loss of body cell mass with subsequent potassium loss	Monitor body weight; weight change > 0.2 kg/day reflects decrease or increase of extracellular fluid.
	Elevated aldosterone levels causing sodium retention	Administer diuretic therapy.
	Altered sodium pump causing excessive intracellular sodium retention	Use formula with lower free-water content if necessary.
	Cardiac, hepatic, or renal insufficiency	
Hypokalemia	Refeeding syndrome in malnourished patients	Monitor serum potassium level daily until stable within normal limits at goal TF rate.
	Depleted body cell mass	Supplement potassium and chloride.
	Effect of antidiuretic hormone and aldosterone	
	Diuretic therapy	
	Excessive losses (e.g., from diarrhea or nasogastric drainage)	
	May induce or be the result of metabolic acidosis	
	Insulin therapy	
	Dilutional state	

Problem	Possible Causes	Prevention or Therapy
Hypophosphatemia	Refeeding syndrome in malnourished patients	Monitor serum phosphorus level daily or every other day until stable within normal limits at goal TF rate.
	Insulin therapy	Supplement phosphorus enterally or parenterally.
	Phosphate-binding antacids	Adjust antacid dose if necessary.
Hypomagnesemia	Refeeding syndrome in malnourished patients	Monitor serum magnesium level daily or every other day until stable within normal limits at goal TF rate.
	Excessive losses from urine, skin, or stool	Supplement magnesium enterally or parenterally.
Hyperkalemia	Metabolic acidosis	Monitor serum potassium level daily or every other day until stable within normal limits at goal TF rate.
	Poor perfusion (e.g., congestive heart failure)	Treat cause of poor perfusion.
	Renal failure	Kayexalate, glucose, and/or insulin therapy.
	Excessive potassium intake from oral diet and/or TF formula	Decrease potassium intake; use formula with lower potassium content.
Hypoglycemia	Sudden cessation of TF for patient receiving oral hypoglycemic agents or insulin therapy	Monitor serum glucose level daily until stable within normal limits at goal TF rate; taper TF gradually.
	Fluid overload	
Hypernatremia	Dilutional state due to elevated antidiuretic hormone level with subsequent parenteral infusion of saline solutions	Monitor serum sodium level daily until stable within normal limits at goal TF rate.
	Cardiac, hepatic, or renal insufficiency	Assess fluid status.
		Administer diuretic therapy, if required.
		Restrict fluids.
		Restrict sodium.
Hypernatremia	Inadequate fluid intake with excessive losses	Monitor daily fluid intake and output; monitor body weight daily; weight change > 0.2 kg/day reflects decrease or increase of extracellular fluid.
	Depletion of total body sodium, extracellular mass, and extracellular fluid	Monitor serum electrolyte values, serum osmolality, urine specific gravity, and BUN and CR levels daily. (BUN/Cr ratio is usually 10:1 in patients with normal hydration status.)
		Assess fluid status; estimate fluid loss (mild loss, 3% body weight decrease; moderate loss, 6% body weight decrease; severe loss, 10% body weight decrease); replace fluid loss in addition to maintenance fluid needs enterally or parenterally for the repletion of extracellular fluid space.
Hyperphosphatemia	Renal insufficiency	Administer phosphate binder therapy.
		Use formula with lower phosphorus content if necessary.
Hypercapnia	Overfeeding	Provide maintenance calorie and protein needs without overfeeding.
	Excessive carbohydrate load in patient with respiratory dysfunction	Use enteral formula with balanced distribution of carbohydrate, protein, and fat.
		Provide 30%–50% of total kcal as fat.
Essential fatty acid deficiency	Inadequate linoleic acid intake (e.g., prolonged use of low-fat enteral formula)	Include at least 4% kcal needs as essential fatty acids (linoleic acid); add modular fat formula to diet regimen; administer 5 ml of enteral safflower oil daily.
Hypozincemia	Excessive losses from diarrhea, wound, or GI losses (Note: serum zinc level may not accurately reflect total body zinc stores.)	Supplement zinc enterally or parenterally.

BUN, blood urea nitrogen; CR, creatinine; GI, gastrointestinal; TF, tube feeding.
Source: Adapted from Ideno KT: Enteral nutrition. In: Gottschlich MM, Matarese LE, Shronts EP, eds. *Nutrition Support for Dietetics Core Curriculum.* 2nd ed. Silver Spring, MD: American Society for Parenteral and Enteral Nutrition; 1993:98–99.

Appendix 22

Mineral Requirements in Adults

Element	RDA/AI (mg)*	Deficiency Symptoms	Toxic Symptoms	Assessment	Dietary Interaction
Calcium	1000	↑ Bone mass, osteoporosis, hypocalcemia, ↑ risk of hypertension	Renal insufficiency, hypercalcemia, respiratory and cardiac failure	Bone density (DEXA) most reliable; 1,25-dihydroxyvitamin D, PTH, and serum calcium helpful	↓ High sodium and protein intake (by ↑ urinary calcium loss), ↓ caffeine
Phosphorus	700	Anorexia, anemia, osteomalacia, rickets, bone pain, muscle weakness, ↑ risk of infection, paresthesia, confusion	↓ Calcium absorption, ↓ urinary calcium excretion, ↑ PTH, ectopic calcification	Serum phosphate	↓ Phosphate, ↓ high protein, ↓ phytate
Magnesium	310–420	Cardiac arrhythmia, neuromuscular hyperexcitability, latent tetany or seizure, hypocalcemia, hypokalemia	Osmotic diarrhea, abdominal cramping, nausea, hypokalemia, metabolic alkalosis	Serum magnesium, ionized Mg^{2+} better	↓ Phytate, ↓ calcium, ↑ animal meat
Iron	8 (men) 18 (women)	Developmental delay, prematurity and stillbirth, cognitive impairment, cold intolerance, koilonychia, glossitis, angular stomatitis, microcytic anemia, ↓ work performance	Acute: vomiting, diarrhea, organ failure Chronic: hemochromatosis, increased risk of ischemic heart disease, zinc deficiency	Ferritin, transferrin, hemoglobin, serum iron	↓ Iron, ↓ calcium, ↓ phosphorus
Zinc	8–11	Retarded growth, poor wound healing, ↓ taste and appetite, alopecia, dermatitis, impotence, birth defects	Acute: nausea, metallic taste, abdominal cramps, diarrhea, nausea, headache Chronic: ↓ immunity, ↓ HDL cholesterol, copper deficiency	Serum zinc	↓ Phytate, ↓ calcium, ↓ phosphorus
Copper	900	Neutropenia, microcytic hypochromic anemia, cardiac arrhythmia, osteoporosis	Acute: abdominal pain, vomiting, ataxia, hepatic necrosis Chronic: cirrhosis, hemolysis, brain, nerve injury	Plasma copper and ceruloplasmin, erythrocyte superoxide dismutase/platelet cytochrome *c* oxidase activity	↓ Antacid, ↓ vitamin C, ↓ Fe, ↓ Zn, ↑ starch as CHO source, ↓ sucrose and fructose as CHO source
Chromium	25–35	Glucose intolerance, ↑ cholesterol and LDL, peripheral neuropathy, weight loss	None reported	Urinary Cr, plasma Cr, glucose tolerance test	↑ Aspirin, ↑ oxalate ↑ ascorbic acid, ↓ zinc, ↓ iron, ↓ antacids, ↓ phytate
Iodine	150	Hypothyroidism, goiter, and cretinism in children	Goiter and hyper- or hypothyroidism	Urine iron concentration, serum T$_3$, T$_4$, TSH	Se (synergistic action)

Mineral	RDA/AI	Deficiency	Toxicity	Assessment	Interactions
Manganese	1.8–2.3	Dermatitis, hypocholesterolemia, bone and cartilage abnormality, anemia	Anorexia, weakness, ataxia, tremor, neurologic irritability	Plasma and whole blood Mn, RBC Mn concentration—no consistent results, MRI	↓ Fe
Molybdenum	45	Intolerance to S-containing amino acids, hypouricemia, mental disturbance, coma	Hyperuricemia, arthritis, gastrointestinal symptoms, growth retardation, anemia	Urine xanthine, plasma Mo	↓ Cu
Selenium	55	Cardiomyopathy, immune deficiency, skeletal myopathy, risk of cancer	Hair and nail loss, tooth decay, neuropathy, mental change	Plasma and RBC Se, selenoprotein in RBCs, glutathione peroxidase	↑ Vitamin E, ↑ iodine
Arsenic	Not set	Unknown	Acute: encephalopathy, GI symptoms Chronic: hepatotoxicity, hematopoietic depression, neuritis, various dermatoses		
Boron	Not set	↓ BUN/creatinine, ↓ serum glucose, ↓ calcitonin, ↑ hemoglobin	DI symptoms, dermatitis, scanty hair, weight loss, anemia, seizures	Plasma boron	↑ Coffee and tea
Nickel	Not set	No reported case of deficiency	Dermatitis, carcinogenesis, nephrotoxicity, immunosuppression	Blood level of nickel	↓ Fe, ↓ Cu
Vanadium	Not set	No reported case of deficiency	Neurotoxicity, hepatotoxicity, nephrotoxicity, green tongue, muscle cramps, diarrhea	No adequate method	
Aluminum	Not set	No reported case of deficiency	Osteomalacia, microcytic hypochromic anemia, encephalopathy (seizures, ataxia, dementia)	Blood and serum aluminum: not accurate	↑ Al containing antacids, ↓ Fe, ↓ Cu, ↓ Zn

Al, aluminum; BUN, blood urea nitrogen; Cr, chromium; Cu, copper; DI, diabetes insipidus; Fe, iron; GI, gastrointestinal; HDL, high-density lipoprotein; LDL, low-density lipoprotein; Mg, magnesium; MRI, magnetic resonance imaging; PTH, parathyroid hormone; RBC, red blood cell; S, sulfur; Se, selenium; T_3, triiodothyronine; T4, thyroxine; TSH, thyroid-stimulating hormone; Zn, zinc.

*Recommended Daily Allowance (RDA) or Adequate Intake (AI).

Source: Reprinted with permission from Recommended Dietary Allowances: 10th Edition © 1989 by the National Academy of Sciences, courtesy of the National Academies Press, Washington, D.C.

Appendix 23

Monitoring and Management of Gastrointestinal Complications in Pediatric Enteral Nutrition Patients

Gastrointestinal Complications	Monitoring	Potential Cause	Management

High gastric residual volumes	Every 2–4 hours	Gastroparesis
		Surgery
		Chemical paralysis
		Neuromuscular blockade
		Sepsis
		High amylin levels
			Stop for residual volumes > 2 times the
			    hourly rate or 80 ml (whichever is greater)
			Elevate head of bed > 30°
			Dilute formulas with high osmolality to half
			    strength and gradually increase
			    concentration over 1–2 days
			Avoid soluble fiber-containing tube feedings
			Provide motility agents
			Place feeding tube postpylorically

Abdominal distention	Before initiation of feedings; daily or more frequently with increased distention	Ileus Obstruction Formula too cold Excessive fiber intake Lactose intolerance	Hold feedings Rule out ileus or obstruction Provide formula at room temperature Evaluate fiber intake based on child's age and diet history Evaluate formula; enteral intake if eating

Nausea/vomiting	Every shift	Feeding intolerance
		Infectious origin
		Medication-related
			Dilute feedings/lower volume of feedings/avoid
			    flavored feedings
			Evaluate infectious etiology
			Evaluate medications, including vitamin/mineral
			    supplements (i.e., zinc, iron)

Diarrhea	Every shift	Medication-related Hyperosmolar feedings Infectious origin Intestinal atrophy due to malnutrition Postpyloric feedings	Evaluate medications, particularly antibiotics; consider probiotic therapy Dilute feedings Check stool cultures Provide elemental feedings until tolerance improves Reduce rate
Constipation	Every shift	High-dose narcotics Immobility Inadequate fiber Inadequate fluid volume Inadequate free water	Initiate bowel regimen immediately with all patients receiving narcotics Fiber may worsen constipation Increase fluid intake if possible

Appendix 24

Nitrogen Balance Calculation

Nitrogen Balance Calculation

Nitrogen balance = Nitrogen intake − nitrogen output

$$\frac{\text{24-hr protein intake (g)}}{6.25^*} - (\text{24-hr UUN (g)} + 4\ \text{g}^\dagger)$$

$$\frac{\text{24-hr protein intake (g)}}{6.25^*} - (\text{24-hr TUN (g)} + 2\ \text{g}^\dagger)$$

TUN, Total urea nitrogen; *UUN,* urinary urea nitrogen.
*Most protein sources contain 16% nitrogen. Check source for exact amount.
†Estimate of fecal, dermal, miscellaneous, and nonurea nitrogen losses.
Source: Adapted from Russell M: Serum proteins and nitrogen balance. Evaluating response to nutrition support. *Support Line,* XVII:3–8, 1995.

Appendix 25

Nutrition Support Algorithm

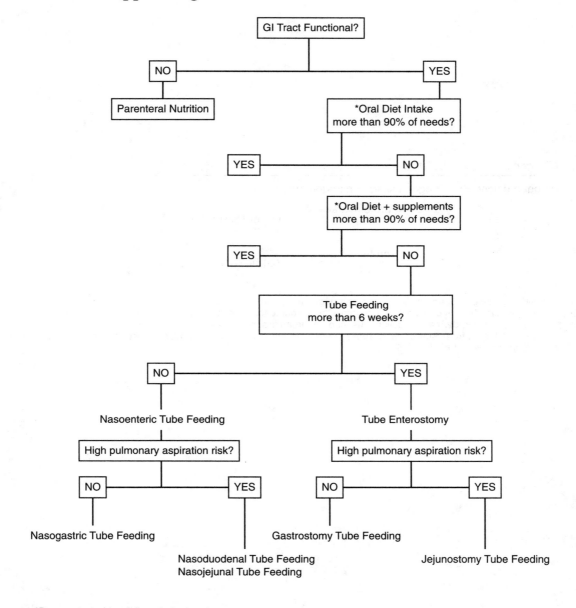

*Demonstrated by daily calorie counts.

Source: Reprinted from Ideno KT. Enteral nutrition. In: Gottschlich MM, Matarese LE, Shronts EP, eds. *Nutrition Support Dietetics Core Curriculum.* 2nd ed. Silver Spring, MD: American Society for Parenteral and Enteral Nutrition; 1993:83 with permission from the American Society for Parenteral and Enteral Nutrition (A.S.P.E.N.).

Appendix 26

Osmolality of Clear Liquids

Item	Mean Osmolality (mOsm/kg)
Cranberry juice	836
Apple juice	705
Orange juice	601
Low-calorie cranberry juice	287
Flavored ice (i.e., Italian ice)	1064
Jell-O	735
Low-calorie Jell-O	57
Cola	714
Diet cola	43
Ginger ale	565
Diet ginger ale	53

Source: Adapted from Bell SJ, Anderson FL, Bistrian BR, et al: Osmolality of beverages commonly provided on clear and full liquid menu. *Nutr Clin Prac.* 1987; 2:241–244.

Appendix 27

Parenteral Electrolyte Recommendations for Adult Patients with Normal Function

	Sheldon	Schlichtig	NAG
Potassium	120–160 mmol/d	70–100 mEq	1–2 mEq/kg
Sodium	125–150 mmol/d	70–100 mEq	1–2 mEq/kg + replacement
Phosphate	12–25 mmol/1000 kcal	20–30 mmol	20–40 mmol
Magnesium	7.5–10 mmol/d	15–20 mEq	8–20 mEq
Calcium		10–20 mmol	10–15 mEq
Chloride			As needed to maintain acid-base balance

Source: Adapted from Sheldon GF, Kudsk KA, Morris JA: Electrolyte requirements in total parenteral nutrition. In: Deitel M, ed. *Nutrition in Clinical Surgery,* Baltimore, MD: Williams and Wilkins, 1985; Schlichtig R, Ayers SM: *Nutritional Support of the Critically Ill.* Chicago, IL: Year Book; 1988:130; National Advisory Group: Safe practices for parenteral nutrition formulations. *JPEN;* 1998;22:49–66.

Appendix 28

Percent of Free Water in Enteral Formulas

Formula Density	Percentage of Free Water
1.0 kcal/ml	84%
1.2 kcal/ml	81%
1.5 kcal/ml	75%
2.0 kcal/ml	70%

Appendix 29

Physical Markers of Hydration Status

Volume deficit
- Decreased moisture in oral cavity
- Decreased skin and tongue turgor (elasticity); skin may remain slightly elevated after being pinched
- Flattened neck and peripheral veins in supine position
- Decreased urinary output ($<$ 30 ml/h without renal failure)
- Postural hypotension (severe deficit)
- Tachycardia
- Acute weight loss ($\geq$ 1 lb/d)

Volume excess
- Clinically apparent edema is usually not present until 12–15 L of fluid has accumulated
- 1 L fluid = 1 kg weight
- Acute weight gain ($\geq$ 1 lb/d)
- Pitting edema (especially in dependent parts of the body, i.e., feet, ankles, and sacrum)
- Distended peripheral and neck veins
- Symptoms of congestive heart failure (CHF) or pulmonary edema
- Central venous pressure (CVP) $>$ 11 cm H_2O

Source: Metheny, *Fluid and Electrolyte Balance,* 1987. Used by permission of Lippincott Williams & Wilkins.

Appendix 30

Physical Signs Related to Nutrient Deficiency or Excess

Nutrient	Deficiency	Excess
PART 1 VITAMINS—FAT SOLUBLE		
Vitamin A	Night blindness Keratomalacia Bitot's spots Xerosis: skin, cornea and/or conjunctiva Follicular hyperkeratosis Crazy paving dermatitis Taste changes	Pruritis Hyperkeratosis Alopedia Painful swelling of bones Syndrome of headache, dizziness, irritability, and drowsiness Hepatomegaly staining of skin (palms and soles) orange, anorexia and vomiting
Vitamin D	Painless costochondral beading Decreased muscle strength Osteomalacia Kyphosis (over lifetime) Bowed legs Pigeon chest and Harrison salcus Prone to fractures Rickets in children Adult osteomalacia	Acute hypercalcemia Nausea Anorexia Abdominal pain Diarrhea
Vitamin E	Sensory loss (R) Decreased vibration sense (R) Impaired position sense (R) Gait sensory ataxia (R) Impaired reflexes (R)	Coagulopathy (vitamin E increases vitamin K requirements) Nausea, flatulence, and diarrhea have been reported
Vitamin K	Ecchymosis Petechia Purpura	
PART 2 VITAMINS—WATER SOLUBLE		
Vitamin C	Petechiae and purpura Perifolliculitis Delayed wound healing Decubitus ulcers Conjunctival hemorrhage Bleeding gums Painful costochondral beading Perifollicular hemorrhages Impaired wound healing	Oxalate stones (R) Gastric irritation Flatulence Diarrhea

continues

Appendix 30 continued

Nutrient	Deficiency	Excess
PART 2 VITAMINS—WATER SOLUBLE (continued)		
Vitamin B$_1$ Thiamin	Edema Muscle wasting Muscle tenderness and cramps Confusion Wernicke-Korsakoff syndrome Decreased vibration sense (#) Paresthesia (#) Ptosis (#) Photophobia (#) Angular blepharoconjunctivitis (#) Amblyopia (#) Dyssebacia (#) Beriberi (wet and dry)	None documented
Vitamin B$_2$ Riboflavin	Flaking, scaly dermatitis Angular blepharoconjunctivitis Magenta tongue Nasolabial seborrheic dermatitis Corneal vascularization Angular stomatitis Cheilosis Filiform papillary atrophy or hypertrophy Glossitis	None documented

Niacin	Pellagra: dermatitis, diarrhea, dementia
	Red/brown scaly dermatitis
	Erythema and swelling on light exposed
	    areas (Casal's necklace, glove and
	    stocking distribution)
	Beefy red/scarlet tongue
	Confusion
	Depression/irritability
	Atrophy of sublingual papillae
	Fissuring edema of the tongue
	Nasolabial seborrheic dermatitis
	Corneal vascularization
	Angular stomatitis
	Cheilosis
	Filiform papillary atrophy or hypertrophy
	Glossitis
		For high doses used to treat
		hyperlipidemia, side effects
		include cutaneous flushing, and
		gastric irritation. Elevated liver
		enzymes, hyperglycemia, and
		gout are less common

Vitamin B$_6$ Pyridoxine	Nasolabial seborrheic dermatitis Angular stomatitis Glossitis Depression Paresthesia Peripheral neuropathy	Sensory neuropathy

Nutrient	Deficiency	Excess
PART 2 VITAMINS—WATER SOLUBLE (continued)		
Vitamin B$_{12}$ Cobalamin	Megaloblastic anemia Lemon-yellow skin pallor Vertiligo Hyperpigmentation Early greying (associated with pernicious anemia only) Vincent's stomatitis (gums) Angular blepharoconjunctivitis Scarlet tongue Pale ventral tongue surface Filiform papillary atrophy or hypertrophy Atrophy of sublingual papillae Glossitis Confusion Dementia Sensory loss; paresthesia and vibration sense Decreased or loss of positive sense Gait sensory ataxia	None documented
Folate	Megaloblastic anemia Skin pallor Pallor of everted lower eyelids Vincent's stomatitis (gums) Filiform papillary atrophy Scarlet tongue Aphthous-like lesions (R) Atrophy of sublingual papillae Glossitis Sensory loss (R)	None documented
Biotin	Flaking, scaly dermatitis Bands of hypopigmentation of the hair shaft Alopecia Coarse hair Pale ventral tongue surface Sensory loss	None documented
PART 3 MINERALS		
Calcium	Trousseau's sign Chvostek's sign Kyphosis (over lifetime) Bowed legs Fractures	Rare: Hypercalcemia may result in mineralization of soft tissue Hypotonia Proximal myopathy

continues

Appendix 30 continued

Nutrient	Deficiency	Excess
PART 3 MINERALS (continued)		
Magnesium	Chvostek's sign Trousseau's sign Tetany Decreased level of consciousness Weakness, muscle cramps Vertigo	Decreased level of consciousness
Phosphorus	Osteomalacia Muscle weakness Malaise	Hyperphosphatemia may result in decreased level of consciousness In renal insufficiency, secondary hyperparathyroidism can occur
Sodium	Hyponatremia Convulsions Diarrhea Anxiety	Sodium and water retention resulting in edema
Potassium	Hypokalemia Motor function weakness Atonia Cardiac arrhythmia	Anxiety
PART 4 TRACE MINERALS		
Copper	Skin pallor Decreased pigmentation of hair shaft (may be banded)	Wilson's disease Blue lunula Kayser-Fleisher rings
Iron	Skin pallor Koilonychia Pallor of everted lower eyelids Angular stomatitis Filiform papillary atrophy Pale ventral tongue surface Glossitis	Hemochromatosis Gray-tan, bronze, blue-grey skin color
Zinc	Diffuse erythema Xerosis Flaking, scaly dermatitis Delayed wound healing Decubitus ulcers Alopedia Night blindness Taste change	

Nutrient	Deficiency	Excess
PART 4 TRACE MINERALS (continued)		
Chromium	Koilonychia	
Iodine	Outer third eyebrow missing Goiter	
Fluoride	Carious teeth Possibly osteomalacia	Fluorosis Paralysis Convulsions GI irritation
		None documented
PART 5 MACRONUTRIENTS		
Protein	Kwashiorkor Fullness, moon-shaped face Brittle, pluckable hair Fine, silky hair Alopecia Decreased pigmentation (hair) Muehrcke's lines (nails) Edema Hyperpigmentation (Sun-exposed skin) Flaky paint or crazy paving dermatitis Delayed wound healing Decubitus ulcers Muscle weakness and wasting	
		None documented
Essential fatty acids	Xerosis Flaking, scaly dermatitis Follicular hyperkeratosis Dry, dull hair	
		Accumulation of adipose tissue
Protein/energy	Marasmus Dry, dull hair Drawn-in cheeks Carious teeth Yellow-brown stained teeth Ascites Impaired grip strength Muscle weakness and wasting Loss of position sense	

(#) Signs associated with B-complex deficiency.
(R) = Rare.
Source: Rombeau et al., *Atlas Nutritional Support Techniques,* 1989. Used by permission of Lippincott Williams & Wilkins.

Appendix 31

Physiologic Impact of Starvation versus Stress

Category	Starvation	Stress
Protein		
Catabolism	+	+++
Carbohydrate		
Glycogenolysis	+	+++
Gluconeogenesis	+	+++
Lipids		
Lipolysis	+++	++/+++
Ketosis	+++	++
Metabolic alterations		
Mobilization of macronutrients	Passive	Active
Energy expenditure	↓	↑
Serum albumin	No change	↓↓
Urine urea nitrogen*	≤ 5 g/day	> 5 g/day

*Assumes initial adequate protein-energy stores.
↑ = increase; ↓ = decrease; ↓↓ = precipitous fall.
Source: Adapted from Daley B, Cahill S, Driscoll DF, Bistrian BR. Parenteral and enteral nutrition. In: Wolfe M, ed. *Gastrointestinal Pharmacology.* Philadelphia, PA: WB Saunders; 1993:293–316.

Appendix 32

Quadrants of the Abdomen

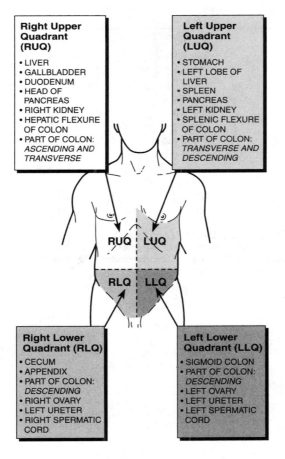

Right Upper Quadrant (RUQ)

- LIVER
- GALLBLADDER
- DUODENUM
- HEAD OF PANCREAS
- RIGHT KIDNEY
- HEPATIC FLEXURE OF COLON
- PART OF COLON: *ASCENDING AND TRANSVERSE*

Left Upper Quadrant (LUQ)

- STOMACH
- LEFT LOBE OF LIVER
- SPLEEN
- PANCREAS
- LEFT KIDNEY
- SPLENIC FLEXURE OF COLON
- PART OF COLON: *TRANSVERSE AND DESCENDING*

Right Lower Quadrant (RLQ)

- CECUM
- APPENDIX
- PART OF COLON: *DESCENDING*
- RIGHT OVARY
- LEFT URETER
- RIGHT SPERMATIC CORD

Left Lower Quadrant (LLQ)

- SIGMOID COLON
- PART OF COLON: *DESCENDING*
- LEFT OVARY
- LEFT URETER
- LEFT SPERMATIC CORD

Source: Reprinted from *Pocket Guide Companion to Contemporary Nutrition Support Practice: A Clinical Guide.* 2nd ed. Philadelphia, PA: Elsevier, Inc.; 2003:60. Used by permission of Elsevier.

Appendix 33

Recommendations for Parenteral Vitamin Intake in Adults

Vitamin	AMA	FDA
Vitamin A	3300 IU	5000 IU
Vitamin D	200 IU	400 IU
Vitamin E	10 IU	30 IU
Vitamin K		150 μg
Ascorbic acid	100 mg	200 mg
Folacin	400 μg	600 μg
Niacin	40 mg	40 mg
Riboflavin	3.6 mg	3.6 mg
Thiamin	3 mg	6 mg
B_6 (pyridoxine)	4 mg	6 mg
B_{12} (cyanocobalamin)	5 μg	5 μg
Pantothenic acid	15 mg	15 mg
Biotin	60 μg	60 μg

AMA, American Medical Association; FDA, Food and Drug Administration.
Source: Adapted from Multivitamin preparations for parenteral use. A statement by the National Advisory Group. *JPEN.* 1979;3:258–262; *Federal Register* April 20, 2000.

Appendix 34

Recommendations for Parenteral Mineral Intake in Adults

Mineral	Amount (mg)
Zinc	2.5–5.0 (additional amounts as follows: 2.0 mg/day in acute catabolism 12.2 mg/L of small bowel fluid losses 17.1 mg/L of stool or ileostomy output)
Copper	0.3–0.5 mg
Chromium	10.0–15.0 μg
Manganese	60–100 μg
Selenium	20–60 μg

Source: Adapted from Guidelines for essential trace element preparations for parenteral use: Statement by an expert panel. *JAMA.* 1979;24:2051–2054; ASPEN Board of Directors: Guidelines for the use of parenteral and enteral nutrition in adult and pediatric patients. *JPEN.* 2002;26(1):1SA–138SA.

Appendix 35

Routine Urinalysis in Nutritional Assessment

Test	Normal Findings	Abnormalities/Deviations
Color	Straw to light amber	Discolor caused by biliary disease (urobilin), hematuria, hemoglobinuria, porphyria, drugs, foods (beets can cause a red color)
Clarity	Clear	Cloudy urine may be due to presence of blood, pus, phosphate, bacteria, fat, vitamin C
pH	4.6–8.0 (average 6.0)	Urine pH (acidic): diabetic ketoacidosis, starvation, uremia, renal acidosis, high-protein or high-fat diet, acidic drugs, intracellular acidosis Urine pH (alkaline): metabolic alkalosis, hyperventilation, vomiting, alkali administration, UTI secondary to *Proteus*
Protein	None to slight trace	Proteinuria: glomerulonephritis, nephrotic syndrome, nephrotoxicity from drugs or chemicals, pregnancy/prostatitis
Glucose	None	Glucosuria: diabetes or low renal threshold for glucose reabsorption (if blood glucose within normal limits)
Ketones	Negative	Ketonuria: diabetic ketoacidosis, starvation, prolonged vomiting, toxemia, Gierke's disease, increased fat or decreased carbohydrate diet, fever, thyrotoxicosis
Sediment (RBCs, WBCs, casts, crystals)	None to little (kidney membranes are effective filters)	RBCs: calculi, tumors, hematuria, hemorrhagic cystitis WBCs: infection, pyelonephritis Casts: infection or damage to renal tubules Crystals: calcium oxalate, hypercalcemia
Specific gravity	1.008–1.030	Value increased: fever, acute glomerulonephritis, nephrosis, toxemia, congestive heart failure (CHF), fluid intake Value decreased: chronic glomerulonephritis, or pyelonephritis, systemic lupus erythematosus (SLE), parenteral nutrition, fluid intake, hypothermia, diabetes insipidus

Source: From Strasinger SK: *Urinalysis and Body Fluids.* Philadelphia, PA: F. A. Davis Company; 1985:54–86, with permission.

Appendix 36

Sample Nutrition Assessment Form for Long-Term Care

Resident Name _____ Admit Date _____

DOB _____ Age at admit _____yrs. Assessment Date _____

Current Diet Order _____

Diagnoses _____

Medications _____ ETOH use ☐ yes ☐ no

Mental Status _____ Ambulatory ☐ yes ☐ no

Diet History

Obtained from _____

Appetite ☐ Good ☐ Fair ☐ Poor

Intake as percent of food served ☐ 75%–100% ☐ 50%–75% ☐ less than 50%

Check those that apply: ☐ Nausea ☐ Constipation ☐ Diarrhea ☐ Difficulty swallowing

☐ Difficulty chewing ☐ Difficulty self-feeding   Explain_____

Allergies/Intolerances _____

Typical Intake:

| Breakfast | Lunch | Dinner |

Snacks

Adequacy of intake

If Tube Fed: Product _____ Frequency/Feeding Method _____

Total water given _____ ml Protein _____ gms Calories _____ 100% RDAs ☐ yes ☐ no

If no, is resident on a vitamin/mineral supplement ☐ yes ☐ no

Adequacy_____

continues

Appendix 36 continued

Anthropometric Data

Height _____ ft. _____ in. Weight _____ lbs Usual weight _____ lbs

% Desirable weight _____ lbs % Usual weight _____ lbs

Other measurements _____

Laboratory Assessment

Date	Albumin	T.Pro	Cholesterol	BUN	Creatinine
	Glucose	Hgb	Hct		

Physical Assessment

Dehydrated □ yes □ no   *Muscle wasting* □ yes □ no   *Edema* □ yes □ no

Pressure ulcers □ yes stage _____ □ no   *Skin turgor* □ good □ poor

Evaluation Summary _____
_____
_____
_____

Plan of Action _____
_____
_____
_____

Recommendations

1. Change diet order: □ yes □ no to: _____

2. Add snack or supplement: □ yes □ no to: _____

3. Parameters to be obtained: _____

4. Other: _____
_____

Signature _____ Title _____ Date _____

Source: Courtesy of Janice Raymond, MS, RD, Seattle, Washington.

Appendix 37

Sample Parenteral Renal Failure Formulas

	Aminosyn-RF	*Aminess*	*NephrAmine*	*RenAmin*
Manufacturer	Abbott	Clintec	B. Braun	Clintec
Concentration (%)	5.2	5.2	5.4	6.5
Nitrogen (g/100 ml)	0.79	0.66	0.65	1
Essential amino acids (mg/100 ml)				
Isoleucine	462	525	560	500
Leucine	726	825	880	600
Lysine	535	600	640	450
Methionine	726	825	880	500
Phenylalanine	726	825	880	490
Threonine	330	375	400	380
Tryptophan	165	188	200	160
Valine	528	600	640	820
Histidine	429	412	250	420
Nonessential amino acids (mg/100 ml)				
Cysteine			<20	
Arginine	600			630
Alanine				560
Proline				350
Glycine				300
Serine				300
Tyrosine				40
Electrolytes (mEq/L)				
Sodium			5	
Acetate	~105	50	~44	60
Potassium	5.4			
Chloride			<3	31
Osmolarity (mOsm/L)	475	416	435	600

Source: Used with permission from Drug Facts and Comparisons, 2005 ed. St. Louis, MO: Wolters Kluwer Health, Inc.

Appendix 38

Screening Reference for Nutrient Deficiencies

Mechanism of Deficiency	If History Of	Suspect Deficiency Of
Inadequate intake	Alcoholism	Calories, protein, thiamin, niacin, folate, pyridoxine, riboflavin
	Avoidance of fruit, vegetables, grains	Vitamin C, thiamin, niacin, folate
	Avoidance of meat, dairy products, eggs	Protein, vitamin B_{12}
	Constipation, hemorrhoids, diverticulosis	Dietary fiber
	Isolation, poverty, dental disease, food idiosyncrasies	Various nutrients
	Weight loss	Energy, other nutrients
Inadequate absorption	Drugs (especially antacids, anticonvulsants, cholestyramine, laxatives, neomycin, alcohol)	Various nutrients, depending on drug/nutrient interaction
	Malabsorption (diarrhea, weight loss, steatorrhea)	Vitamins A, D, K; energy; protein; calcium; magnesium; zinc
	Parasites	Iron, vitamin B_{12} (fish tapeworm)
	Pernicious anemia	Vitamin B_{12}
	Surgery	
	Gastrectomy	Vitamin B_{12}, iron
	Small bowel resection	Vitamin B_{12} (if distal ileum), others as in malabsorption
Decreased utilization	Drugs (especially anticonvulsants, antimetabolites, oral contraceptives, isoniazid, alcohol)	Various nutrients, depending on drug/nutrient interaction
	Inborn errors of metabolism (by family history)	Various nutrients
Increased losses	Alcohol abuse	Magnesium, zinc
	Blood loss	Iron
	Centesis (ascitic, pleural taps)	Protein
	Diabetes, uncontrolled	Energy
	Diarrhea	Protein, zinc, electrolytes
	Draining abscesses, wounds	Protein, zinc
	Nephrotic syndrome	Protein, zinc
	Peritoneal dialysis or hemodialysis	Protein, water-soluble vitamins, zinc
Increased requirements	Fever	Energy
	Hyperthyroidism	Energy
	Physiologic demands (infancy, adolescence, pregnancy, lactation)	Various nutrients
	Surgery, trauma, burns, infection	Energy, protein, vitamin C, zinc
	Tissue hypoxia	Energy (inefficient utilization)
	Cigarette smoking	Vitamin C, folic acid

Source: Adapted from Weinsier RL, Morgan SL, Perrin VG. *Fundamentals of Clinical Nutrition.* St. Louis, MO: Mosby; 1993.

Appendix 39

Selected Doses of Antidiarrheal Medications

Medication	Adult Dose
Antimotility	
Lomotil	5 mg qid, do not exceed 20 mg/day
Loperamide	Initially 4 mg, then 2 mg after each loose stool; do not exceed 16 mg/day
Paregoric	5–10 ml 1–4 times daily
Opium tincture	0.6 ml qid
Adsorbents	
Kaolin and pectin	30–120 ml after each loose stool
Antisecretory	
Bismuth	Two tablets or 30 ml every 30 min to 1 hr as needed; up to 8 doses/day
Octreotide	Initial: 100 μg subcutaneously tid

Source: Adapted from Spruill WJ, Wade WE: GI disorders. In: DiPiro JT, Talbert RL, Yee GC, et al, eds. *Pharmacotherapy: A Pathological Approach.* 5th ed. New York: McGraw-Hill; 2002:660.

Appendix 40

Selected ICD-9 Codes for Diagnoses Pertinent to the Need for Enteral Nutrition

Code	Anatomic Conditions
145.9	Carcinoma of the mouth
141.9	Carcinoma of the tongue
151.9	Carcinoma of the stomach
195.0	Carcinoma of the head, face, neck
230.0	Carcinoma of the oral cavity
230.1	Carcinoma of the esophagus
230.2	Carcinoma of the larynx
230.7	Carcinoma of the intestine
530.3	Esophageal stricture/stenosis
530.84	Tracheo-esophageal fistula
537.3	Duodenal obstruction
537.4	Gastro-jejunocolic fistula
569.81	Intestinal fistula
802.2	Mandible fracture

Code	Cognitive, Neurologic, and Neuromuscular Conditions
191.0	Brain tumor
290.0	Senile dementia
331.0	Alzheimer's disease
332.0	Parkinson's disease
335.2	Amyotrophic lateral sclerosis
336.9	Spinal cord compression
340.0	Multiple sclerosis
343.2	Quadriplegia
343.9	Cerebral palsy
358	Myasthenia gravis
434.9	Cerebral infarct
436.0	Cerebral vascular accident
780.0	Coma
780.03	Persistent vegetative state

Code	Motility Disorders
478.3	Vocal cord paralysis
507	Aspiration pneumonia
530.81	Esophageal reflux
536.3	Gastroparesis
536.9	Unspecified functional disorder of the intestine
560.9	Pyloric obstruction
564.2	Postgastrectomy dumping syndrome
643	Hyperemesis gravidarum
787.2	Dysphagia

Code	Intestinal Disease/Malabsorptive Disorders
157	Cancer of the pancreas
277.0	Cystic fibrosis
555.0	Regional enteritis/Crohn's disease
577.0	Acute pancreatitis
577.1	Chronic pancreatitis
579.30	Short bowel syndrome
579.4	Pancreatic steatorrhea
579.9	Intestinal malabsorption

Code	Malnutrition
261.0	Severe malnutrition
262.0	Protein-calorie malnutrition
263.0	Moderate malnutrition
263.1	Mild malnutrition
783.4	Lack of normal physiologic development
783.41	Failure to thrive—child
783.7	Failure to thrive—adult

Code	Inborn Errors of Metabolism
270.1	Phenylketonuria
270.2	Tyrosinemia
270.3	Maple syrup urine disease
270.4	Homocystinuria
270.5	Histidinemia

Appendix 41

Severity of Weight Loss

Time	Significant Weight Loss (%)*	Severe Weight Loss (%)*
1 week	1–2	> 2
1 month	5	> 5
3 months	7.5	> 7.5
6 months	10	> 10

*Percent weight change = [(Usual Weight minus Actual Weight) ÷ (Usual Weight)] × 100

Source: Reprinted from Blackburn GL, Bistrian GR, Haini BS, Schlamm HT, Smith MF. Nutritional and metabolic assessment of the hospitalized patient. *JPEN.* 1977;1:17 with permission from the American Society for Parenteral and Enteral Nutrition (A.S.P.E.N.).

Appendix 42

Subjective Nutritional Global Assessment for Adult Liver Transplant Candidates

Patient name _____ I.D. number _____

Age _____ Diagnosis(es) _____

Duration of disease _____ Referring physician _____

I. **HISTORY**

    A. *Weight**

        Height _____ Current wt. _____ Preillness wt. _____ Ideal wt. _____

        Weight in past 6 months: High _____ Low _____

        Overall change in past 6 months: _____% [(High wt – low wt)/low wt] × 100%

        _____ 1%–5% change   _____ 6%–10% change   _____ > 10% change

        _____ Weight loss   _____ Weight gain   _____ Fluctuation

        *Weight change is significant when due to weight loss or ascites/edema

    B. *Appetite*

        1. Dietary intake change—relative to normal

            Appetite in past two weeks

            _____ Good   _____ Fair   _____ Poor

        2. Early satiety

            _____ None   _____ 1–2 weeks   _____ > 2 weeks

        3. Taste changes

            _____ None   _____ 1–2 weeks   _____ > 2 weeks

    C. *Current intake per recall*

        Calories _____ Grams protein _____ Grams sodium _____

        BEE _____ REE _____ Based on weight of _____

        Calorie needs _____ Protein needs _____

    D. *Gastrointestinal symptoms*

        1. Nausea

            _____ None   _____ 1–2 weeks   _____ > 2 weeks

        2. Vomiting

            _____ None   _____ 1 week   _____ > 1 week

        3. Diarrhea (loose stools, > 3 per day)

            Number stools day _____ Consistency _____

            _____ None   _____ 1 week   _____ > 1 week

        4. Constipation

            _____ None   _____ 1–2 weeks   _____ > 2 weeks

continues

Appendix 42 continued

    5.   Difficulty chewing

    _____ None   _____ 1–2 weeks   _____ > 2 weeks

    6.   Difficulty swallowing

    _____ None   _____ 1–2 weeks   _____ > 2 weeks

  E. *Functional capacity*

    Occupation _____ # hours still working _____

    Increase in fatigue? _____ Type of activities/exercise _____

        No dysfunction _____   Dysfunction _____

                                        _____ weeks

                                        _____ working suboptimally

                                        _____ ambulatory

                                        _____ bedridden

II. PHYSICAL

  A. *Status of subcutaneous fat (triceps, chest)*

    _____ good stores   _____ fair stores   _____ poor stores

  B. *Muscle wasting (quadriceps, deltoids, shoulders)*

    _____ none   _____ mild to moderate   _____ severe

  C. *Edema and ascites*

    _____ none   _____ mild to moderate   _____ severe

III. EXISTING CONDITIONS

  A. *Encephalopathy*

    _____ none _____ Stage I–II _____ Stage III _____ Stage IV

  B. *Other conditions affecting nutritional status*

    _____

    _____

IV. SUBJECTIVE NUTRITIONAL ASSESSMENT RATING (based on sections I, II, III)

  A. _____ *Well nourished*

  B. _____ *Moderately (or suspected of being malnourished)*

  C. _____ *Severely malnourished*

V. ADDITIONAL INFORMATION

  A. *History of Diabetes Mellitus* _____

  B. *Vitamin/Mineral supplements* _____

  C. *Other dietary supplements* _____

  D. *ETOH* _____

  E. *Current diet* _____

  F. *Compliance to diet based on hx* _____

  G. *Food intolerances/allergies* _____

  H. *Medications* _____

Source: Courtesy of Baylor University Medical Center, Dallas, Texas.

Appendix 43

Classification of Obesity

Underweight	BMI <18.5 kg/m^2	Associated health risk low
Normal range	BMI 18.5–24.9 kg/m^2	Associated health risk low
Overweight	BMI 25–29.9 kg/m^2	Associated health risk increased
Class I obesity	BMI 30–34.9 kg/m^2	Associated health risk moderate
Class II obesity	BMI 35–39.9 kg/m^2	Associated health risk severe
Class III obesity	BMI ≥40 kg/m^2	Associated health risk very severe

Source: From National Institutes of Health: Clinical guidelines on the identification and treatment of overweight and obesity in adults—the evidence report. *Obes Res.* 1998;6:515–2095.

Index